Farr's Physics for Medical Imaging

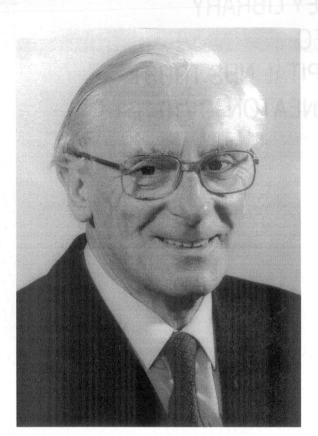

Frank Farr (1922–1998)
FRCR physics teacher and examiner

May his wit and wisdom long be remembered

Commissioning Editor: Timothy Horne
Project Development Manager: Lulu Stader
Project Manager: Emma Riley
Designer: Erik Bigland
Illustrator: David Graham

Farr's Physics for Medical Imaging

Second Edition

Penelope Allisy-Roberts OBE FIPEM FInstP

Section Head, Ionizing Radiations, Bureau International des Poids et Mesures, Sèvres, France

Jerry Williams MSc FIPEM

Consultant Medical Physicist, Royal Infirmary of Edinburgh, Edinburgh, UK

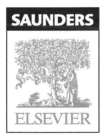

SAUNDERS

ELSEVIER

EDINBURGH LONDON NEW YORK OXFORD PHILADELPHIA ST LOUIS SYDNEY TORONTO 2008

SAUNDERS
ELSEVIER

First edition 1996
Second edition 2008

ISBN: 978-0-7020-2844-1

British Library Cataloguing in Publication Data
A catalogue record for this book is available from the British Library

Library of Congress Cataloging in Publication Data
A catalog record for this book is available from the Library of Congress

Notice
Neither the Publisher nor the Authors assume any responsibility for any loss or
injury and/or damage to persons or property arising out of or related to any use
of the material contained in this book. It is the responsibility of the treating
practitioner, relying on independent expertise and knowledge of the patient, to
determine the best treatment and method of application for the patient.

The Publisher

The
Publisher's
policy is to use
paper manufactured
from sustainable forests

Printed and bound by CPI Group (UK) Ltd, Croydon, CR0 4YY

Transferred to digital print 2013

Contents

Preface

The second edition of this book, while still based on the physics lectures given by Frank Farr in Birmingham, UK, has been updated in line with the new syllabus for the FRCR examination, particularly in terms of radiation protection legislation and to reflect current clinical imaging practice and technology. As for the first edition, it has been written primarily for trainee radiologists studying for the FRCR and the Preface is addressed to them, but we expect that the text will be helpful to others interested in medical imaging.

We have avoided complex formulae but some simplified equations are used to aid the memory. Much of the data in the text is simply illustrative and often only approximate or typical values are given. Imaging technology is advancing continually so the values applicable to equipment and methods in current use in the local radiology department should be known.

Details of the construction of radiology imaging equipment are only given as necessary to understand the nature of the radiation beams and the creation of images. It is important to relate our basic line diagrams to the specific equipment used in the local department. The purpose of various controls and how they affect the image should be understood. Practical knowledge and experience are essential. For every imaging procedure, relevant aspects of equipment design, machine settings and the recording media used locally should be noted.

Each method of medical imaging is a compromise between the conflicting requirements of maximizing the information carried by the image (its quality) while minimizing the risk it carries to the patient. This is the theme of the book. Chapter 2 includes current thinking on radiation hazards and legislative requirements for radiation protection, knowledge of which subjects are a hallmark of the radiologist. Throughout Chapters 3 to 7, there are references to factors that affect the patient dose and how it can be minimized.

Although quality assurance is included in Chapter 2, various measures of image quality such as spatial resolution, contrast and quantum noise are introduced in Chapters 3 and 4 for 'conventional' analogue radiography with films and screens. They are developed further in Chapters 5, 6 and 7 as the effects are progressively more limiting for digital, and particularly in Chapter 8, for radionuclide images. Image quality is also covered in Chapters 9 and 10. This stepwise approach seemed preferable to a portmanteau chapter devoted to image quality.

A common theme of the later chapters is the production and processing of digital images. Digital images are first encountered in Chapter 5 and recur in the chapters on computed tomography, radionuclide imaging, ultrasound and magnetic resonance imaging (MRI), each of which is relatively self-contained, so that they can be studied in any order. Our descriptions of the various artefacts in digital images should be related to those seen in real diagnostic images. In Chapters 5, 6 and 7, some background concepts have been placed in boxes. The more complex imaging procedures in Chapters 8, 9 and 10 are really the realm of the FRCR Part II examination although a trainee needs to understand the basic concepts. Technological developments in PET scanners and in PET radionuclide production have been dramatic in recent years and are likely to continue with the increasing use of PET/CT. MRI too is a rapidly developing technique. The physics is somewhat complex and whole books are devoted to the topic. Consequently, we have concentrated on the basic principles, common pulse sequences, the use of gradient fields and safety aspects. MRI is a topic that repays reading several times.

Each of the methods of digital imaging depends on two procedures: sampling and Fourier transform. These are essentially mathematical ideas but we have used analogies and graphs in preference to equations. The fusion of different imaging modalities has not been covered but trainees should be aware of these possibilities.

Medical imaging continues to develop through collaboration between radiologists, scientists and engineers from many countries. This can lead to differences in approach and there are often several alternative names and acronyms for the same or similar quantities. We mention most of these to make recognition easier when answering multiple choice questions.

In changing the title of the book and including his photograph, we intend to honour the memory of Frank Farr without whom this project would not have been possible. We are indebted too, to all our colleagues, particularly Dr Maggie Flower, Dr Valda Gazzard, Dr Liz Moore and Dr Nick Weir for their corrections and helpful guidance. Any imperfections that remain are ours alone. We express our sincere thanks to our publisher, Lulu Stader for nursing us through the update process, to the Elsevier editorial staff; and not least, to generations of past and present students with whose help we have learned so much.

P J Allisy-Roberts
J R Williams

2007

Chapter 1

Radiation physics

Diagnostic imaging employs radiations – X, gamma, radiofrequency and sound – to which the body is partly but not completely transparent, and it exploits the special properties of a number of elements and compounds. As *ionizing* radiations (X-rays and gamma rays) are used most, it is best to start by discussing the structure of the atom and the production of X-rays. Some properties of the particles making up the atom and described elsewhere in this text are given in Table 1.1.

1.1 STRUCTURE OF THE ATOM

An atom consists mainly of empty space. Its mass is concentrated in a central nucleus that contains a number A of nucleons (protons and neutrons), where A is called the mass number. The nucleus comprises Z protons, where Z is the atomic number of the element, and $(A - Z)$ neutrons. A nuclide is a species of nucleus characterized by the two numbers Z and A. The atomic number is synonymous with the name of the element. Thus, $^{12}_{6}C$ refers to a carbon atom with

Table 1.1 Some fundamental particles

	Relative mass	Relative charge	Symbol
Nucleons			
Neutron	1	0	n
Proton	1	+1	p
Extranuclear			
Electron	0.00054	−1	e^-, β^-
Other			
Positron	0.00054	+1	e^+, β^+
Alpha particle	4	+2	α

$A = 12$ and $Z = 6$ and is often shortened to ^{12}C and called carbon-12. On the other hand, carbon-14 still has $Z = 6$ but has two more neutrons. The combination of six protons plus eight neutrons is unstable and therefore radioactive. It is called a radionuclide.

Orbiting in specific shells around the positively charged nucleus, like planets around the sun, are Z electrons. The shells are designated K, L, M, N, ... outwards from the centre. Figure 1.1 illustrates the structure of a sodium atom with two electrons in the K-shell, eight in the L-shell and one in the outermost M-shell.

In each atom, the outermost or *valence* shell is concerned with the chemical, thermal, optical and electrical properties of the element. The properties of X-rays and their interaction with materials concern the orbiting electrons, particularly those in the inner shell. Radioactivity concerns the nucleus. Radioactivity is described in Chapter 8.1, where alpha and beta particles and gamma rays are discussed further.

No valence shell can have more than eight electrons. Metals have one, two or three valence electrons, one of which is easily detached from the atom and is described as being free. This accounts for their good conduction of heat and electricity.

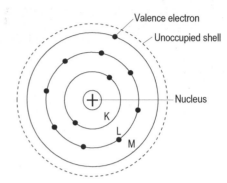

Figure 1.1 Electron shells in a sodium atom.

Box 1.1 SI units

The SI system of units (le Système International d'Unités) for measurement uses a base set of quantities and units.

Mass	kilogram (kg)
Length	metre (m)
Time	second (s)
Amount of a substance	mole (mol)
Electric current	ampere (A)
Temperature	kelvin (K)
Luminous intensity	candela (cd)

All other units are derived from these. For example, the unit of energy is $1 \text{ kg m}^2\text{s}^{-2}$ and is given the special name joule (J), and the unit of power (watt, W) is equal to 1 J s^{-1}. The unit of electrical charge, the coulomb (C), is likewise derived from the base units and is the quantity of charge transported by a current of 1 A flowing for 1 s, $1 \text{ C} = 1 \text{ A.s}$. The unit of electrical potential and electromotive force (EMF), the volt (V), is the EMF required for a charge of 1 C to acquire 1 J of energy, $1 \text{ V} = 1 \text{ J C}^{-1}$.

In describing the energy of photons, it is common to use a derived unit that is not strictly defined in accordance to the SI convention that does not allow more or less arbitrary multipliers to be applied to the base units. The electronvolt (eV) is the energy acquired by an electron when it is accelerated through a potential difference of 1 V. Because the charge of an electron is 1.6×10^{-19} C, the eV is equal to 1.6×10^{-19} J. It is convenient to use the eV as a unit to describe the very small quantity of energy represented by a photon. In addition, it has direct relevance to the energy of X-rays generated by stopping electrons that have been accelerated to the kilovoltage (kV) applied across the X-ray tube. The maximum photon energy (keV_{max}) is simply numerically equal to the applied kV.

Other units derived from the SI base units will be introduced later in this text. These include the unit for absorbed dose, gray (Gy), $1 \text{ Gy} = 1 \text{ J kg}^{-1}$ and the unit of activity, becquerel (Bq), $1 \text{ Bq} = 1 \text{ s}^{-1}$.

Units may also have multiplying factors that can be used conveniently to describe very large or small amounts of any quantity. These are as follow.

pico (p)	10^{-12}
nano (n)	10^{-9}
micro (µ)	10^{-6}
milli (m)	10^{-3}
kilo (k)	10^{3}
mega (M)	10^{6}
giga (G)	10^{9}
tera (T)	10^{12}

Silver bromide is an example of an *ionic crystal*, and consists of equal numbers of positive silver ions (silver atoms that have each lost their single valence electron) and negative bromine ions (bromine atoms that have each gained an outer shell electron). The two kinds of ion hold each other, by electrostatic attraction, in a highly regular three-dimensional lattice. This accounts for the well-known properties of such crystals. Other examples encountered in imaging equipment are sodium iodide and caesium iodide.

Binding energy

An atom is described as *ionized* when one of its electrons has been completely removed. The detached electron is a negative ion and the remnant atom a positive ion. Together, they form an ion pair.

The binding energy (E) of an electron in an atom is the energy expended in completely removing the electron from the atom against the attractive force of the positive nucleus. This energy is expressed in electronvolts (eV), explained in Box 1.1.

The binding energy depends on the shell ($E_K > E_L > E_M$ ...) and on the element, increasing as the atomic number increases. For example, for tungsten (W; $Z = 74$) the binding energies of different shells are $E_K = 70$, $E_L = 11$, and $E_M = 2\,keV$.

The K-shell binding energies of various elements encountered in X-ray imaging are given in Table 1.2.

An atom is *excited* when an electron is raised from one shell to another further out. This involves the expenditure of energy; the atom as a whole has more energy than normal and so is said to be excited. For example, a valence electron can be raised to one of the unoccupied shells further out, shown dashed in Figure 1.1. When it falls back, the energy is re-emitted as a single 'packet' of energy or photon of light (visible or ultraviolet). This is an example of the quantum aspects of electromagnetic radiation.

1.2 ELECTROMAGNETIC RADIATION

This is the term given to energy travelling across empty space. All forms of electromagnetic radiation travel with the same velocity (c) as light when in vacuo, very close to $3 \times 10^8\,ms^{-1}$ and not significantly less in air. They are named according to the way in which they are produced and the special properties they possess. X-rays (emitted by X-ray tubes) and gamma rays (emitted by radioactive nuclei) have essentially the same properties and differ only in their origin.

Quantum aspects

Electromagnetic radiation can be regarded as having particle-like properties. But rather than being composed of particles, the radiation is represented as a stream of packets or quanta of energy, called photons, that travel in straight lines.

Wave aspects

Electromagnetic radiation can also be regarded as sinusoidally varying electric and magnetic fields, travelling with velocity c when in vacuo. They are transverse waves: the electric and magnetic field vectors point at right angles to each other and to the direction of travel of the wave.

At any point, the graph of field strength against *time* is a sine wave, depicted as a solid curve in Figure 1.2a. The peak field strength is called the amplitude (A). The interval between successive crests of the wave is called the period (T). The frequency (f) is the number of crests passing a point in a second, and $f = 1/T$. The dashed curve refers to a later instant, showing how the wave has travelled forwards with velocity c.

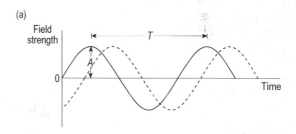

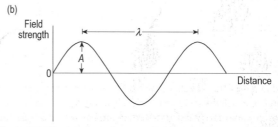

Figure 1.2 Electromagnetic wave. Field strength versus (a) time and (b) distance.

Table 1.2 Atomic number (Z) and K-shell binding energy (E_K) of various elements

Element	Z	E_K (keV)
Aluminium	13	1.6
Calcium	20	4
Molybdenum	42	20
Iodine	53	33
Barium	56	37
Gadolinium	64	50
Tungsten	74	70
Lead	82	88

Table 1.3 Electromagnetic spectrum

Radiation	Wavelength	Frequency	Energy
Radiowaves	1000–0.1 m	**0.3–3000 MHz**	0.001–10 μeV
Microwaves	100–1 mm	**3–300 GHz**	10–1000 μeV
Infrared	**100–1 μm**	3–300 THz	10–1000 meV
Visible light	**700–400 nm**	430–750 THz	1.8–3 eV
Ultraviolet	**400–10 nm**	750–30 000 THz	1.8–100 eV
X- and gamma rays	1 nm–0.1 pm	$3 \times 10^5 - 3 \times 10^9$ THz	**1 keV–10 MeV**

At any instant, the graph of field strength against *distance* is also a sine wave, as shown in Figure 1.2b. The distance between successive crests of the wave is called the wavelength (λ).

Wavelength and frequency are inversely proportional to each other:

$$\text{wavelength} \times \text{frequency} = \text{constant.}$$

Their product is equal to the velocity (λf = c). This relation is true of all kinds of wave motion, including sound, although for sound the velocity is about a million times less.

The types of electromagnetic radiation are listed in Table 1.3, in order of increasing photon energy, increasing frequency, and decreasing wavelength. The values are rounded and the boundaries between the types of radiation are not well defined, other than for visible light, for which the boundaries are defined by the properties of the receptor, i.e. the human eye. The nomenclature that is most commonly used in practice is emphasized in bold in the table.

Wave and quantum theories combined

Photon energy is proportional to the frequency. The constant of proportionality is called *Planck's constant* (*h*). Thus $E = hf$.

More usefully, because frequency is inversely proportional to wavelength, so also is photon energy:

$$E \text{ (in keV)} = 1.24/\lambda \text{ (in nm).}$$

For example:

Blue light	λ = 400 nm	E ≈ 3 eV
Typical X- and gamma rays	E = 140 keV	λ ≈ 0.1 nm.

Intensity

Radiation travels in straight lines called rays that radiate in all directions from a point source. A collimated set of rays is called a beam. A beam of radiation can be visualized by taking at some point a cross-section at right angles to the beam (Fig. 1.3a).

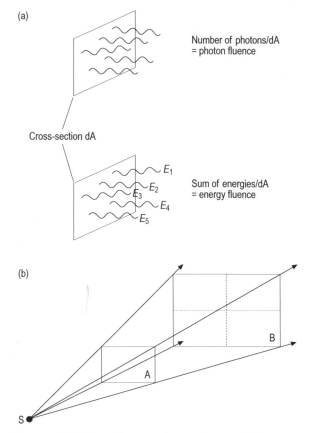

Figure 1.3 (a) Photon fluence and energy fluence. (b) The inverse square law applying to a point source S.

Suppose the beam is switched on for a given (exposure) time. Simply counting the photons allows the number per unit area passing through the cross-section in the time to be determined, and is called the *photon fluence* at the point. A beam may contain photons of different energies. Adding up the energies of all the individual photons gives the total amount of energy per unit area passing through the cross-section in the time, and is called the energy fluence at the point.

The total amount of energy per unit area passing through the cross-section *per unit time* (watts per square millimetre) is called the energy fluence rate at the point, and is also referred to as the beam *intensity*. In wave theory, intensity is proportional to the square of the amplitude (*A*, see Fig. 1.2), measured from the peak of the wave to the axis.

Energy fluence and intensity are not easy to measure directly. As explained in section 1.6.2, in the case of X- and gamma rays an easier indirect measurement of energy fluence is usually made, namely *air kerma*, and, instead of intensity, air kerma rate. The relationship between these quantities is discussed later in section 1.6.4.

Inverse square law

Because electromagnetic radiation travels in straight lines, it follows that the dimensions of the beam are proportional to the distance from a point source S, as is shown in Figure 1.3b. As a result, the area of the beam is proportional to the square of the distance from a point source. Therefore the air kerma is inversely proportional to the square of the distance from the source.

With reference to Figure 1.3b:

$$\frac{\text{air kerma at B}}{\text{air kerma at A}} = \frac{(\text{distance to A})^2}{(\text{distance to B})^2}$$

For the inverse square law to hold, it is essential that the radiation comes from a point source and that there is no absorption or scatter of radiation between the source and the points of measurement. Figure 1.3b has been drawn such that the distance from the source doubles in going from A to B. In this instance, the air kerma reduces by a factor of 4.

1.3 PRODUCTION OF X-RAYS

The X-ray tube

X-rays are produced when fast-moving electrons are suddenly stopped by impact on a metal *target*. The kinetic energy of the electrons is converted into X-rays (no more than 1%) and into heat ($\geqslant$99%).

An X-ray tube, depicted in Figure 1.4, consists of two electrodes sealed into an evacuated *glass envelope*:

- a negative electrode (*cathode*) that incorporates a fine tungsten coil or filament
- a positive electrode (*anode*) that incorporates a smooth flat metal target, usually of tungsten.

The *filament* is heated by passing an electrical current through it to a temperature at which it is white hot (incandescent). In this state, it emits electrons by the process of thermionic emission. At such high

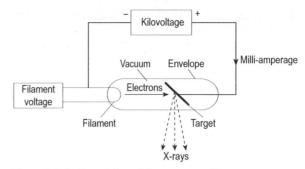

Figure 1.4 An X-ray tube and its power supplies.

temperatures (~2200°C), the atomic and electronic motion in a metal is sufficiently violent to enable a fraction of the free electrons to leave the surface despite the net attractive pull of the lattice of positive ions.

The electrons are then repelled by the negative cathode and attracted by the positive anode. Because of the *vacuum*, they are not hindered in any way and bombard the target with a velocity around half the speed of light.

Kilovoltage and milliamperage

Two sources of electrical energy are required and are derived from the alternating current (AC) mains by means of transformers. Figure 1.4 shows:

- the filament heating voltage (about 10 V) and current (about 10 A)
- the accelerating voltage (typically 30–150 kV) between the anode and cathode (referred to as tube potential, high voltage, kilovoltage or kV); this drives the current of electrons (typically 0.5–1000 mA) flowing between the anode and cathode (referred to as tube current, milliamperage or mA).

The mA is controlled by adjusting the filament voltage and current and thus filament temperature. A small increase in temperature produces a large increase in tube current.

An X-ray set is designed so that, unlike most electrical components, increasing or decreasing the tube voltage does not affect the tube current. It is also designed so that the kV is unaffected by changes in the mA. The two factors can therefore be varied independently.

The *waveform* of a high-voltage generator can be described graphically to demonstrate how voltage varies with time. Figure 1.5 depicts the waveforms of four types of high-tension voltage supply. These are explained in Box 1.2.

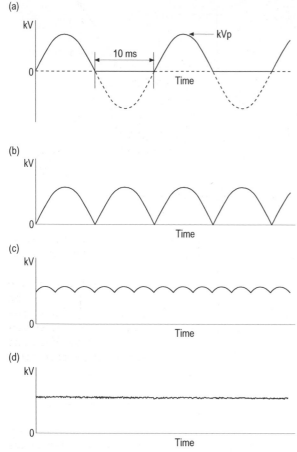

Figure 1.5 Waveforms of high-voltage generators: (a) single-phase, half wave–rectified; (b) single-phase, full wave–rectified; (c) three-phase, six-pulse; and (d) high-frequency generator.

Processes occurring in the target of an X-ray tube

Each electron arrives at the surface of the target with a kinetic energy (expressed in units of kiloelectronvolts, keV) equivalent to the kV between the anode and cathode at that instant. The electrons penetrate several micrometres into the target and lose their energy by a combination of processes:

- as a large number of very small energy losses, by interaction with the outer electrons of the atoms, constituting unwanted *heat* and causing a rise in temperature

- as large-energy losses producing *X-rays*, by interaction with either the inner shells of the atoms or the field of the nucleus.

Interaction with the K-shell: line spectrum, characteristic radiation

As depicted in Figure 1.6, when an electron (a) from the filament collides with an electron in the K-shell of an atom, an electron (b) will be ejected from the atom, provided that the energy of the bombarding electron is greater than the binding energy of the shell.

The vacancy or hole then created in the K-shell is most likely to be filled by an electron (c) falling down from the L-shell with the emission of a single X-ray photon (d) of energy equal to the difference in the binding energies of the two shells, $E_K - E_L$. The photon is referred to as K_α radiation.

Alternatively, but less likely, the hole may be filled by an electron falling in from the M-shell with the

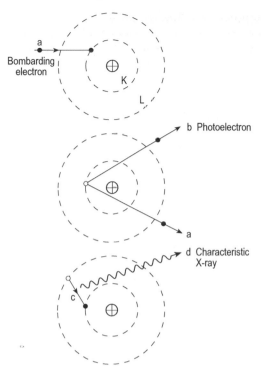

Figure 1.6 Production of characteristic radiation.

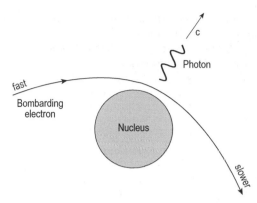

Figure 1.7 Production of bremsstrahlung.

emission of a single X-ray photon of energy, $E_K - E_M$, referred to as K_β radiation.

In the case of tungsten ($Z = 74$), the standard target material used in medical X-ray tubes,

$$E_K = 70\,\text{keV}, E_L = 12\,\text{keV, and } E_M = 2\,\text{keV}.$$

Thus, the K_α radiation has a photon energy of 58 keV and the K_β radiation has a photon energy of 68 keV. There is also L-radiation, produced when a hole created in the L-shell is filled by an electron falling in from further out. Even in the case of tungsten, these photons have only 10 keV of energy, insufficient to leave the X-ray tube assembly, and so they play no part in radiology.

The X-ray photons produced in an X-ray tube in this way have a few discrete or separate photon energies and constitute a *line spectrum*.

In the case of molybdenum ($Z = 42$), the target material most commonly used in mammography,

$$E_K = 20\,\text{keV and } E_L = 2.5\,\text{keV},$$

and so the K_α radiation has a photon energy of 17.5 keV and the K_β radiation has a photon energy of nearly 20 keV.

The photon energy of the K-radiation therefore increases as the atomic number of the target increases.

It is referred to as *characteristic radiation*, because its energy is determined by the target material and is unaffected by the tube voltage.

A K-electron cannot be ejected from the atom if the tube voltage and thus the maximum energy of the electrons crossing the tube is less than E_K. For a tungsten target, therefore, K-characteristic radiation cannot be produced in a tube operating below 70 kV. The rate of production of characteristic radiation increases as the kV is increased above this value.

Interaction with the nucleus: bremsstrahlung, continuous spectrum

As depicted in Figure 1.7, if a bombarding electron penetrates the K-shell and approaches close to the nucleus it is deflected. It approaches fast and leaves less quickly, losing some or all of its energy. The lost energy is carried away as a single photon of X-rays or bremsstrahlung (literally, 'braking radiation'). Except in mammography, 80% or more of the X-rays emitted by a diagnostic X-ray tube are bremsstrahlung.

Very rarely, an electron arriving at the target is immediately and completely stopped in this way and produces a single photon of energy equivalent to the applied kV. This is the largest photon energy that can be produced at this kV.

It is more likely that the bombarding electron first loses some of its energy as heat and then, when it interacts with the nucleus, it loses only part of its remaining energy, with the emission of bremsstrahlung of lower photon energy.

The X-rays may be emitted in any direction (although mainly sideways to the electron beam) and with any energy up to the maximum. Figure 1.8 plots the relative number of photons having each photon energy (keV). The bremsstrahlung forms a *continuous spectrum* (A). The maximum photon energy (in keV) is numerically equal to the kV.

The dashed line (B) in Figure 1.8 shows the spectrum of bremsstrahlung produced near the target nuclei. In fact, the target itself, the glass wall of the tube, and other materials collectively referred to as the filtration, substantially absorb the lower-energy photons. There is therefore a low-energy cut-off, at about 20 keV, as well as a maximum energy. The latter depends only on the kV and the former on the filtration added to the tube (see section 1.5).

For the X-rays emerging from an X-ray tube operated at constant potential, the peak of the continuous spectrum (i.e. the most common photon energy) is typically between one-third and one-half of the kV. The average or *effective energy* is greater, between 50 and 60% of the maximum. Thus an X-ray tube operated at 90 kV can be thought of as emitting, effectively, 45-keV X-rays. As the operating kV is greater than the K-shell binding energy, characteristic X-rays are also produced. They are shown in Figure 1.8 as lines superimposed on the continuous spectrum.

The area of the spectrum represents the total output of all X-ray photons emitted. Figure 1.9 compares the spectrum from a tube with a tungsten target, operating at three different kV values. As the tube voltage is increased, both the width and height of the spectrum increase.

In the range 60–120 kV, the intensity of the emitted X-rays is approximately proportional to $kV^2 \times mA$, the exact exponent being dependent on the filtration. This may be compared with the electrical power supplied, which is proportional to $kV \times mA$. The *efficiency* of X-ray production is the ratio

$$\frac{\text{X-ray output}}{\text{electrical power supplied}}$$

and increases with the kV. The efficiency is also greater the higher the atomic number of the target.

Controlling the X-ray spectrum

To summarize, there are five factors that affect the X-ray spectrum. The following are the effects of altering each in turn, the other four remaining constant.

- Increasing the kV shifts the spectrum upwards and to the right, as shown in Figure 1.9. It increases the maximum and effective energies and the total number of X-ray photons. Below a certain kV (70 kV for a tungsten target), the characteristic K-radiation is not produced.

- Increasing the mA does not affect the shape of the spectrum but increases the output of both bremsstrahlung and characteristic radiation proportionately.

- Changing the target to one of lower *atomic number* reduces the output of bremsstrahlung but does not otherwise affect its spectrum, unless the filtration is also changed. The photon energy of the characteristic lines will also be less.

- Whatever the kV *waveform* (see Fig. 1.5), the maximum and minimum photon energies are unchanged. However, a constant potential or three-phase generator produces more X-rays and at higher energies than those produced by a single-phase pulsating potential generator when operated with the same values of kV and mA. Both the output and the effective energy of the beam are therefore greater. This is because in Figure 1.5c,d the tube voltage is at the same peak value throughout the exposure. In Figure 1.5a,b, it is below peak value during the greater part of each half cycle.

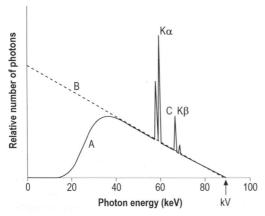

Figure 1.8 An X-ray spectrum.

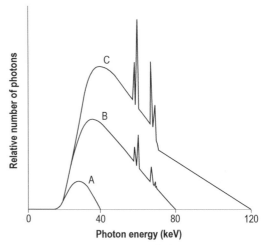

Figure 1.9 Effect of tube kilovoltage (kV) on X-ray spectra for three tube potentials: A, 40 kV; B, 80 kV; and C, 120 kV.

A half wave–rectified, single-phase generator (Fig. 1.5a) produces useful X-rays in pulses, each lasting about 3 ms during the middle of each 20-ms cycle of the mains.

For the effect of the fifth factor, *filtration*, see section 1.5.

1.4 THE INTERACTION OF X- AND GAMMA RAYS WITH MATTER

Where the following refers to X-rays, it applies equally well to gamma rays. Figure 1.10 illustrates the three possible fates of the individual photons when a beam of X- or gamma rays travels through matter. They may be any of the following.

- *Transmitted*: pass through unaffected, as primary or direct radiation.

- *Absorbed*: transferring to the matter all of their energy (the photon disappearing completely).

- *Scattered*: diverted in a new direction, with or without loss of energy transferring to the matter, and so may leave the material as scattered or secondary radiation.

X-ray absorption and scattering processes are stochastic processes governed by the statistical laws of chance. It is impossible to predict which of the individual photons in a beam will be transmitted by 1 mm of a material, but it is possible to be quite precise about the fraction of them that will be, on account of the large numbers of photons the beam contains.

The X-ray image is formed by the transmitted photons. Those that are absorbed or scattered represent attenuation by matter. An understanding of how the properties of X-rays and the materials through which they travel affect the relative amounts of attenuation and transmission gives an understanding of how the X-ray image is formed.

1.4.1 Attenuation

Attenuation refers to the fact that there are fewer photons in the emerging beam than in the beam entering the material. It is represented by the photons that are completely absorbed and those that are scattered.

It is helpful to consider first the attenuation in a simple case.

A narrow, monoenergetic beam of X-rays
The fundamental law of X-ray attenuation states that, for a monoenergetic beam, equal thicknesses of an absorber transmit equal fractions (percentages) of the radiation entering them. This is illustrated in Figure 1.11a, where each sheet reduces the beam by 20%.

In particular, the *half-value layer* (HVL) is the thickness of stated material that will reduce the intensity of a narrow beam of X-radiation to one-half of its original value. For example, as is shown in Figure 1.11b, two successive HVLs reduce the intensity of the beam by a factor $2^2 = 4$ from 1024 to 256. Ten HVLs would reduce the intensity of the beam by a factor $2^{10} = 1024$, i.e. down to 1 in this example.

The HVL is a measure of the penetrating power or effective energy of the beam. It is useful to have a parameter that quantifies the attenuating properties of the material. This is the *linear attenuation coefficient* (μ), which is inversely proportional to the HVL:

$$\mu = 0.693/\text{HVL}$$

More precisely, the linear attenuation coefficient measures the probability that a photon interacts (i.e. is absorbed or scattered) per unit length of the path it travels in a specified material.

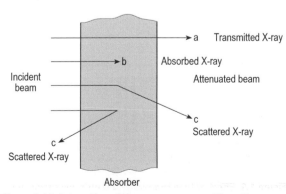

Figure 1.10 Interaction of X- or gamma rays with matter.

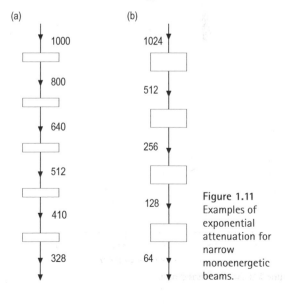

Figure 1.11 Examples of exponential attenuation for narrow monoenergetic beams.

However, the linear attenuation coefficient applies only to narrow monoenergetic beams. The HVL can be used for beams that are not monoenergetic but applies only to narrow beams.

The HVL decreases and the linear attenuation coefficient therefore increases as:

- the density of the material increases
- the atomic number of the material increases
- the photon energy of the radiation decreases.

For example, lead is more effective than either aluminium or tissue at absorbing X-rays, because of its higher density and atomic number. X-rays of 140 keV are more penetrating and are said to be 'harder' than those of 20 keV.

The mass attenuation coefficient (μ/ρ) is obtained by dividing the linear coefficient by the density of the material. It is therefore independent of density and depends only on the atomic number of the material and photon energy.

Exponential graph

However thick the absorber, it is never possible to absorb an X-ray beam completely. This is shown, in Figure 1.12a, by the shape of the graph of percentage transmission versus thickness d, both being plotted on linear scales. This is an exponential curve described by the equation

$$I = I_0 e^{-\mu d},$$

in which I_0 is the intensity of X-rays incident on the absorber with a linear attenuation coefficient equal to μ and thickness d and I is the intensity transmitted through it.

If, as in Figure 1.12b, the percentage transmission is plotted on a logarithmic scale, a linear graph results, making it easier to read off the HVL and calculate μ.

The experimental arrangement for measuring HVL and the attenuation coefficient is illustrated in Figure 1.13a. The beam is restricted by means of a lead diaphragm or collimator to just cover a small detector. The diaphragm B and sheets of the absorbing material C are positioned halfway between the source A and detector D. This arrangement minimizes the amount of scattered radiation S entering the detector.

Attenuation of a wide beam

The measured percentage transmission depends on the width of the beam. For the narrow beam in Figure 1.13a, a relatively small amount of scatter is produced in the absorbing material. However, the amount of scatter produced, and thus detected, is very much greater for the broader beam illustrated in Figure 1.13b. In the latter case, the measured HVL would be increased.

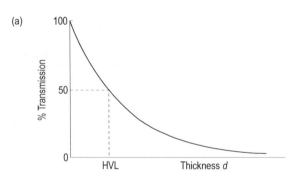

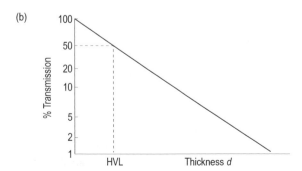

Figure 1.12 Exponential attenuation, half-value layers: (a) linear scale, (b) logarithmic scale. HVL, half-value layer.

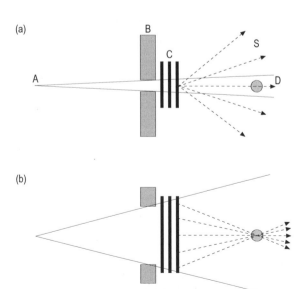

Figure 1.13 (a) A narrow beam is used for the measurement of the half-value layer. (b) Transmission of a wide beam.

Attenuation of a heterogeneous beam

The beams produced by X-ray tubes are heterogeneous (polyenergetic), i.e. they comprise photons of a wide range of energies, as shown in the spectrum in Figure 1.8. As the beam travels through an attenuating material, the lower-energy photons are attenuated proportionally more than the higher-energy photons. The exponential law does not therefore apply exactly. It is still, however, correct to refer to the HVL of the beam. The HVL of a typical diagnostic beam is 30 mm in tissue, 12 mm in bone and 0.15 mm in lead.

As the beam penetrates the material, it becomes progressively more homogeneous. The proportion of higher-energy photons in the beam increases, a process described as beam hardening.

The average energy of the photons increases – the beam becomes harder or more penetrating. The second HVL, which would reduce the beam intensity from 50 to 25%, is thus greater than the first HVL, which reduces it from 100 to 50%.

The X-ray beams used in practice are usually both wide and heterogeneous, and the exponential law of absorption does not strictly apply. However, it is still possible to use the exponential law of X-ray attenuation in approximate calculations together with an effective attenuation coefficient.

Interaction processes

Three processes of interaction between X-rays and matter contribute to attenuation:

- interaction with a loosely bound or free electron – usually referred to as the Compton effect but also described as inelastic or non-coherent scattering scatter (see section 1.4.2)
- interaction with an inner shell or 'bound' electron – photoelectric absorption, a process in which the photon is totally absorbed (section 1.4.3)

and, less importantly,

- interaction with a bound electron – elastic scatter (see Box 1.4).

1.4.2 Compton effect

As depicted in Figure 1.14, the photon passing through the material bounces off a free electron, which recoils and takes away some of the energy of the photon as kinetic energy. The photon is scattered, i.e. diverted in a new direction, with reduced energy.

The angle of scatter θ is the angle between the scattered ray and the incident ray. Photons may be scattered in all directions. The electrons are projected only in sideways and forwards directions.

Effect of the angle of scattering

Figure 1.14 illustrates three different angles of scattering. The lengths of the arrows indicate the relative energies of the recoil electrons. It will be seen that the greater the angle of scatter,

- the greater the energy and range of the recoil electron, and also
- the greater the loss of energy (and increase of wavelength) of the scattered photon.

Thus a back-scattered photon ($\theta = 180°$) is less energetic or is 'softer' than a side-scattered photon ($\theta = 90°$), which in turn is softer than a forward-scattered photon ($\theta = 0$).

Effect of initial photon energy

The higher the initial photon energy,

- the greater the remaining photon energy of the scattered radiation and the more penetrating it is, and also
- the greater the energy that is carried off by the recoil electron and the greater its range.

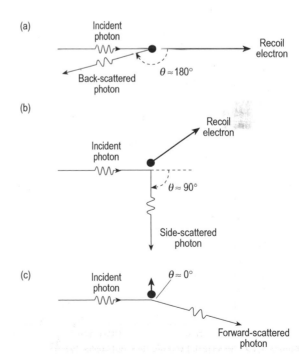

Figure 1.14 Compton scattering by a free electron.

Box 1.3 Electron density

The probability of the Compton effect occurring (which is proportional to σ) depends on the number of electrons per unit *volume* while being otherwise independent of atomic number. It therefore depends on

(mass per unit volume) $\times$ (number of electrons per unit mass).

The former is the usual physical density, and the latter is called the electron density.

Because the number of atoms per unit mass is proportional to $1/A$, and the number of electrons per atom is proportional to Z, the number of electrons per unit mass must be proportional to Z/A.

Apart from hydrogen (for which $Z/A = 1$), almost all light elements relevant to radiology have $Z/A = 0.5$. As a result, hydrogenous materials have slightly more electrons per gram than materials without a hydrogen content. The electron density of bone, air, fat, muscle and water does not vary by more than 10%. On account of this small variation, we often simply say that Compton attenuation is proportional to physical density.

Air-equivalent materials and tissue-equivalent materials must have the same electron density as air and soft tissue, respectively, as well as having the properties stated in section 1.6.3.

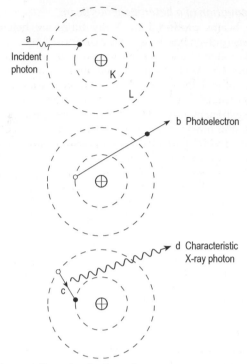

Figure 1.15 Photoelectric absorption.

This is seen in the following examples.

Incident photon	Back–scattered photon	Recoil electron
25 keV	22 keV	3 keV
150 keV	100 keV	50 keV

The softening effect of Compton scatter is therefore greatest with large scattering angles as well as with high-energy X-rays.

The Compton effect contributes to the total linear attenuation coefficient μ an amount σ that is called the Compton linear attenuation coefficient. The probability that the Compton process will occur is proportional to the physical density (mass per unit volume) of the material, as with all attenuation processes. It is also proportional to electron density, as explained in Box 1.3. It is independent of the atomic number of the material, as it concerns only free electrons for which the binding energy is negligible in comparison with the photon energy. Finally, it decreases only slightly over the range of photon energies encountered in diagnostic radiology, and may be thought of as being very approximately proportional to $1/E$.

To summarize, σ is proportional to ρ/E and is independent of Z.

The mass attenuation coefficient for the Compton effect, σ/ρ, is the same within 10% for such diverse materials as air, tissue, bone, contrast media and lead. They are all represented by a single dashed curve in Figure 1.16, which shows how σ/ρ varies with photon energy.

The energy carried off by the recoil electron is said to have been absorbed by the material, and the remainder, carried by the photon, to have been scattered. The Compton effect therefore represents only a partial absorption of the photon energy. In the diagnostic energy range, no more than 20% of the energy is absorbed, the rest being scattered.

1.4.3 Photoelectric effect

When, as in Figure 1.15, an X- or gamma ray photon (a) collides with an electron in (say) the K-shell of an atom, it can, if its energy is greater than the binding energy of the shell, eject the electron (b) from the atom. The energy of the photon is completely absorbed in the process, i.e. the photon disappears. Part of its energy, equal to the binding energy of the

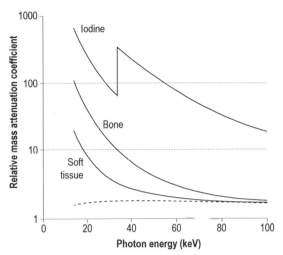

Figure 1.16 Mass attenuation coefficients as a function of energy. Photoelectric effect (τ/ρ, solid lines) for soft tissue, bone and iodine) and Compton effect (σ/ρ, dashed line) averaged for all tissues.

K-shell, is expended in removing the electron from the atom, and the remainder becomes the kinetic energy of that electron:

kinetic energy of the electron = photon energy $- E_K$.

Less often, the X- or gamma ray photon may interact with an electron in the L-shell of an atom. The electron is then ejected from the atom with kinetic energy = photon energy $- E_L$.

The electrons so ejected are called photoelectrons. In each case, the 'holes' created in the atomic shell are filled by electrons falling in from a shell further out (e.g. electron (c) in Fig. 1.15), with the emission of a series of photons of characteristic radiation such as photon (d) in Figure 1.15. The whole of the original photon energy is accounted for in this way.

In contrast to the characteristic radiation produced in the tungsten target of the X-ray tube, in low Z materials such as tissue, the characteristic radiation has very low energy. It is absorbed immediately with the ejection of a further, low-energy or Auger electron. Thus all the original photon energy is converted into the energy of electronic motion and is said to have been absorbed by the material. Photoelectric absorption in such materials is complete absorption.

On the other hand, the characteristic rays from barium and iodine in contrast media may be sufficiently energetic to leave the patient. In this respect, they act like Compton scattered rays.

Photoelectric absorption contributes to the total linear attenuation coefficient μ an amount τ that is called the photoelectric linear attenuation coefficient. Thus $\mu = \sigma + \tau$.

The more tightly the electron is bound to the atom and the nearer the photon energy is to its binding energy, the more likely photoelectric absorption is to happen (so long as the photon energy is greater than the binding energy). So the probability that photoelectric absorption will occur decreases markedly as the photon energy of the radiation increases, being inversely proportional to the cube of the photon energy E. It increases markedly as the atomic number of the material increases, being proportional to the cube of the atomic number Z. Finally, it is proportional to the density of the material, as with all attenuation processes.

To summarize:

$$\tau \propto \rho Z^3/E^3.$$

The foregoing is illustrated in Figure 1.16, which shows how the mass photoelectric attenuation coefficient τ/ρ varies with photon energy in the case of soft tissue (T), having $Z = 7.4$, bone (B), with $Z = 13$, and iodine (I), with $Z = 53$.

Effective atomic number
A mixture or compound has an effective atomic number that is a (weighted) average of the atomic numbers of the constituent elements. To take account of the photoelectric absorption, the effective atomic number is defined as the cube root of the weighted sum of the cubes of the atomic numbers of the constituents. Some examples are:

Fat	Air	Water, muscle	Bone
6.4	7.6	7.4	13.3

The Compton and photoelectric interactions depend on the effective atomic number but not on the molecular configuration.

Absorption edges
For photon energies between the L- and K-shell binding energies (E_L and E_K), the photoelectric attenuation decreases according to the $1/E^3$ relation as the photon energy is increased. When the photon energy reaches E_K, interaction with the K-shell electron becomes possible and the probability of photoelectric absorption jumps up to a higher value. It then decreases again as the photon energy increases further. Called the K-absorption edge, this jump is illustrated for the case of iodine in Figure 1.16 ($E_K = 33$ keV).

The sudden change of attenuation coefficient, the K-absorption edge, occurs at different photon energies with different materials. The higher the atomic number of the material, the greater is E_K and the greater is the photon energy at which the edge occurs.

For example, in the case of iodine, photons of energy 31 keV are attenuated much less than photons of energy 35 keV. The K-edges of low atomic number materials such as air, water, tissue and aluminium have no significance, as they occur at $E_K = 1$ keV or less. The absorption edge is important in choosing materials for X-ray beam filters (see section 1.5), contrast media (see Ch. 3.2.1) and imaging phosphors (see Ch. 4.1.2). Because the photon energy of the K-radiation of any material is somewhat less than its E_K, a material is relatively transparent to its own characteristic radiation.

1.4.4 Relative importance of Compton and photoelectric effects

The photoelectric coefficient is proportional to Z^3/E^3 and is particularly high when the photon energy is just greater than E_K. The Compton coefficient is independent of Z and little affected by E. Accordingly, photoelectric absorption is more important than the Compton process with high-Z materials as well as with relatively low-energy photons. Conversely, the Compton process is more important than photoelectric absorption with low-Z materials as well as with high-energy photons. This is illustrated in Figure 1.17, in which, for the combination of photon energies and atomic numbers above and to the left of the line, the photoelectric effect is the prominent interaction, whereas Compton scatter predominates below and to the right of the line. The photon energy at which the two processes are equally important is about 30 keV for air, water and tissue, 50 keV for aluminium and bone, 300 keV for iodine and barium, and 500 keV for lead.

For example, there is about a 2% probability that a 30 keV photon traversing 1 mm of soft tissue undergoes a photoelectric interaction. The probability that a photon of this energy undergoes a Compton interaction also happens to be 2%. If a 30-keV photon traverses 1 mm of bone, the probabilities are about 12% and 3%, respectively.

Figure 1.16 compares the attenuation coefficients for three materials over a range of photon energies. The component of the coefficient due to Compton scatter in tissue is also shown.

As regards diagnostic imaging with X-rays, therefore:

- the Compton process is the predominant process for air, water and soft tissues

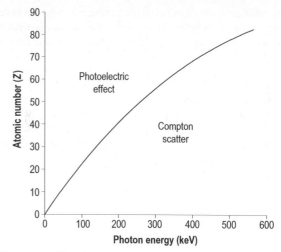

Figure 1.17 The relation between atomic number and the energy at which there is equal probability of a photon interaction through the Compton and photoelectric effects.

Box 1.4 Elastic scatter

There is a third process whereby X- and gamma rays interact with matter. The photon bounces off an electron that is firmly bound to its parent atom. The effect occurs if the photon energy is less than the binding energy of the electron and with diminishing probability at increased energies. No secondary electron is set moving and no ionization or other effect is produced in the material. The process is associated with small angles of scatter and has little significance in radiology. It may also be known as coherent, classical, unmodified or Rayleigh scattering.

- photoelectric absorption predominates for contrast media, lead and the materials used in films, screens and other imaging devices
- while both are important for bone.

A third interaction process, known as elastic or coherent scatter, is also possible at low photon energies. It is less important than Compton scatter or the photoelectric effect. It is described briefly in Box 1.4.

1.4.5 Secondary electrons and ionization

The term *secondary radiation* refers to Compton-scattered radiation, and *secondary electrons* to the recoil electrons and photoelectrons set moving in the material by the two processes. As they travel through the material, the secondary electrons interact with the outer shells of the atoms they pass nearby and excite or ionize them. The track of the electron is therefore dotted with ion pairs. When travelling through air, the electron loses an average of 34 eV per ion pair formed. This is accounted for by about 3 eV being needed to excite an atom and about 10 eV to ionize it, and there being about eight times as many excitations as ionizations.

When it has lost the whole of its initial energy in this way, the electron comes to the end of its *range*. The greater the initial energy of the electron, the greater is its range. The range is inversely proportional to the density of the material.

For example, when 140 keV photons are absorbed in soft tissue, some of the secondary electrons are photoelectrons having an energy of 140 keV, able to produce some 4000 ion pairs with a range of about 0.2 mm in tissue. However, most of the secondary electrons are Compton recoil electrons with a spectrum of energies averaging 25 keV and an average range of about 0.02 mm. The ranges in air are some 800 times greater than in tissue. Because of their continual collisions with the atoms, the tracks of secondary electrons are somewhat tortuous.

It is the excitations and ionizations produced by the secondary electrons that account for various properties of X- and gamma rays.

- The ionization of air and other gases makes them electrically conducting: used in the measurement of X- and gamma rays (see section 1.6.3).

- The ionization of atoms in the constituents of living cells causes biological damage: responsible for the hazards of radiation exposure to patients and staff and necessitating protection against radiation (see Ch. 2).

- The excitation of atoms of certain materials (phosphors) makes them emit light (luminescence, scintillation or fluorescence): used in the measurement of X- and gamma rays and as a basis of radiological imaging (see section 1.7 and Chs 4–8).

- The effect on the atoms of silver and bromine in a photographic film leads to blackening (photographic effect): used in the measurement of X- and gamma rays (see Ch. 2) and as a basis of conventional radiography (see Ch. 4).

- The greater part of the energy absorbed from an X- or gamma ray beam is converted into increased molecular motion, i.e. heat in the material, and produces an extremely small rise in temperature.

Other ionizing radiations

Some ultraviolet radiation has a sufficiently high photon energy to ionize air. Beta particles emitted by many radioactive substances, and other moving electrons (in a TV monitor, for example) also possess the above properties. Alpha particles (helium nuclei, ^{4}He), which are particularly stable combinations of two neutrons and two protons, are also emitted by some radioactive substances. Both alpha and beta particles are charged particles and are *directly ionizing*.

X- and gamma rays are *indirectly ionizing*, through their secondary electrons; the secondary ions produced along the track of a secondary electron being many times more than the single primary ionization caused by the initial Compton or photoelectric interaction. Neutrons also ionize tissue indirectly through collisions with hydrogen nuclei.

1.5 FILTRATION

When a radiograph is taken, the lower-energy photons in the X-ray beam are mainly absorbed by and deposit dose in the patient. Only a small fraction, if any, reaches the film and contributes to the image. The object of filtration is to remove a large proportion of the lower-energy photons before they reach the skin. This reduces the dose received by the patient while hardly affecting the radiation reaching the film, and so the resulting image.

This dose reduction is achieved by interposing between the X-ray tube and patient a uniform flat sheet of metal, usually aluminium, and called the *added* or *additional filtration*. The predominant attenuation process in this filter should be photoelectric absorption. Because this varies inversely as the cube of the photon energy, the filter will attenuate the lower-energy photons (which mainly contribute to patient dose) much more than it does the higher-energy photons (which are mainly responsible for the image).

The X-ray photons produced in the target are initially filtered within the target itself, because they may be generated below its surface, and then by the window of the tube housing, the insulating oil and the glass insert. The combined effect of these disparate components is expressed as an equivalent thickness of aluminium, typically 1 mm Al, and is called the *inherent filtration*. The light beam diaphragm mirror also adds to the filtration, as does the dose area product (DAP) chamber (see section 1.6.3). When inherent filtration must be minimized, a tube with a window of beryllium ($Z = 4$) instead of glass may be used.

The *total filtration* is the sum of the added filtration and the inherent filtration. For general diagnostic radiology, it should be at least 2.5 mm Al equivalent. This will produce an HVL of about 2.5 mm Al at 70 kV and 4.0 mm at 120 kV. The amount of added filtration is therefore typically 1.5 mm Al.

Choice of filter material

The atomic number should be sufficiently high to make the energy-dependent attenuating process, photoelectric absorption, predominate. It should not be too high, because the whole of the useful X-ray spectrum should lie on the high-energy side of the absorption edge. If not, the filter might actually soften the beam.

Aluminium ($Z = 13$, $E_K = 1.6\,keV$) is generally used, as it has a sufficiently high atomic number to be suitable for most diagnostic X-ray beams. The most common alternative is copper ($Z = 29$), with added filter thicknesses in the range of 0.1–0.3 mm being typical. Copper is a more efficient filter, but it emits 9 keV characteristic X-rays. These must be absorbed by a backing filter of aluminium on the patient side of the compound filter.

Effects of filtration

Figure 1.18 shows the spectrum of X-rays generated at 60 kV after passing through 1, 2 and 3 mm Al. A filter attenuates the lower-energy X-rays more in proportion than the higher-energy X-rays. It therefore increases the penetrating power (HVL) of the beam at the cost of reducing its intensity. It reduces the skin dose to the patient while having little effect on the radiological image. It is responsible for the low-energy cut-off of the X-ray spectrum, depicted in Figure 1.18.

Increasing the filtration has the following effects. It causes the continuous X-ray spectrum to shrink and move to the right, as seen in Figure 1.18. It increases the minimum and effective photon energies but does not affect the maximum photon energy. It reduces the area of the spectrum and the total output of X-rays. Finally, it increases the exit dose:entry dose ratio or film dose:skin dose ratio.

Above a certain thickness, there is no gain from increasing the filtration, as the output is further reduced with little further improvement in patient dose or HVL. In addition, the reduction in total output of X-rays may require the exposure time for a radiograph to be increased to an extent that patient movement becomes a problem. It may also require an increase in tube current during fluoroscopy that cannot be sustained because of excess heat production.

K-edge filters

Filter materials with K-edges in the higher-energy part of the X-ray spectrum can be used. These remove both high- and low-energy X-rays but are relatively transparent to the energies just below the K-edge. An example of an 80-kV beam filtered with a 0.1-mm erbium filter ($Z = 68$, $E_K = 57\,keV$) is shown in Figure 1.19. K-edge filters are rarely used except in mammography (Ch. 4.6).

Compensating or wedge filter

A shaped filter may be attached to the tube to make the exposure across the film more uniform and compensate for the large difference in transmission by, for example, the upper and lower thorax, neck and shoulder, or foot and ankle. In fluoroscopy equipment, the filter may be incorporated into the beam diaphragm and can be driven into the beam to prevent flaring of the image at the edges of the body while not totally obscuring the underlying anatomy. These filters may be referred to as soft or wedge filters.

1.6 RADIATION DOSIMETRY

1.6.1 Absorbed dose

The effects of ionizing radiations described above may be correlated with the energy deposited as ionization and excitation of the atoms of the material

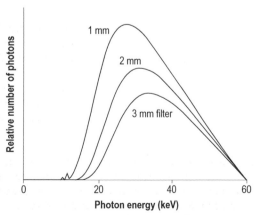

Figure 1.18 Effect of increasing aluminium filtration on the X-ray spectrum.

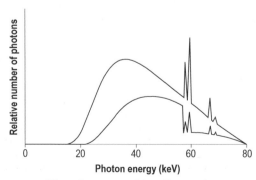

Figure 1.19 Effect of a 0.1 mm erbium filter on the spectrum at 80 kV compared with the same beam filtered by 2.5 mm Al.

irradiated. The absorbed dose is the energy deposited per unit mass of the stated material (in joules per kilogram). The SI unit of absorbed dose is the gray (Gy); $1\,Gy = 1\,J\,kg^{-1}$. Absorbed dose rate is measured in grays per second, with the usual multiples and submultiples. Absorbed dose is commonly used to define the quantity of radiation delivered at a specified point in the radiation field. Its definition is therefore concerned with the vanishingly small quantities of energy absorbed and of mass of material. It can be thought of as the concentration of energy delivered to the position of measurement.

The concept of absorbed dose applies to all directly and indirectly ionizing radiations and to any material. It is particularly valuable when considering tissue and biological effects. The term *dose* is applied loosely to several dosimetric quantities used to describe radiation fields and their effects on biological systems. When encountering the word 'dose', it is necessary to decide on the quantity being referred to from the context. Within this text, whenever 'dose' is used alone, it is taken to mean absorbed dose in the material specified.

Before 1980, the international unit of absorbed dose was the rad. It is used in some old textbooks. The conversion factor is $1\,Gy = 100\,rad$; $1\,rad = 1\,cGy = 10\,mGy$.

1.6.2 Kerma

Another quantity sometimes used is kerma, which is also measured in grays. The difference between kerma and absorbed dose is subtle. Kerma is an acronym for *kinetic energy released to matter*. It is the energy *transferred* per unit mass of irradiated material, from photons to electrons at the specified position. In contrast, absorbed dose is the energy *deposited* (as ionization and excitation) by secondary electrons at that position. The only practical difference between the two is that at high energies (greater than about 1 MeV) a small part of the energy of the electrons may produce bremsstrahlung radiation, and the energy transferred to electrons at a specific location will be deposited away from that location because of the increased electron range. For diagnostic energies, they are effectively equal and, in the subject matter of this text, absorbed dose and kerma can be used interchangeably.

The reader should be aware that there is an obsolete quantity, *exposure*, that may be encountered in some older publications. Unlike kerma, it applies to X- and gamma rays only (kerma also applies to neutrons). Exposure describes the quantity of ionization produced by a photon beam per unit mass of air. Its units are therefore $C\,kg^{-1}$. Exposure was historically useful, because it could be measured directly (although only for photon energies up to about 500 keV). Before the adoption of SI units, exposure had the special unit, roentgen (R). In reading older literature, the roentgen can be taken to be approximately equal to 10 mGy.

1.6.3 Measurement of X- and gamma ray dose

It is extremely difficult to measure absorbed dose in solids or liquids directly. In theory, this can be done by measuring temperature rise, but in practice, because the temperature change for a relatively high absorbed dose of 1 Gy would lead to a temperature rise not much greater than $10^{-4\circ}C$ (0.1 mK), it is impractical. It is more usual to measure the dose delivered to air (or air kerma) under the same conditions and to multiply it by a conversion factor to obtain the dose in the specified material such as tissue. The conversion factor depends on the relative amounts of energy absorbed in air and the material.

Like the mass attenuation coefficients, the factor depends on the effective atomic number of the material and on the effective energy of the X- or gamma rays. For X-rays used in radiology, the following are approximate values of the conversion factor:

- for muscle, the atomic number of which is not very different to that of air and in which the Compton process predominates, the ratio is close to unity and varies only between 1.0 and 1.1 over the whole kV range

- for compact bone, with its higher atomic number and in which photoelectric absorption is important, the ratio varies from about 5 at low keV to 1.2 at 150 keV

- for fat, with its lower atomic number, the ratio varies in the opposite direction, from about 0.6 at low keV to 1.1 at high keV.

Ionization chamber

Air kerma is commonly determined by measuring the amount of ionization produced by the photon beam in air. The instrument used is known as an *ionization chamber*, and a simple version of it is the *thimble* chamber shown in Figure 1.20. The chamber consists of a plastic thimble-shaped outer wall (A) surrounding an air-filled cavity (B), and with an insulator separating it from a thin central electrode (C). It is positioned at the point of interest.

Each X-ray photon (X) absorbed in the wall liberates a secondary electron (e^-), which produces ion pairs along its track. (Although in the diagram the track is for simplicity idealized as a straight line, it is in fact quite tortuous.) For each ion pair, approximately 34 eV of energy is deposited. Therefore for each

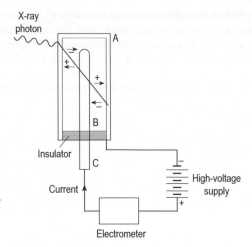

Figure 1.20 Ionization chamber.

coulomb of charge (and remembering the definition of electron volt as being the energy in J multiplied by the electron charge, Box 1.1), 34 J of energy will have been deposited. Theoretically therefore, the air kerma is 34/mass of air in the chamber.

To measure the charge, the ions are separated before they can recombine by applying a polarizing voltage (typically in the range of 100–300 V) between the outer thimble wall and the central electrode. The positive ions are attracted to the negative electrode and the negative ions (electrons) to the positive electrode. The ionization current is measured by a device known as an electrometer. It is proportional to air kerma rate and the total charge collected to air kerma.

The chamber wall must be made of a suitable material. As Figure 1.20 shows, the air in the thimble is ionized by secondary electrons that have been set moving by X-rays absorbed in the wall and electrode. So far as the X-rays and their secondary electrons are concerned, these components should be indistinguishable from air, except in density. They must be made of *air-equivalent material* that matches air in terms of its effective atomic number, and so absorbs energy from an X-ray beam, whatever its energy, to the same extent as the same mass of air. The density is not important. There are other conditions to be fulfilled, such as electrical conductivity and mechanical stability. Generally, a compromise is made with a plastic material being used ($Z \approx 6$) with graphite deposited on its inner wall to make it electrically conducting.

The chamber wall must be sufficiently thick so that the electrons produced outside the chamber will not penetrate the wall to deposit ionization in the cavity; 0.2 mm is sufficient for photoelectrons from 140 keV X-rays, for example. If the wall is too thick, it will attenuate unduly the radiation being measured. This is of particular concern in mammography beams, for which thinner walled chambers are used.

Another correction has to be applied if the ambient temperature or pressure differs from standard values. At high pressures and/or low temperature, the chamber will over-read because of increased density and therefore mass of air in the cavity. However, the correction is small and is generally ignored.

As indicated above, there is a theoretical relationship between the measured charge and air kerma. In practice, however, there would be a need to apply several corrections, in particular to account for the non-air equivalence of the chamber and the attenuation in the chamber wall. Ionization chambers and their associated electronics are therefore sent to a standards laboratory for calibration at the energies at which they are to be used.

Figure 1.20 illustrates a particular shape of ionization chamber. In principle, any shape of cavity could be used, but the commonest chambers are either cylindrical (as illustrated here) or consist of parallel electrodes. The so-called parallel plate chamber typically has two outer electrodes (generally circular) defining the cavity, with a central collecting plate between the two, the three plates being separated by insulators.

The sensitivity of an ionization chamber (charge per unit of air kerma) is proportional to volume. In general, for diagnostic radiology chambers with a volume of approximately 10–30 cm^3 are used for measurements in the radiation beam, with chambers of 150 cm^3 or bigger being suitable for the measurement of scatter radiation.

Air is chosen as the standard material for dosimetry because:

- it has an effective atomic number (7.6) close to that of tissue (7.4), so that the factor used to convert absorbed dose in air to absorbed dose in tissue can be made easily and accurately
- it is applicable for measurement over a wide range of X- and gamma ray energies
- large and small doses and large and small dose rates are easily and accurately measured
- it is universally available with an invariable composition.

Dose area product meters

Dose area product meters are used for the assessment of patient dose (DAP). They use an ionization chamber mounted on the collimator of the X-ray tube. The chamber is a parallel plate type, generally with square plates. It has an area bigger than the maximum beam size at the position at which it is mounted. It is a sealed chamber so as to avoid changes in calibration caused by changes in temperature and pressure. The amount of ionization produced within the chamber is proportional not just to dose but also to the area of beam. Thus it is measuring the product of dose and area with unit of Gy cm^2. Different submultiples may be used by different manufacturers, two common examples being cGy cm^2 and µGy m^2. Use of DAP for patient dose audits is discussed in Chapter 2.8.3.

Other dosimeters
It is often convenient to measure radiation dose by means of:

- lithium fluoride thermoluminescence dosimeters used for both personal dosimetry (see Ch. 2.5.5) and patient dosimetry (see Ch. 2.8.3)

- the photographic effect in silver bromide, used in a film badge (see Ch. 2.5.5)

- photoconductivity in silicon diodes to be used in direct reading electronic personal dosimeters and dosimeters used for quality assurance.

Films and diodes use high atomic number materials, so that factors to correct their readings to air kerma are critically dependent on the energy spectrum. To provide meaningful results, they are used with filters so that their readings can be correctly interpreted.

1.6.4 Radiation quantity and quality

In this text, the amount or quantity of radiation has been discussed in terms of intensity (energy fluence rate) or air kerma rate. It has been shown that they are:

- approximately proportional to the square of the kV
- proportional to the mA
- inversely proportional to the square of the distance F from a point source.

Thus air kerma rate is proportional to kV^2 × mA/F^2. The energy fluence or air kerma is, in addition,

- proportional to the exposure time: air kerma is proportional to kV^2 × mAs/F^2, where mAs is the product of mA and exposure time (in seconds).

In addition, these quantities are:

- decreased as the filtration is increased
- greater for a constant potential than a pulsating potential
- greater for high rather than low atomic number targets.

Quality is a term used to describe the penetrating power of an X-ray beam. The most complete description of quality is the spectrum of X-ray energies, but in practice a simpler, single-figure description is preferred. It may be specified as the HVL of the beam in a stated material, usually aluminium for diagnostic X-rays. Alternatively, it may be described by the average or *effective energy* of the spectrum. This may be deduced from the measured HVL. The greater is the HVL, the greater the effective energy. The effective energy can be defined as the photon energy of monoenergetic X-rays that have the same HVL as the polyenergetic beam being assessed. For example, 100-kV X-rays filtered with 2 mm Al have the same HVL (3 mm Al) as 30-keV photons. When filtered with 10 mm Al, the effective energy is increased to 50 keV.

The HVL and effective energy of an X-ray beam:

- increase as the applied kV is increased
- are greater for constant potential than pulsating potential
- are unaffected by the mA or exposure time
- increase as the filtration is increased
- are unaffected by the distance from the target.

Further descriptive terms may be applied. A hard X-ray beam is produced by a high kV and a thick filter, a soft beam by a low kV and a thin filter. Because the two principal factors affecting HVL or effective energy are kV and filtration, and because the latter is normally not changed, it is common in radiography to describe the quality of X-rays simply by stating the tube kV.

1.7 LUMINESCENCE

Luminescence is a general term to describe the process in which a material absorbs energy from an external source and re-emits that energy in the form of visible light. The external energy source may be one of many including chemical, biological and physical sources, but in the context of radiology we are concerned only with radiation sources for which the term *photoluminescence* may be used.

Luminescence can be divided into two types:

- *fluorescence*, which is (more or less) the instantaneous emission of light following energy input
- *phosphorescence*, which describes delayed light emission referred to as afterglow.

The distinction between the two is somewhat arbitrary, with the delay time being of the order of 10^{-6} s. A material that has luminescent properties is described as a *phosphor*. It should be noted that crystalline materials with luminescent properties that are used for the detection of gamma radiations are commonly referred to as *scintillants*.

Box 1.5 Luminescence

In Figure 1.1, the structure of the sodium atom is shown, in which the electrons occupy shells with discrete binding energies. In a solid, the atoms are closely packed together and the allowed energy levels are spread into energy bands as shown in Figure 1.21. Commonly, the individual atoms will be combined into molecules such that the *valence band*, i.e. the outermost band that is occupied with electrons, will be completely filled. The next higher energy band will be vacant and is referred to as the *conduction band*. Between the two energy bands, there is the *forbidden zone* that describes the energy levels that cannot be occupied by an electron in that material.

Within the material, there will be impurities (deliberately introduced in the case of a commercial phosphor). These impurity materials have energy levels that differ from those of the phosphor itself and may introduce discrete energy shells within the forbidden zone that are unoccupied. These are referred to as *electron traps*.

On irradiation of the material, Compton recoil and photoelectrons will be produced as described in section 1.4. These will cause excitation in the molecules of the material. Excitation is the process that results in electrons being raised from the valence into the conduction band, as is illustrated by arrow A in Figure 1.21. Once in the conduction band, the electron is able to move freely within the material. Should the electron come within the vicinity of an impurity atom, it can move down into the electron trap, as shown by arrow B. The electron in the electron trap cannot return to the valence band unless there is a space or *hole* available for it to drop back into. However, holes are being created in the valence band while the material is being irradiated and the holes are able to travel within the valence band. When a hole is created in the vicinity of the electron trap, the electron will then fall back into the valence band D, generally via the conduction band C, and the energy thus liberated is given out in the form of light. The intensity of the light emitted from the phosphor is proportional to the amount of energy it absorbs from the X-ray beam and is thus proportional to the intensity of the X-ray beam.

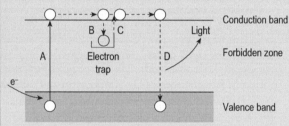

Figure 1.21 Luminescence caused by ionizing radiation.

A further distinction can be made between those phosphors that emit light spontaneously and those that require a further energy input before light is given out. Two such processes of significance in radiology are *thermoluminescence*, in which light is emitted only following heating of the irradiated material, and *photostimulable* luminescence, in which light is emitted when the irradiated phosphor is exposed to light. Either process can be used for the measurement of radiation dose (*thermoluminescent dosimetry and optically stimulated luminescence*, see Ch. 2.5.5), and the latter is the basis for *computed radiography* (see Ch. 5.3).

The process of luminescence is described in more detail in Box 1.5. The intensity of light emitted from a phosphor is proportional to the energy absorbed from the X-ray or gamma beam, which itself is proportional to the intensity of the radiation beam itself. Because the intensity of light is relatively easy to measure or to record, the process of luminescence is the most important effect that is used in X- and gamma ray

imaging and is common to most detectors used for that purpose.

1.8 SUMMARY

- X-rays and gamma rays are electromagnetic radiations.

- X-rays are produced by stopping high-energy electrons in a tungsten target.

- X-rays are emitted in a continuous spectrum (bremsstrahlung) with a maximum energy equal to the peak accelerating potential of the X-ray tube and at discrete energies dependent on the binding energies of electrons in the target atom.

- The X-ray beam is filtered (usually with aluminium) to remove low-energy photons that contribute to patient dose but not to the image.

- The intensity of the beam falls off in accordance with the inverse square law.

- X-rays are attenuated and scattered within a material, with the image being formed by those X-rays transmitted through the body.

- There are two principal interaction processes.
  — Compton scatter is an interaction with a free electron and depends on the electron density of the material. It is only weakly dependent on photon energy in the diagnostic range.
  — Photoelectric effect is an interaction with a bound electron and is strongly dependent on the atomic number of the material and photon energy.

- X-rays and gamma rays ionize matter through the secondary electrons generated in the interaction processes.

- Absorbed dose is the energy deposited in a material from the interaction of ionizing radiations.

- Absorbed dose is expressed in the unit gray (Gy).

- Absorbed dose is commonly measured using ionization chambers.

- X-rays and gamma rays cause luminescence in certain materials, which can be used for image formation and also for radiation measurement.

Chapter 2

Radiation hazards and protection

2.1 IONIZING RADIATION INTERACTIONS WITH TISSUE

When ionizing radiations such as X- and gamma rays interact with living tissue, it is the absorption of radiation energy in the tissues that causes damage. If the radiation passed through the tissue without absorption, there would be no biological effects and no radiological image would be produced. Whenever radiation is absorbed, chemical changes are produced virtually immediately, and subsequent molecular damage follows in a short space of time (seconds to minutes). It is after this, during a much longer time span of hours to decades, that the biological damage becomes evident (Fig. 2.1).

There are many examples of *radiation-induced damage*: to the skin and hands suffered by the early radiologists, excess leukaemias in patients treated with radiation for ankylosing spondylitis, and radiation accidents in various parts of the world. However, the current estimates of radiation risk for cancer induction have been mostly derived from the outcomes, since 1945, of those exposed to nuclear explosions, particularly the 90 000 survivors of the atomic bomb attacks on Hiroshima and Nagasaki.

The principal radiation source for medical exposures is diagnostic X-rays; other important sources include gamma-emitting radionuclides in nuclear medicine and radiotherapy sources including beta emitters, electron beams, and gamma and X-ray sources (and in very rare cases neutron and proton beams).

Whenever a beta particle or an electron passes through tissue, ionizations and excitations occur repeatedly until eventually the particle comes to rest, giving up all its energy. Being relatively light, such electrons are easily deflected by the negatively charged orbital electrons of the tissue atoms that they

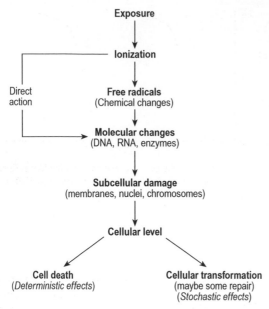

Figure 2.1 Chain of events following exposure to ionizing radiation.

encounter, and so follow a very tortuous path. The total range involved in tissue interactions is of the order of a few millimetres at most. Hence electrons are easily absorbed by a shield of a few millimetres of perspex or by thin sheets of metal, depending on their initial energy.

Unlike beta particles, X- and gamma radiations do not have a maximum depth of penetration associated with them, but they simply undergo progressive attenuation. That is, the intensity of the radiation beam continues to fall as it interacts with tissue but at any given depth a residual beam always remains, however much less intense (see Ch. 1.4.1).

During radiation exposures, it is the *ionization* process that causes the majority of immediate chemical changes in tissue. The critical molecules for radiation damage are believed to be the proteins (such as enzymes) and nucleic acid (principally DNA). The damage occurs in two basic ways: by producing lesions in solute molecules directly (e.g. by rupturing a covalent bond) or by an indirect action between the solute molecules and the free radicals produced during the ionization of water.

Indirect damage arises more commonly, because living tissue is about 70–90% water. If a pure water molecule is irradiated, it emits a free electron and produces a positively charged water ion, which immediately decomposes:

$$H_2O + radiation \rightarrow H_2O^+ + e^-$$

$$H_2O^+ \ decomposes \rightarrow H^+ + OH.$$

The hydroxyl free radical OH is a highly reactive and powerful oxidizing agent that produces chemical modifications in solute organic molecules. These interactions, which occur in microseconds or less after exposure, are one way in which a sequence of complex chemical events can be started, but the free radical species formed can lead to many biologically harmful products and can produce damaging chain reactions in tissue.

The exact mechanism of these complex events is incompletely understood, but biological damage following exposure to ionizing radiations has been well documented at a variety of levels. Figure 2.1 shows the chain of events. At a *molecular level*, macromolecules such as DNA, RNA and enzymes are damaged; at the *subcellular level*, cell membranes, nuclei, chromosomes, etc. are affected; and at the *cellular level*, cell division can be inhibited, cell death brought about, or transformation to a malignant state induced. Cell repair can also occur, and is an important mechanism when there is sufficient time for recovery between irradiation events.

2.2 RADIATION DOSES AND UNITS

To study the effects of radiation, it is necessary to quantify the amount of radiation received. In Chapter 1.6, the physical quantities *kerma* and *absorbed dose* were introduced, as well as their unit, the gray (Gy). These are measurable quantities related to the energy transferred (kerma) or absorbed (absorbed dose) from the radiation beam. While it is reasonable to assume that biological effects will be related to energy absorption, there are biological factors that need to be considered, in particular the influence of radiation type and the relative radiosensitivities of the different organs and tissues within the body. Two further dosimetry quantities to account for these effects are therefore introduced: *equivalent dose* and *effective dose*. These incorporate empirical weighting factors based on observations of radiation effects.

Equivalent dose

X- and gamma rays are indirectly ionizing radiations, ionization being produced by electrons generated in the photon interactions with tissue. Electrons produce ionization over a distance that is relatively large compared with cellular dimensions and are considered to have a low ionization density. This is described by the quantity *linear energy transfer* (LET), being the sum of the energy deposited in tissue per unit path length. In contrast, alpha particles, being the nucleus of the helium atom with two protons plus two neutrons, are very much heavier. For the same initial energy as an electron, an alpha particle travels a much shorter distance. For these high-LET particles, ionizing events are much more closely spaced and within distances comparable with the dimensions of a single strand of DNA. For this reason, the damage caused by high-LET radiations is much more likely to be non-repairable than is the case for electrons (low-LET radiation). This difference in radiation effects is described by the term *relative biological effectiveness* (RBE), which is the ratio of absorbed doses required to induce the same biological end point for two radiation types. RBE is generally expressed in terms of a comparison with a reference beam of X-rays. It is highly dependent on a number of factors, including biological end point, and may be 20 or greater for alpha particles, implying that they produce the same biological end point as X-rays with 5% or less absorbed dose.

Equivalent dose is a quantity used only in radiation protection, i.e. for relatively low levels of dose. It is derived from absorbed dose multiplied by a radiation weighting factor w_R. The factor depends on radiation type and is defined as being unity for X- and gamma rays, electrons and beta particles. For alpha particles, it is set equal to 20, and for protons and neutrons equal to 5, 10 or 20 depending on radiation energy. The SI unit of equivalent dose is $J kg^{-1}$ given the special name sievert (Sv) to distinguish it from absorbed dose.

Effective dose is a second radiation protection dosimetry quantity that incorporates factors to account for the variable radiosensitivities of organs and tissues in the body. It also has the unit sievert. Effective dose is considered in more detail in section 2.3.2.

This text is concerned with the diagnostic use of ionizing radiations and deals exclusively with the use of X- and gamma rays for which the radiation weighting factor w_R is unity. Absorbed dose and equivalent dose are therefore numerically equal. To avoid confusion caused by the use of the same unit (Sv) for two distinct radiation protection dose quantities, when reference is made to the dose to specific organs or tissues (sometimes referred to as *organ dose*) doses are given in terms of the absorbed dose in Gy. The exception to this is for the dose limits (see section 2.5.2). These apply to all types of radiation, and it is necessary to use equivalent dose (in Sv) for those limits that apply to specific organs or tissues and effective dose (in Sv) for the whole body limits.

2.3 EFFECTS OF RADIATION

There are two categories of radiation effect: *somatic* effects, which occur in the individual exposed, and *genetic* or *hereditary* effects, which occur in the

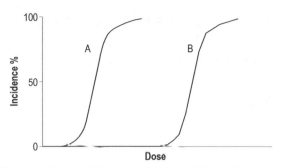

Figure 2.2 Dose–incident curves for deterministic effects. Curve A represents a relatively mild, low-dose effect compared with the effect represented by curve B.

descendants of those individuals as a result of lesions in the germinal cells. These effects may be further described as being either *deterministic* or *stochastic* in nature.

2.3.1 Deterministic effects

Threshold dose
Deterministic effects (sometimes called non-stochastic) are characterized as having a threshold dose below which the effect will not occur. The value of the threshold may vary to a small extent from individual to individual. Once the threshold dose is exceeded, the likelihood of the effect occurring increases rapidly with dose up to a level at which the effect will invariably occur. This is illustrated in Figure 2.2, in which two dose–incidence curves are shown. Curve A might represent relatively mild damage, for example skin erythema, for which the threshold dose is relatively low. Curve B in Figure 2.2 represents more severe damage, such as irreversible ulceration of the skin, with a very much higher dose threshold. Some examples of deterministic effects and approximate threshold doses are given in Table 2.1.

Cataracts are produced above a threshold of about 5 Gy to the lens of the eye. The damage to the eye is cumulative. Attention therefore has to be paid to the lifetime dose for those working in radiation-intense areas such as interventional radiology. This is considered further in section 2.5.2.

Unlike damage to the eye, most deterministic effects have repair mechanisms such that the rate at which the dose is delivered influences the threshold dose. For example, the threshold dose for skin erythema is in the region of 2–5 Gy. If somebody were to receive 20 mGy week^{-1} to the skin over

Table 2.1 Threshold doses for deterministic effects

Effect	Threshold dose (Gy)[a]
Skin erythema	2–5
Irreversible skin damage	20–40
Hair loss	2–5
Sterility	2–3
Cataracts (lens of eye)	5
Lethality (whole body)	3–5
Fetal abnormality	0.1–0.5

[a]Threshold doses are given in terms of the absorbed dose (in Gy). They could be given in terms of the equivalent dose (Sv) and be applicable to all types of ionizing radiation. In this text, which is concerned only with medical radiations (X- and gamma rays) for which the radiation weighting factor is unity, absorbed dose is used to clarify the distinction with effective dose used for whole body exposures.

Table 2.2 Typical absorbed doses in diagnostic radiology

	Dose
Radiographic examination (skin dose)	
PA chest	0.15 mGy
AP abdomen	5 mGy
Lateral lumbar spine	12 mGy
Fluoroscopy skin dose rate	5–50 mGy min^{-1}
CT scan (within examined region)	10–30 mGy
Fetal dose (pregnant patient)	
AP pelvis	1.5 mGy
Barium enema	5 mGy
CT pelvis	10–30 mGy

AP, anteroposterior; CT, computed tomography; PA, posteroanterior.

a period of many years, the effect would not be seen even although the accumulated dose at 5 years would be 5 Gy.

Deterministic effects and the developing fetus

For women who are pregnant, there is a particular concern regarding potential harm to the developing fetus. The potential for fetal abnormalities to be caused by irradiation in utero is greatest in the third to eighth week of pregnancy. The damage may be sufficient to cause spontaneous abortion, or it may induce birth defects or abnormalities such as Down's syndrome. Threshold doses for deterministic effects on the developing fetus are in the range 100–500 mGy.

Absorbed doses in radiology

To understand the significance of deterministic effects in diagnostic radiology, it is necessary to know the doses patients or staff might receive. Table 2.2 shows some typical doses. It can be seen that, in general, the doses are no more than a few tens of mGy, indicating little significance of threshold doses in diagnostic radiology. Computed tomography (CT) scans can result in relatively high eye doses in the region of several tens of mGy. Although this may be much less than the threshold dose, the possibility of the patient having several scans over their lifetime linked to the cumulative nature of the effect makes it good practice to use techniques that will minimize the dose to the lens. Skin doses in fluoroscopy may be as high as 50 mGy min^{-1}. Some complex interventional procedures are associated with protracted screening times, up to 60 min or more. In these instances, the risk of occurrence of effects such as skin erythema or hair loss cannot be discounted.

2.3.2 Stochastic effects

Stochastic means statistical in nature, and stochastic effects are those that arise by chance. The fact that ionizing radiations can cause cancer or genetic abnormalities is not a matter of debate; however, the shape of the dose–effect curve is. It is the conventional wisdom on which radiation protection principles are based that there is no threshold dose for stochastic effects, and that the risk increases linearly with dose. This is known as the *linear no threshold theory*. Although the risk increases with dose, the severity of the effect does not; the irradiated person will either develop cancer or will be unaffected.

Carcinogenesis and organ risk

The evidence for radiation-induced cancer and for risk factors is derived from many sources. These include populations irradiated following atomic weapons tests, occupationally exposed workers (including radiologists from earlier times when minimal precautions were taken), medical irradiations (e.g. radiotherapy for non-malignant conditions such as ankylosing spondylitis) and radiation accidents. In analysing cancer incidence for such populations, deriving radiation-specific risk factors is beset by uncertainties caused by the underlying high natural incidence of the disease.

The most significant studies of the stochastic effects of radiation come from the lifetime study of the approximately 90 000 survivors of the atomic bombs dropped over the Japanese cities Hiroshima and Nagasaki in 1945. The studies considered survivors who received whole body doses from photons and neutrons greater than about 0.2 Sv. Following analysis of excess cancers in this population and from

Table 2.3 Organ- and tissue-specific radiation risk factors and tissue weighting factors, w_T

Organ or tissue	Risk factor (% per Sv)	Weighting factor (w_T)
Gonads	–	0.20
Stomach	1.10	0.12
Colon	0.85	0.12
Lung	0.85	0.12
Red bone marrow	0.50	0.12
Bladder	0.30	0.05
Oesophagus	0.30	0.05
Breast	0.20	0.05
Liver	0.15	0.05
Thyroid	0.08	0.05
Ovaries	0.10	–
Bone surface	0.05	0.01
Skin	0.02	0.01
Remainder	0.50	0.05
Total	5.0	1

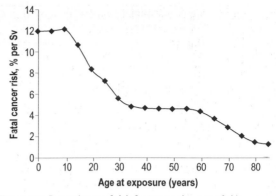

Figure 2.3 Dependence of risk factor on the age of the irradiated person.

other studies, the organ-specific risk factors shown in Table 2.3 have been derived. It should be noted that the risk factors are specified for fatal cancers and not for incidence. In particular, the risk factor for the thyroid is relatively low because, although the probability of induction is relatively high, the mortality is low. Overall, for a uniform whole body irradiation, the risk of fatal cancer is 5% per Sv or 1 in 20000 per mSv for the general population. This is the risk to the irradiated individual. The logical outcome of linear no threshold theory is that irradiating a population of 20000 people to a uniform, whole body dose of 1mSv would result (on average) in one excess cancer death in that population.

One of the problems in quantifying risk is the latency period between irradiation and the clinical manifestation of the disease. Leukaemias arising from irradiation of the red bone marrow have a latency period of several years, with a peak in incidence occurring at about 7–10 years following irradiation. In contrast, solid tumours have a latency period of 40 years or more. This has two consequences. First, the estimation of risk following the irradiation of a population becomes difficult to assess. Second, the risk to the younger population with a long life expectancy is greater than that to the older population, as shown in Figure 2.3. In particular, the risk to children is more than double the value averaged over the whole population.

Genetic effects

It is difficult to assess the genetic risk in humans. Even the descendants of the survivors of the atom bombs dropped on Hiroshima and Nagasaki have not shown any excess of genetic disorders: the frequency of congenital defects, fecundity and life expectancy appear to be no different than for the children of non-irradiated parents. Similarly, surveys of descendants of radiotherapy patients show no increase in congenital defects. However, in view of the paucity of data, a safety margin is included in all risk estimates. The risk of hereditary ill health in subsequent children and future generations is estimated to be 1 in 70000 for an exposure of 1mGy to the gonads. This is the risk averaged over the whole population. For the reproductive population, i.e. those who will have children at some time following exposure, the risk is obviously greater and is estimated as 1 in 40000.

Effective dose

The risk factors given in Table 2.3 are for single organs or tissues and quantify the risk of developing fatal cancer following the irradiation of that specific organ or tissue. The carcinogenic risk has been summed over all organs to provide an overall risk factor for the situation in which the individual has been irradiated to a uniform whole body dose. In practice, the individual is rarely irradiated uniformly, for example the patient having an X-ray examination will receive a significant dose only in the region being examined; the radiologist conducting the examination will receive much higher doses on the side of the body facing the patient.

To compare risks from different irradiation geometries, an averaging procedure is used. The average equivalent dose to each organ and tissue in the body is multiplied by a tissue weighting factor, w_T, and the values are summed over the whole body. The summed value of the weighted organ dose is the *effective dose* with the same unit as equivalent dose, i.e. the

Table 2.4 Calculation of effective dose for anteroposterior radiograph of thoracic spine

Organ	Equivalent dose (H_T mSv^{-1})	Weighting factor (w_T)	$w_T \bullet H_T$ mSv^{-1}
Gonads	0.001	0.2	<0.001
Stomach	0.34	0.12	0.041
Colon	0.001	0.12	<0.001
Lung	0.56	0.12	0.067
Red bone marrow	0.12	0.12	0.014
Bladder	0.0004	0.05	<0.001
Oesophagus	0.40	0.05	0.020
Breast	0.56	0.05	0.028
Liver	0.38	0.05	0.019
Thyroid	0.63	0.05	0.032
Bone surface	0.26	0.01	0.003
Skin	0.15	0.01	0.002
Remainder	0.15	0.05	0.008
Effective dose per mSv	–	–	0.234

sievert (Sv). The values of the tissue weighting factors are shown in Table 2.3. It can be seen that for carcinogenic risks the tissues have been grouped, with those having a high risk being assigned a value of 0.12; moderate risk, 0.05; and low risk, 0.01. In calculating effective dose, the risk of genetic effects is included, with a weighting factor of 0.20 being assigned to the gonads. It will be noted that the sum of the weighting factors is 1.

Mathematically, effective dose is expressed as:

$$E = \sum_T w_T \bullet H_T ,$$

in which H_T is the equivalent dose to tissue T and $\sum_T$ represents the sum over the range of tissues T. Included in the calculation is a factor for those tissues to which a weighting factor is not assigned, the *remainder* tissues. The factor is applied to the average dose to nine additional tissues (adrenals, brain, kidney, muscle, small intestine, pancreas, spleen, thymus and uterus) for which there is some evidence of cancer induction but insufficient data to provide a specific risk factor.

Having calculated effective dose for a non-homogeneous irradiation, the risk can be calculated from the risk factor for fatal cancer, i.e. 1 in 20 000 per mSv.

An example of the calculation of effective dose is shown in Table 2.4 for an anteroposterior (AP) radiograph of the thoracic spine. The effective dose for the examination is 0.23 mSv. The assumption implicit in the formulation of effective dose is the risk to the patient would be the same if a numerically equal absorbed dose was delivered uniformly to the whole body.

Risk of childhood cancer

Irradiation in utero increases the risk of childhood cancer. A risk factor has been derived from cancer incidence data in the children of mothers who were X-rayed as part of their obstetric management in the years before ultrasound became the imaging modality of choice. The risk of developing fatal childhood cancer is 3% per Gy or 1 in 33 000 per mGy. Again, the radiation quantity is absorbed dose to indicate that it is the average dose to the developing fetus and because we are concerned only with X- and gamma rays with a radiation weighting factor of 1. The risk is probably less than this in the first few weeks of pregnancy. The radiation risk factor may be compared with the incidence of fatal childhood cancer, which is approximately 1 in 1800, so that a dose of about 17 mGy would be required to double the natural risk. This is comparable with the dose that would be received should the mother have a CT scan of the pelvis (see Table 2.5).

2.3.3 Population dose

We are all exposed to natural sources of radiation to an extent that depends on where we live and what we eat. There are four categories of natural sources.

- *Cosmic radiation* is generated in space, for example from the sun. It is a mixture of particulate radiations and a broad spectrum of X- and gamma rays. Most of the radiation is attenuated by the atmosphere, and at sea level the amount is about 320 μSv year^{-1}. The levels rise with altitude, to the

Table 2.5 Approximate dose to the fetus from radiological examinations

Examination	Fetal dose (mGy)
Chest PA	<0.01
Abdomen or pelvis AP	1
Lumbar spine (AP and lateral)	1.5
Barium follow-through	2
Barium enema	8
CT chest	0.1
CT pelvis	25
Tc-99 m bone scan	4
Tc-99 m thyroid scan	0.5
Tc-99 m lung perfusion scan	0.3

AP, anteroposterior; CT, computed tomography; PA, posteroanterior; Tc-99 m, technetium-99 m.

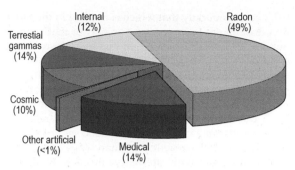

Figure 2.4 The relative proportions of natural and artificial sources of radiation to the UK population dose average of 2.2 mSv year^{-1}.

extent that air travellers receive approximately 4 μSv h^{-1} due to the reduced effect of attenuation in the atmosphere.

- *Terrestrial gamma rays* are emitted from radioactive materials in the earth's crust. We are exposed to an average of 350 μSv year^{-1}, the amount depending on where we live and on the materials used in the construction of the buildings we inhabit.

- *Internal sources* of radiation contribute a further 270 μSv year^{-1}. One atom of potassium in 10 000 is the naturally occurring radioisotope potassium-40. Potassium is an essential part of our diet, and we cannot avoid this source of exposure. Potassium-40 contributes about 60% of our internal radiation exposure. There are other natural radionuclides in the food we eat, and the extent to which we are exposed to them depends on our diet and where our food comes from.

- *Radon* is produced in the decay chain of uranium. Like all elements with atomic numbers greater than 82, it is radioactive and its decay is associated with the emission of alpha particles. Radon is an inert gas and may permeate through the ground and into buildings. It represents the largest source of radiation to which we are exposed (an average of 1.3 mSv year^{-1} in the UK) and the most variable, with average doses in some regions of the country being about four times greater, with doses in individual houses being as high as 50 mSv year^{-1} due to the precise geology of the underlying ground.

From all natural sources, the average dose to the UK population is 2.2 mSv year^{-1}, rising to about 7 mSv in Cornwall due to radon. In addition to this, we receive an average of approximately 0.4 mSv from artificial sources of radiation. Artificial sources include fallout from nuclear weapons tests (4 μSv), miscellaneous sources such as those used in smoke detectors (0.1 μSv), nuclear discharges (0.3 μSv) and occupational exposure (6 μSv). The largest artificial source is medical radiation from diagnostic procedures, which, averaged over the whole population, contributes about 370 μSv. The contribution of different sources to annual dose is illustrated in Figure 2.4.

Applying the risk factor given in section 2.3.2 to the dose from medical irradiations implies that diagnostic radiology in the UK, with a population of nearly 60 million, results in over 1000 cancer deaths each year. This is an overestimate, because the irradiated population is skewed towards a higher age range than the general population, but it does underline the imperative for applying the principles of radiation protection to the patient.

2.4 PRINCIPLES OF RADIATION PROTECTION

The system of radiation protection proposed by the International Commission on Radiological Protection (ICRP) has long been incorporated into UK legislation. Recommendations of the ICRP published in 1991 were the basis of the European directives that form the basis of current UK legislation. The ICRP introduced three basic principles to be applied to radiation protection: justification, optimization and a system of dose limits.

2.4.1 Justification

Ionizing radiations should not be used unless it can be demonstrated that the benefit exceeds the risk to those who are liable to be exposed. In general terms, the benefit may be to society as a whole because the use of radiation, for example in an industrial process, might make that process more economic or effective and there may be a benefit to those working with radiation because they have employment. On the risk side of the balance sits not only that which is implicit in the radiation dose likely to be received as part of that process, but also the risk of much larger radiation doses due to accidents and unexpected or unusual occurrences.

Justification is most easily understood within the medical context. An extreme example is the treatment of non-malignant conditions using radiotherapy. High doses of radiation give symptomatic relief for certain inflammatory conditions such as ankylosing spondylitis. With present day knowledge of the risks of radiation, and with alternative forms of treatment, the benefit is clearly outweighed by the risk. In diagnostic radiology, the risks are much less. Justification must consider the likelihood of the examination influencing the management of the patient and the clinical outcome. It should consider the alternatives, such as the use of magnetic resonance imaging or ultrasound. In determining whether an examination is justified, various factors should be considered.

- Risk is proportional to dose, and doses for diagnostic examinations vary over almost five orders of magnitude (i.e. by a factor of up to 100000; see section 2.8.3).
- Risk is significantly greater for children than for adults.
- The possibility of pregnancy and the consequent risk to the developing fetus have to be considered for female patients having examinations of the pelvis or lower abdomen.
- It is easier to justify the use of X-rays for the patient who is seriously ill and for whom an accurate diagnosis could significantly affect clinical outcome than it is for a relatively minor condition.
- Great care is needed for the justification of an exposure of a healthy individual, for example a woman having a screening mammogram or a normal volunteer participating in a medical research programme.

Justification of medical exposures is principally concerned with the exposure of the patient. There may also be situations in which doses received by staff have to be considered. An example could be the placement of biopsy needles using real-time CT imaging. This technique can be associated with high doses, particularly to the operator's fingers. Although the benefit to the patient may be significant, the risk to the operator must also be considered.

2.4.2 Optimization

The principle of optimization as stated by the ICRP is that in using ionizing radiations the dose should be *as low as reasonably achievable*, economic and social factors

being taken into account. This is commonly referred to as the ALARA principle and is incorporated into radiation protection legislation, although *as low as reasonably practicable* (*ALARP*) is the UK legal phraseology. Optimization is built into radiology at a number of levels.

- It is incorporated into the design of equipment, for example the control of X-ray output during fluoroscopy.
- The selection of technique designed to produce diagnostic images at the lowest possible dose, for example the selection of kV in radiography.
- Operator technique, for example use of the minimum screening times in fluoroscopy.
- Quality assurance programmes to ensure equipment performance.

2.4.3 Dose limitation

Notwithstanding the requirements for justification and optimization, there should be a system of dose limits such that doses in excess of those values are deemed not to be justified no matter how great the benefit. It should at the same time be recognized that compliance with dose limits is not in itself sufficient because of the imperative for optimization.

Dose limits apply to those who are employed to work with radiation and to members of the public who are liable to be exposed to radiation as a result of a work activity. The limits are different because the person working with radiation is deemed to receive benefit in terms of employment for that activity, whereas the member of the public does not. Dose limits do not apply to patients; the control of patient dose is based solely on the principles of justification and optimization.

The dose limits in the UK (and European) legislation are based on the recommendations of the ICRP; they are given in section 2.5.2. They include limits on effective dose to restrict the risk of stochastic effects. Implicit in the limits is a judgement on the *tolerable risk*, that is the boundary between a risk that may be acceptable and that which is unacceptable. In proposing dose limits, the ICRP took account of the latency period of radiation risks and that the health detriment is not immediate. Risk increases with time and reaches a maximum value some 20 years after the period of employment.

2.4.4 UK legislation

UK regulations concerning safety at work are issued under the umbrella of the Health and Safety at Work Act (1974). The Act established an advisory body, the Health and Safety Commission (HSC), and the Health and Safety Executive (HSE). Regulations issued under the Health and Safety at Work Act are a part of the criminal law, and the HSE are effectively the body policing compliance with the law, having powers of inspection and prosecution.

UK legislation on health and safety is determined by European directives. Regulations concerned with ionizing radiations take account of the recommendations of the ICRP and, in particular, the principles of radiation protection outlined above. The current regulations governing the safety of staff and public are the Ionising Radiations Regulations 1999 (IRR99). These apply to all workplace use of ionizing radiations, although certain exemptions may be granted to the Ministry of Defence. In conjunction with the regulations, the HSC have published an Approved Code of Practice (ACOP). This outlines a means of compliance with IRR99 that the HSE would consider sufficient. Although compliance with the ACOP is not itself a legal requirement, the employer would need to demonstrate to the HSE how alternative methods fulfil the requirements of the legislation. In addition to the ACOP, the HSC have published guidance representing good practice. This has a lesser status than the ACOP, and failure to comply is less likely to be used as evidence of breach of the regulations. The HSC have published the three documents (IRR99, ACOP and guidance) in a single publication, Work with Ionising Regulations (L121), which is presented in such a way that the relevant parts of the ACOP and guidance are linked directly to the relevant regulation.

The IRR99 is not concerned with the radiation protection of patients other than for requirements regarding equipment for medical exposures. There is a separate European directive concerned with patient protection introduced into UK law in the Ionising Radiation (Medical Exposure) Regulations 2000 (IRMER). Although the regulations come under the Health and Safety at Work Act, the enforcing authority is not the HSE. In England and Wales, it is the Healthcare Commission and is the appropriate national executive in the devolved administrations of the UK.

The HSE encourage professional bodies to produce sector specific guidance to regulations. The Institute of Physics and Engineering in Medicine, in consultation with other professional organizations and specialist bodies, has published Medical and Dental Guidance Notes: a Good Practice Guide on All Aspects of Ionising Radiation Protection in the Clinical Environment. It is specific to the healthcare use of ionizing radiations and considers the means of compliance with all relevant legislation.

The application of IRR99 and IRMER in radiology is considered in the following two sections.

2.5 THE IONISING RADIATIONS REGULATIONS 1999

2.5.1 General requirements

The regulations place a number of general requirements on the employer.

Notification
The employer has to notify the HSE of its intention to use ionizing radiation for the first time, including details of the premises where the work is to be carried out and the type of work.

Radiation protection adviser
The radiation employer is required to consult a radiation protection adviser (RPA) on compliance with the regulations. The RPA must satisfy the HSE's requirements for competence and should have experience of the employer's business. In the health service, the RPA is almost invariably a medical physicist who commonly will combine radiation protection duties with those of the medical physics expert (see section 2.6.3). The RPA may be an employee of the organization or an external consultant.

Prior risk assessment
A prior risk assessment is required before any new activity involving ionizing radiation, for example installation of new X-ray equipment or the introduction of a new radiopharmaceutical. The assessment is generally carried out by the RPA and is used to identify risks to staff, public and patients and to consider necessary control measures.

The prior risk assessment should consider *contingency plans* for potential situations in which things may go wrong. With an X-ray set, such plans may be very simple. Should there be a failure in the system such that X-rays are emitted outside the operator's control, then the instruction is simply to turn the set off and not to use it again until a qualified person has corrected the fault. For radioactive materials, there are a wider range of possibilities concerned with the loss or spillage of sources. Contingency plans should be written into the local rules (see section 2.5.3).

2.5.2 Dose limits

Annual dose limits are given in Table 2.6. The effective dose (sometimes referred to as the whole body dose) limit is concerned with carcinogenic risk, whereas

Table 2.6 Annual dose limits

	Employees (mSv)	Public (mSv)
Effective dose	20	1
Equivalent dose		
Lens of the eye	150	15
Skin, hands, forearms, feet, ankles	500	50
Abdomen of woman of reproductive capacity	13[a]	–
Fetus of pregnant employee	1[b]	–

[a]In any consecutive 3-month period.
[b]Over declared term of pregnancy.

the equivalent dose limits are designed to ensure that individual doses are kept below the dose thresholds for deterministic effects. The dose limit for the skin applies to the dose averaged over an area of $1\,cm^2$.

It may be noted that the annual limit to the eye lens (150 mSv) is related directly to the threshold dose for cataracts (approximately 5 Sv). A person at work who received a dose at or close to the dose limit would exceed the dose threshold after about 35 years.

The dose limits for employees are for those aged 18 or above. There are additional limits (set as three-tenths of those given in Table 2.6) for employees between the ages of 16 and 18. These are generally irrelevant in healthcare. In practical terms, a distinction is made between employees who work with ionizing radiations (i.e. those required to enter controlled or supervised areas; see section 2.5.3) and those who do not. It is normal practice to consider that the public dose limit applies to those other staff.

Pregnant staff
There is a requirement to ensure that the fetus of a pregnant employee is not exposed to a significant risk. A dose limit is set that is equal to the limit for a member of the public. The limit applies over the declared term of the pregnancy; that is, from the date that the employee informs her employer in writing that she is pregnant. For diagnostic X-rays, it can be assumed that the fetal dose is no greater than 50% of the dose on the surface of the abdomen, i.e. of the dose recorded on the dose monitor. For higher-energy radiations, including those used for radionuclide imaging, it is assumed that the fetal dose is equal to the dose monitor reading.

There is an additional dose limit for female staff restricting the average dose to the abdomen to 13 mSv over any consecutive 3-month period. The limit is intended to ensure that the work pattern of the employee is not scheduled in such a way that she would be liable to receive a major part of the annual dose limit over a short time period that might

be coincident with the interval between conception and the confirmation of pregnancy. This dose limit is generally of no relevance in healthcare employment, because doses are relatively low and are generally spread more or less evenly over the year.

Comforters and carers
There are certain exceptional situations in medicine in which a person who is not working with radiation might incur a radiation dose in excess of the public dose limit. An example is associated with the treatment of neuroectodermal tumours with iodine-131-meta-iodobenzylguanidine. These tumours occur in children and involve administration of activities of 10 GBq or more, delivering therapeutic doses of 1 or 2 Gy. The child has to remain for a period of a few weeks (iodine-131 has a half life of 8 days) in a special facility designed to ensure the containment of contamination and to afford adequate protection from external radiations. Medical staff work to local rules to restrict their exposures, with minimum close contact time with their patient. In these circumstances, it is unreasonable to deny children, particularly if very young and unable to understand what is happening, close contact with their parents on the basis of a dose limit based on a tolerable risk to people who do not benefit from the work activity.

The IRR99 permits the dose limit to be relaxed for comforters and carers who knowingly and willingly are exposed to doses in excess of the limit. The employer is required to set a dose constraint for these situations, which might be as high as 5 mSv, to explain to the person (almost invariably the parent) the doses and risks involved, and to provide guidance on precautions to be taken to ensure that the dose constraint is not exceeded. The relaxation of the dose limit for comforters and carers cannot be applied to employees. The circumstances in which it is needed are rare and would hardly ever apply to the diagnostic use of X-rays. A parent holding his or her young child in position while an X-ray is taken is not a comforter and carer in terms of the legislation; the dose to the parent in these circumstances should be only a tiny fraction of the public dose limit.

2.5.3 Designation of areas and control of working practices

Protection begins at the source of the radiation, for example the X-ray tube or the syringe of radiopharmaceutical, and requires shielding to reduce the radiation exposure from the source. Where this cannot be reduced to a reasonable level, further controls are required. Three sets of control can be identified:

- designation of radiation areas
- written working procedures
- identification of day to day responsibility for radiation protection.

Controlled area

The employer is required to designate as a controlled area any area in which:

- a person working in that area is likely to receive a radiation dose greater than three-tenths of any dose limit, or
- there is a requirement to follow special working procedures in order to restrict exposure, or
- the external dose rate could exceed $7.5\,\mu Sv\,h^{-1}$ averaged over the working day.

Examples of controlled areas include the X-ray room or the injection room used for radionuclide imaging. The walls of the room should have sufficient shielding to ensure that there is no requirement to designate the adjacent rooms as controlled areas. Access should be restricted to staff who are required to be present and to the patient. Control on access may be the responsibility of the person operating the X-ray set but, in the case of radioactive materials where the source of radiation cannot be switched off, may require a door lock. It is the purpose of the prior risk assessment to determine the appropriate form of control. Controlled areas must be clearly marked with warning signs describing the nature of the source (e.g. X-rays, radioactive materials) and of the risk (e.g. external radiation, contamination).

For mobile X-ray equipment, designation of the whole room (e.g. the ward) as a controlled area is generally impractical, and it is standard practice to designate the area within 2 m of the X-ray tube and patient as the controlled area. In these circumstances, it is the responsibility of the radiographer to ensure that when the X-ray is taken no member of staff is closer to the patient unless they are wearing a lead apron.

Box 2.1 Possible contents of local rules

Local rules are written instructions for people working in controlled or supervised areas and should describe safe working methods. Items that might be included are:

- description of controlled and supervised areas
- names of radiation protection supervisor and radiation protection adviser
- identification of responsibility for radiation protection during, for example, an X-ray examination
- identification of who is permitted to operate the equipment (usually by title)
- identification of those who may remain in the controlled area, for example while X-rays are used
- requirements for the use of personal dosimeters
- requirements for the wearing and storage of personal protective equipment
- practical instructions, for example on where to stand in the room, on the use of additional radiation shields (e.g. ceiling mounted screens in X-ray rooms, syringe shields) and on the significance of warning lights
- Contingency plans
- For radioactive sources, instructions on contamination monitoring
- Arrangements for pregnant staff

Supervised area

There are areas in which there is a possibility of exposure of staff or the public, but the doses are insufficient to require designation as a controlled area. Such an area has to be designated as a supervised area if:

- it is necessary to keep the exposure conditions under review to determine whether designation as a controlled area may be required in the future, or
- it is likely that any person could exceed the dose limit for a member of the public ($1\,mSv\,year^{-1}$).

An example of a supervised area is the waiting room for patients who have been injected with a radiopharmaceutical in preparation for an imaging study.

Local rules

Local rules describe safe methods of working with ionizing radiations. They are required whenever the employer has designated a controlled area and may be needed for supervised areas. Typical contents of local rules are listed in Box 2.1.

Radiation protection supervisor

Overall responsibility for radiation protection rests with the employer. However, for the day to day management of radiation protection, the employer is required to appoint one or more radiation protection supervisors (RPSs). RPSs should have a management role in the area for which their appointment covers. The RPS is required to oversee the work being performed so as to ensure that it is in accordance with the relevant local rules. Specific responsibilities must be clearly defined and might include:

- preparation and review of local rules
- supervision of staff dose monitoring
- investigation of instances of excessive dose
- risk assessments (e.g. for pregnant staff)
- contamination monitoring when radioactive sources are used
- testing personal protective equipment
- ensuring that an effective quality assurance programme for X-ray equipment is in place.

The exact duties depend on local circumstances. Although the RPS may have specific responsibilities for ensuring that particular tasks are performed, the actual performance of those duties may be delegated to other staff.

It is common practice for an employer to establish a radiation protection committee. This might include representatives of the organization's management and of radiation-using departments, RPAs, RPSs and health and safety advisers. The remit of the committee could include radiation protection policies, approval of local rules, and receipt of reports from the RPA. It also provides a reporting route for RPAs to senior management.

2.5.4 Equipment

There is a general requirement that the design and construction of radiation equipment should be such as to ensure that the risk of exposure to staff and other persons is minimized. In this regard, there is a requirement for a *critical examination* to be carried out before the equipment is used. The critical examination is concerned with radiation safety and must be carried out in conjunction with an RPA. Responsibility for the critical examination rests with the installer. However, the RPA is not necessarily appointed by the installer; prior to installation, it can be agreed that the hospital's own RPA will carry out this role.

For X-ray equipment, the RPA will check that the equipment complies with the requirements of the Medical and Dental Guidance Notes, as shown in Box 2.2.

There are specific requirements for equipment used for medical exposures, in particular that they are subject to a *quality assurance programme* to include commissioning tests before the equipment is first used and performance tests at appropriate intervals thereafter. The requirement for quality assurance extends to ancillary equipment whose performance may affect the magnitude of the radiation dose received by patients (e.g. automatic exposure control devices, image intensifiers and radionuclide calibrators). The quality assurance programme should include periodic assessment of patient doses. A further critical examination and commissioning test may be required following major repair or modification (including software upgrade). Further general information on quality assurance is given in Box 2.3 and in the chapters on particular imaging systems.

2.5.5 Classification of staff and dose monitoring

Designation of staff as *classified persons* is a means of identifying and monitoring individual employees who are at particular risk from ionizing radiations. Designation is required for those employees whose dose is likely to exceed three-tenths of any dose limit. To work as a classified person, the individual must be:

- 18 years old or over, and
- certified as being medically fit to work as a classified person.

Before employment as a classified person, the individual should be seen by an *appointed doctor* or employment medical adviser. The appointed doctor is commonly an occupational health physician whose appointment for this purpose is made by the HSE. The classified person must be subject to dose monitoring and annual health checks, the records of these to be kept for 50 years beyond the date that the individual stops working as a classified person.

Classification is rarely needed for health service personnel. Less than about 1% of staff whose dose is monitored receive more than 1 mSv in any year, and in normal circumstances none of those would be expected to exceed 5 mSv. The highest doses tend to be those received by radiographers or technicians working in radionuclide imaging, by radiopharmacy staff, and by interventional radiologists and cardiologists. The most likely basis for classification is in respect of finger dose. For radiologists carrying out certain interventional procedures, such as biliary drainage, which require the hands to be very close to the area of the body being imaged, finger doses may approach 150 mSv year^{-1} (three-tenths the dose limit for the skin). Other healthcare staff who may receive high

Box 2.2 Medical and Dental Guidance Notes: standards for X-ray equipment

The recommendations in the Medical and Dental Guidance Notes are not strictly legal requirements in themselves, but they represent standards that are considered to be compliant with the overall requirement of the Ionising Radiations Regulations 1999 that equipment should be designed and constructed so as to ensure that radiation doses to staff and patients are kept as low as reasonably practicable. These are some of the principal recommendations.

X-ray tube
- Leakage radiation from the tube should be less than 1 mGy in 1 h at a distance of 1 m from the focus.
- The total filtration of the tube and tube assembly should be stated on the tube casing. It should not be less than the equivalent of 2.5 mm of aluminium (1.5 mm in the case of dental X-ray equipment operating at 70 kV or below).
- The position of the focus should be marked on the tube casing.

Warnings signals
- There should be an indicator light on the control panel to show that the X-ray beam is switched on, which should be visible for the shortest exposure times.

Collimation
- Maximum beam size should be restricted to the maximum image size required.
- For fluoroscopy equipment:
  - collimators should preferably adjust automatically to the field of view on magnification and with changes in focus to intensifier distance
  - the maximum beam size should be restricted to the area of the image receptor
  - the collimators should be capable of restricting field size down to $5 \times 5\,cm^2$.

Exposure switches
- They should require positive pressure to be maintained for continuous exposures. An exception is made for computed tomography scanners in which the scan sequence can be started with a single button press or keyboard action.
- For mobile equipment, the position of the exposure switch should be designed so that the operator can stand at least 2 m from the tube and X-ray beam, i.e. outside the controlled area. This is generally achieved by having the switch on an extending cable.
- Footswitches for fluoroscopy equipment should be designed so as prevent inadvertent production of X-rays, for example to prevent:
  - fluids from entering the switch (a particular hazard for equipment used for urodynamics studies)
  - screening should they be accidentally overturned
  - pressure being placed on the switch while being stored.
- There should be a key-operated switch on mobile equipment to prevent unauthorized use.

Shielding
- The housing and support plate for the image intensifier should have shielding of at least 2 mm lead equivalence.
- For an undercouch fluoroscopy system, there should be a lead apron suspended from the intensifier support that should be not less than 45 cm wide and 40 cm long, with at least 0.5 mm lead equivalence.

Fluoroscopy dose rates
- Skin entrance dose rates should not exceed 100 mGy min^{-1} for any field size, and remedial action is needed if it is greater than 50 mGy min^{-1} for the largest available field of view for a standard-sized patient.

finger doses include those who prepare or administer radiopharmaceuticals.

The IRR99 only makes it mandatory to monitor the dose to classified staff. However, there is a requirement for the employer to be able to demonstrate that the dose to other staff working in controlled areas is adequately controlled and that they do not require to be designated. Therefore, in practice, the majority of staff working in controlled areas are issued with individual dosimeters. Personal dosimetry systems are described in more detail in Box 2.4. Dosimeters should be provided by an *approved dosimetry service*, approval in the UK being given by the HSE. Most

approved dosimetry services also have approval for dose record-keeping purposes to comply with the record-keeping requirements for classified staff.

The monitoring period for classified staff would generally be 1 month, but for staff exposed to only very low doses it could be extended to 3 months.

There are certain situations in which an individual could be subcontracted to work with more than one radiation employer during the year. By the nature of the work, the employee may be designated as a classified worker. The employer in whose premises the work is carried out has responsibility for compliance with IRR99 and monitoring doses to people working in

Box 2.3 Quality assurance

Quality assurance is a term used quite loosely and commonly taken to mean the performance of tests to determine whether a piece of equipment or process is working in accordance with its design specification. However, quality assurance should encompass all actions required to ensure that the outcome of a process meets the quality criteria set for that process.

We can consider an example in radiology. Radiographers may carry out a simple performance test on an image intensifier system to determine whether the automatic exposure control is consistent with a baseline measurement made when the equipment was first installed. This is an important test, because quite significant changes in performance could occur without the operator being aware of them, leading to the dose to the patient being much greater than necessary.

In this example, the quality assurance programme should ensure that:

- tests are done in a consistent manner in accordance with a written protocol
- there are action levels to indicate significant deviation from a baseline value
- a system is in place to ensure that when action levels are exceeded then this is reported to the appropriate manager with responsibility for initiating remedial action
- equipment used for testing is calibrated
- the process is reviewed at agreed time intervals to check that the tests are being carried out in accordance with the protocol, that appropriate action has been taken when action levels have been exceeded, and that the test methods and frequency remain appropriate for the purpose.

To illustrate that quality assurance is not simply concerned with the testing of equipment, it may be noted that the Ionising Radiation (Medical Exposure) Regulations 2000 (IRMER) have a requirement for quality assurance with no direct relevance to equipment. IRMER requires written procedures to be in place to ensure the protection of the patient. In this context, quality assurance is concerned with ensuring that those procedures and operating protocols are reviewed and revised as necessary, that there are adequate management systems in place to ensure adherence to those procedures, and that there is audit.

Box 2.4 Personal dosimetry systems

Dose limits are specified in terms of the effective dose, and for skin, extremities and the lens of the eye, equivalent dose. Effective dose cannot be measured directly. Instead, the dosimetry services measure the personal dose equivalent H_p, which is the equivalent dose at a depth of d mm in a standard phantom. The personal dose equivalent at a depth of 10 mm, H_p, sometimes referred to as the *deep dose*, is taken to be a measure of effective dose, and the *shallow dose*, H_p, as a measure of the skin dose. The standard body badge is used to measure both quantities and therefore includes filters so that an estimate of radiation energy to which the person has been exposed can be made and for the two quantities to be calculated.

Several types of dosimeters may be used.

- *Film* is the traditional material of choice. Increasing dose results in increasing blackening of the film (the optical density; see Ch. 4.1.1), thus providing an indicator of dose. Film is used because it needs relatively simple equipment for processing and reading and it provides a permanent record of exposure. It does have several disadvantages, however, including the following.
  - The sensitivity of the film (optical density as a function of dose) is highly energy-dependent because of the high atomic numbers of silver and bromine in the emulsion. This is particularly apparent at diagnostic X-ray energies.
  - The overall sensitivity is no better than 0.1–0.2 mSv.
  - It cannot be used for the assessment of finger dose.
  - It is subject to environmental effects, not just radiation but also heat, making it unsuitable for monitoring over periods greater than 1 month.

The film used for personal dosimeters has different emulsions on each side of the film, with different sensitivities. The fast (most sensitive) emulsion is used routinely, but if the badge has received a particularly high dose it will be too black to provide a meaningful

Box 2.4 (Continued)

result. This emulsion can then be removed and the less sensitive side of the film is used to extend the useful range of the badge.

- *Thermoluminescent dosimeters* (*TLDs*; see section 2.8.3) are used in conjunction with filters set in the badge holder to measure deep and shallow dose. Their response has minimal energy dependence, but the overall sensitivity is not significantly better than film. They are much less susceptible to environmental effects. TLD chips are relatively expensive, but they can be reused many times. TLDs are the most common dosimeter to be used for assessment of finger dose. They have the disadvantage that they can be read only once.
- *Optical simulated luminescent dosimeters* are used by one dosimetry provider. The material (aluminium oxide) has similar properties to the phosphors used for computed radiography (see Ch. 5.3). Following irradiation by X-rays, the material emits light in proportion to the dose when it is exposed to light. The light source in the reader used for optical simulated luminescent dosimetry systems is a laser. The advantage of this system is increased sensitivity, giving readings down to 0.01 mSv. Also, the reading process does not fully clear the signal from the phosphor, so that there is a possibility of a second reading should the first result be queried.

An alternative to the recording systems described above is the use of *electronic dosimeters*. These direct reading devices are generally based on Geiger–Müller tubes or silicon diode detectors. Their response is highly energy-dependent, but if placed behind suitable filters they can provide reasonably accurate dose measurements down to 20 keV. They have a high sensitivity, being able to measure to the nearest 1 μSv. Because they provide a direct reading, electronic dosimeters are very useful in identifying methods of dose reduction for procedures in which there is the potential for high doses to staff, and for teaching. They have the disadvantage of being expensive.

controlled areas. However, if more than one employer is involved, it is possible that the sum of the individual's doses could exceed a dose limit without that being recognized. This is addressed in IRR99 for *outside workers*, who are required to have a passbook issued by HSE into which the doses from each employer can be entered. These are summed over the year so as to provide a record that can be used to ensure that the individual does not exceed any dose limit.

2.5.6 Radiation incidents

The employer has to notify the HSE should the following type of incident occur.

- An individual receives a dose greater than any relevant dose limit. This would include not only a person working with radiation who receives more than the annual dose limit, but also a member of the public or the fetus of a pregnant worker.
- A radiation source is spilt, causing significant contamination, or it has been lost or stolen. The IRR99 specifies the activities of radioactive material for which notification might be required. For technetium-99 m, for example, notification would be required only if the loss involved more than 100 MBq.

- A patient has received a radiation dose much greater than intended because of an equipment fault, for example the failure of an X-ray exposure to terminate because of a fault in the automatic exposure control. HSE have provided guidance on what is meant by 'much greater than intended', using multiplying factors dependent on the dose from the examination (see Table 2.7).

Notwithstanding the requirement for notification, the employer must have in place a system for the investigation of all incidents in which somebody may have been inadvertently exposed to radiation. This would normally involve the RPS and RPA.

2.5.7 Personal protective equipment

The employer has to provide personal protective equipment. In the case of X-rays, this might include lead aprons, thyroid shields, and leaded glasses or goggles. One of the functions of the prior risk assessment is to determine what personal protective equipment is appropriate for the particular circumstances. The employer is required to ensure that personal protective equipment is properly used, and IRR99 places the same obligation on the employee.

Table 2.7 Health and Safety Executive guidance figures concerning patient overexposures involving radiation equipment

Type of diagnostic examination	Guideline multiplying factor applied to intended dose
• Interventional radiology • Radiographic and fluoroscopic procedures involving contrast agents • Nuclear medicine with intended effective dose >5 mSv • CT examinations	1.5
• Mammography • Nuclear medicine with intended effective dose <5 mSv but >0.5 mSv • All other radiographic examinations not referred to elsewhere in this table	10
• Radiography of extremities, skull, dentition, shoulder, chest, elbow and knee • Nuclear medicine with intended effective dose <0.5 mSv	20

2.6 IONISING RADIATION (MEDICAL EXPOSURE) REGULATIONS 2000

In the UK, IRMER replaced earlier patient protection legislation, the Ionising Radiation (Protection of Persons Undergoing Medical Examination or Treatment) Regulations 1988, commonly referred to as POPUMET. The emphasis in IRMER is on the responsibilities of the employer and the requirements for justification and optimization of individual exposures.

2.6.1 Justification and optimization

In addition to the employer, IRMER identifies three key persons who have a role in an individual medical exposure. These roles are described in respect of diagnostic X-ray examinations.

- The *referrer* is the person who initiates the X-ray request.
- The *practitioner* is required to consider whether the examination requested is justified in terms of the clinical benefit set against the radiation risk and, if justified, to authorize the examination to proceed.
- The *operator* carries out the practical aspects of the exposure following authorization.

Entitlement to act in any one of these three roles is determined by the employer within certain constraints set in IRMER: both referrer and practitioner must be registered medical or dental practitioners or other healthcare professionals, and both practitioner and operator must have had adequate training in radiation protection and in the relevant clinical applications of ionizing radiation.

The three roles will be considered in more detail.

Referrer

The employer should define not only who may act as referrer but also any restrictions on examinations that may be requested. For example, although medical practitioners may be given an automatic entitlement to be a referrer, there might be certain restrictions placed such that, for example, general practitioners may not be permitted to request a CT scan. Such restrictions apply particularly to other healthcare professionals. For example, nurse practitioners in areas such as accident and emergency may be permitted to request X-rays, but this may be limited to particular clinical circumstances and examinations (e.g. to examinations of extremities).

The employer is required to provide the referrer with recommendations on referral criteria. It is common practice to adopt the recommendations of the Royal College of Radiologists for this purpose: Making the Best of a Department of Clinical Radiology – Guidelines for Doctors.

In making the request, the referrer is required to provide sufficient clinical information for the IRMER practitioner to be best able to determine whether the examination is justified.

Practitioner

It is unfortunate that the term *practitioner* is used in IRMER to designate the person who has a single role under the legislation, i.e. the justification of individual exposures, when the title *practitioner* is used by many healthcare professionals who may not be entitled to fulfil this role. To avoid confusion, the term *IRMER practitioner* will be used in this text.

Training to be an IRMER practitioner requires both theoretical knowledge of radiation protection and imaging techniques and practical experience in the specific area of clinical practice. Generally, radiologists and radiographers are considered to have had the required training for this role. The theoretical knowledge required by the IRMER practitioner is contained within part 1 of the FRCR training syllabus, with the practical experience being gained over the subsequent period of training. The extent to which a radiographer may act as an IRMER practitioner depends on the employer, but it would be unusual, for example, to have a radiographer fulfil this role for high-dose examinations such as CT scanning.

Other healthcare practitioners who are generally entitled to act as IRMER practitioners are as follow.

- Dentists: dental radiology is an essential part of their practice and is included in their training.

- Cardiologists in respect of cardiac catheterizations: they have to make the clinical decision on the appropriate intervention in individual cases.

- Administration of Radioactive Substances Advisory Committee (ARSAC) certificate holders in respect of radionuclide studies (see section 2.7.2).

Authorization is the outcome of justification and is generally given by the IRMER practitioner. However, there may be circumstances in which this is not practicable, and the IRMER practitioner may provide written justification guidelines to permit the operator to authorize an examination in particular clinical circumstances.

Operator

Unlike that of the IRMER practitioner, the role of the operator is very broad. It encompasses all practical aspects of the medical exposure that might affect patient dose or image quality. Such practical aspects might include confirmation of the identity of the patient, carrying out the examination, processing the image, providing an evaluation of the image, calibration and maintenance of the equipment, and preparation and administration of radiopharmaceuticals. The breadth of the operator role means that, for a single exposure, there may be several individuals with an operator responsibility. It is also the reason that IRMER does not require the operator to be a registered healthcare professional, for example this would not be appropriate for the service engineer. IRMER does, however, require the operator to be adequately trained for the particular role. For example, proper maintenance of the processor used for conventional film–screen radiography is essential for image quality. However, minimal training in radiation protection is required for this role; the training need only be concerned with the practical aspects.

> **Box 2.5** Employer's procedures required by the Ionising Radiation (Medical Exposure) Regulations 2000
>
> - Patient identification: to ensure that the correct patient is examined or treated
> - Entitlement to act as referrer, practitioner or operator
> - For medico-legal exposures
> - Female patients: to establish whether the patient might be pregnant or breast feeding (radionuclide studies)
> - For quality assurance programmes (that is quality assurance of procedures and protocols)
> - For the assessment of patient dose and administered activity
> - For diagnostic reference levels
> - In relation to the use of ionizing radiations in medical research programmes, particularly in respect of healthy volunteers
> - Provision of information to patients who have been administered with a radiopharmaceutical, in order to minimize the radiation risks to others
> - For the evaluation of a medical exposure and recording dose
> - To minimize the risk of accidental or unintended exposure of patients

In contrast, the training and practical experience required to carry out the examination of the patient so as to produce images of the required diagnostic quality while ensuring that the dose to the patient is kept ALARP is extensive and is generally the level of training given to radiographers and radiologists.

2.6.2 Duties of the employer

IRMER makes it clear that the employer has overall responsibility for compliance with the regulations, in particular that there should be written procedures in place. The regulations specify matters to be included, and these are summarized in Box 2.5. These are distinct from operating procedures for standard radiological practices that are also required. The standard operating procedures might include, for example, exposure factors to be used by radiographers for every radiographic examination.

2.6.3 Other requirements of IRMER

Diagnostic reference levels

Diagnostic reference levels (DRL) are defined as doses for typical examinations for standard-sized patients.

The DRL can be considered as a performance standard against which individual patient doses can be judged. They are used as an aid to optimization. DRLs should be set locally, that is by the employer, and should reflect local practice. In general, this is through patient dose audit with the DRL being set equal to the dose for a standard-sized patient averaged for all rooms in the organization. In setting the local DRL, it is a requirement to take account of national or European DRLs. The local value should not be greater than the national DRL unless it can be justified on clinical grounds; the use of ageing equipment would not be sufficient justification. Setting a DRL for a specific examination requires that doses are audited for that examination, and therefore the examinations for DRLs should be chosen with care. Because of the requirement for audit, DRLs should be set in terms of measurable quantities such as dose area product (DAP). Section 2.8.3 discusses patient dose assessment in more detail. For radionuclide imaging, the DRL would be given in terms of activity administered.

Exposure not for direct health benefit (medico-legal, research, screening)

There are certain examinations in which the patient is unlikely to receive any direct health benefit. These might include:

- medico-legal exposures
- health-screening programmes for healthy individuals
- research programmes involving healthy volunteers.

These situations are explicitly included in IRMER but with few specific requirements other than that there should be procedures in place. For research programmes, there is a general requirement to ensure that there is approval from the appropriate research ethics committee. Participation is voluntary, and participants are informed of the risks of the exposure. In addition, for healthy volunteers there should be dose constraints.

Special attention areas

IRMER also provides a somewhat unspecific requirement for practitioners and operators to pay special attention to certain specified situations including the first two bulleted points above as well as medical exposures of children, high-dose procedures, examinations of female patients in whom the possibility of pregnancy cannot be excluded, and, in the case of radionuclide studies, examinations of women who are breast feeding. Procedures that may be adopted to minimize the risk to the developing fetus and the young children of female patients are summarized in Box 2.6.

Box 2.6 Examination of female patients

When examining a female patient, consideration has to be given to the possibility of pregnancy, in particular if the examination involves the lower abdomen or pelvis. If the patient is pregnant, the examination may not be justified because of the additional risk to the developing fetus.

Two approaches may be taken, both being applied to female patients of a reproductive age (generally taken to be between about 12 and 55 years old) and to examinations involving the examination of lower abdomen or pelvis.

- *The 10-day rule.* Establish the date of the last menstrual period and schedule the examination to be no more than 10 days from that date. The basis of the rule is that pregnancy is very unlikely at that stage of the cycle.
- *The 28-day rule.* Ask the patient whether she is or might be pregnant. If the patient rules out the possibility of pregnancy, proceed with the examination. If she says that she is pregnant or that her period is overdue, the IRMER practitioner should reconsider the justification for the examination taking account of the additional risk to the developing fetus.

The 10-day rule has been considered to be unnecessarily restrictive, because it applies to all women no matter what their personal circumstances and introduces precautions disproportionate to the risk. It has largely been abandoned in favour of the 28-day rule, although for particularly high-dose examinations, such as computed tomography scans, a policy may be adopted to reschedule the examination for the first half of the menstrual cycle in those circumstances in which the possibility of pregnancy cannot be excluded.

The possibility of pregnancy has also to be considered for most radionuclide imaging studies, because the radiopharmaceutical is excreted through the kidneys and therefore collects in the bladder to deliver a relatively high dose to the uterus (see Table 2.5).

In addition, in radionuclide imaging the possibility that the woman might be breast feeding should be considered. The radiopharmaceutical may be taken up in the breast milk. If the woman is to have a scan, she must be informed in advance of her appointment so that she can make arrangements to interrupt breast feeding in the first day or two following the examination.

Quality assurance

Quality assurance of radiation equipment is a requirement of IRR99 (see section 2.5.4). The quality assurance requirements of IRMER are concerned with procedures and include regular review of procedures and protocols and periodic audit of compliance.

Medical physics expert

The employer is required to have expert advice and ensure that a medical physics expert (MPE) is involved with medical exposures. For diagnostic radiology, this involvement is likely to be with optimization including patient dosimetry and quality assurance. The role of the MPE and RPA are usually closely linked.

Inventory

IRMER specifies that the employer should keep an inventory of equipment used for medical exposures.

Notification and enforcement

There is a requirement to notify the appropriate authority if the dose to the patient is much greater than intended. This does not include incidents involving equipment faults for which notification to HSE is required under IRR99 (see section 2.5.6). Notifiable incidents include those in which the wrong patient was examined, typically because of a failure to correctly identify the patient. In England and Wales, the enforcement authority is the Healthcare Commission. There are separate reporting arrangements in the devolved administrations in the UK.

2.7 OTHER LEGISLATION

There are other pieces of legislation in the UK that govern the use of ionizing radiations, two of which will be briefly considered here.

2.7.1 Radioactive Substances Act 1993

In contrast to IRR99, which is concerned with the protection of individuals, the Radioactive Substances Act 1993 is concerned with the protection of the population as a whole and the protection of the environment. It introduces a system in which users of radionuclide sources must be licensed or registered to hold radioactive sources and must be authorized for their disposal through licensed disposal routes. Hospitals are regularly inspected by the enforcing authorities (the Environment Agency in England and Wales and equivalent organizations in Scotland and Northern Ireland) to ensure compliance with the conditions for registration and authorization.

2.7.2 Medicines (Administration of Radioactive Substances) Regulations 1978

The Medicines (Administration of Radioactive Substances) Regulations 1978 (MARS), like IRMER, are concerned with the protection of the patient. For doctors to be able to administer a radioactive product to a patient, they must have been granted a certificate licensing them for that particular procedure, or in exceptional circumstances, for a particular patient. The certificate will only be issued on the basis of evidence that the applicant has received adequate training and has sufficient experience. The licence is specific to the hospital and will be issued only if there are adequate facilities. Certificates are granted by a committee set up under the regulations, the Administration of Radioactive Substances Advisory Committee (ARSAC), and the terminology *ARSAC certificate* is commonly used. ARSAC issues guidance on approved tests and normal and maximum levels of activity to be used. These maximum levels are generally considered to be the national DRLs for these procedures.

2.8 PRACTICAL ASPECTS OF RADIATION PROTECTION

2.8.1 Protection of staff

Room design

The most effective form of protection of staff is to exclude them from the controlled area. X-ray rooms are designed so that the radiation doses in adjacent areas are sufficiently low for staff in those areas to receive doses no greater, and generally very much less, than the public dose limit. The use of a dose constraint of 0.3 mSv is common practice, although account may be taken of occupancy of the adjacent area (less shielding is required, for example, for a storage area than for an office). Protection is achieved through shielding incorporated into the walls. In general, sufficient shielding is achieved through the use of 1–2 mm of lead. In a modern construction, with timber frame partition walls (generally referred to as stud partition), lead is incorporated using plasterboard on to which lead sheet has been bonded. In older buildings, there may be brick or concrete block internal walls with sufficient shielding properties, for example a single thickness of solid brick (approximately 120 mm) will provide protection equivalent to 1 mm of lead. An alternative protection material is barium plaster, which exploits the photoelectric effect by substituting barium with its high atomic number for calcium in standard plaster. However, barium plaster is rarely used for new installations. Doors to X-ray rooms also incorporate lead.

Within the room, there is likely to be a lead screen to protect staff operating the equipment. This has panels incorporating, almost invariably, 2 mm of lead and viewing windows made of lead glass, which incorporates lead salts to provide an equal amount of protection as the solid panels.

The requirement to exclude staff from the controlled area may be written into local rules, for example to prevent the use of the room as a passageway through the department, to discourage storage of items not required in the room, or to ensure that non-essential staff are not present when the patient is examined. However, exclusion from the room cannot be applied to all staff, and it is important to consider the precautions that may be taken by those who have to remain in the unprotected part of the room.

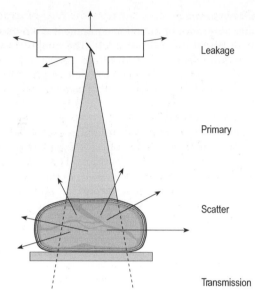

Figure 2.5 Radiation sources in the X-ray room.

Radiation sources

Within the room, there are several sources of radiation to which one might be exposed (Fig. 2.5).

- The *primary beam* is collimated to the region being examined and, in the case of fluoroscopy, is no greater than the size of the image receptor and no more than about 10% larger than the field of view on the monitor. Exposure to the primary beam could be of the operator's fingers; these would then be seen on the monitor if they are being exposed, and protective gloves should be worn. Using an undercouch tube is obviously preferable in terms of staff doses, both finger and whole body.

- *Transmitted radiation* at the exit side of the patient is generally no greater than 2% of the primary. In fluoroscopy, because the beam is confined to within the area of the image receptor, the transmitted radiation at the back of the image intensifier is negligible. The two concerns are: that the operator's fingers may be inserted between the patient and image intensifier; and, in radiography when a patient has to be supported and a lateral beam is used (for example patient in accident and emergency with a neck injury), there should be nobody standing in the direct line of the beam.

- *Leakage radiation* from the X-ray tube is restricted to 1 mGy h^{-1} at a distance of 1 m under worst conditions, i.e. maximum kV. In practice, it is very much less than this and is generally less than 2% of the dose due to scatter.

- *Scatter radiation* arises from Compton interactions principally from within the patient but also from the collimator. It is important to recognize that the main radiation source in the X-ray room to which staff are likely to be exposed is that part of the patient being examined.

Most fluoroscopy equipment is fitted with a DAP meter to monitor patient dose (see section 2.8.3). The amount of scatter is dependent on both the amount of radiation (dose) and the area of patient irradiated. Scatter is therefore proportional to DAP for a particular radiation geometry. As a rule of thumb, the maximum amount of scatter at a distance of 1 m from the patient is about 5 μGy/(Gy cm^2). Thus for a typical barium enema examination (see Table 2.9) with a patient dose of 2500 cGy cm^2, the operator standing at a distance of 1 m is liable to be exposed to a dose of 125 μGy. This factor increases with kV, but more importantly it is a function of scattering angle. For scatter towards the X-ray tube arising from the entrance side of the patient where the primary dose is high, the scatter factor is increased by a factor of 2 or 3, whereas on the exit side (image intensifier side) of the patient it is almost halved.

Protection in practice

Distance and the use of the *inverse square law* can easily be overlooked. A single step back from the patient may double the distance and reduce dose by a factor of 4. This can be combined with the *time* of exposure. Reducing exposure time is clearly important for patient protection, but staff should also minimize the time standing close to the patient.

Because of the substantial difference in scatter from the entrance and exit sides of the patient, it is always better to have the X-ray tube below the patient, because the maximum dose to the operator will then be to the lower part of the body rather than to the upper part including the tissues with the greater radiosensitivities. Overcouch screening tables (with the X-ray tube above the table) should only be used routinely with remote screening from behind a protective screen; they are not suitable for interventional studies. It is also important to ensure that for oblique views the X-ray tube is angled away from the operator so as to minimize exposure to X-rays scattered from the entrance side of the patient.

Protective clothing is invariably required for staff working in the unprotected part of the controlled area while the X-ray beam is on. *Lead apron* specifications are generally 0.25, 0.35 or 0.5 mm lead equivalent. These transmit approximately 5%, 3% and 1.5%, respectively. The thickness to be used depends on local risk assessments, but as a general rule a radiologist would use a 0.35-mm lead apron for general work and a 0.5-mm lead apron for interventional procedures. A major issue is comfort, and this will be the biggest factor in selecting the style of apron to be used. One important protection issue is to select an apron that can be fully closed at the side; a right-handed radiologist will often have that arm raised and that side of the body turned towards the patient. The weight of the apron can be reduced by having thinner lead on the back; it is unusual for operators to turn their back on the patient. There are also so-called lightweight materials used in lead aprons. These incorporate lower atomic number materials such as barium and tin with K-edges in the mid to lower part of the X-ray spectrum, making them more effective in attenuating X-rays with energies below the K-edge of lead (88 keV). A weight reduction of about 30% is claimed to provide the same protection as a standard lead apron.

Most lead aprons leave the thyroid unprotected because of the added discomfort introduced with a high collar. For high-dose procedures, there may then be a requirement to wear a separate thyroid collar, usually with 0.5 mm lead equivalence. The requirement will be based on a risk assessment and will be included in the local rules. In addition, interventional radiologists may be required to use lead glasses or goggles. It is important that these incorporate protection on the sides, as it is common practice for radiologists to have their head turned away from the patient to watch the monitor. It is possible to get prescription lead glasses.

Of almost equal importance to personal protective equipment is other shielding incorporated in the X-ray installation. Undercouch fluoroscopy installations have a lead apron attached to the explorator or image intensifier mounting. If the explorator is lowered to the maximum extent and the apron is correctly positioned, the amount of radiation reaching the operator should be minimal. In rooms with fixed C-arm installations, it is common practice to have a lead screen attached to the side of the table to reduce scatter radiation to the legs and feet and to have a shield (incorporating a lead glass screen) mounted on the ceiling. When using these screens, it is important to remember that the source of radiation is scatter from the patient. The screen should be positioned directly between the region being examined and the operator. If a ceiling-mounted screen is used with a lead glass panel and the radiologist is able always to see the part of the patient being examined through that panel, then there should be no need to use lead glasses.

2.8.2 Protection of the patient

The most important consideration in protecting the patient is to ensure that images of sufficient quality for accurate diagnosis are produced without the need for any repeat. The means to achieve this are the design and maintenance of equipment, training and experience of staff, robust operating procedures and clinical protocols. These matters are controlled by the requirements of IRR99 and IRMER, which need not be discussed further here. There are certain practical methods for further dose reduction.

- *Collimation* should always be to the region of interest. Visualization of the collimator edges on the image confirms that there is no unidentified region of the patient being exposed.

- During fluoroscopy, the use of *magnified fields of view* may reduce dose. It may seem that magnification should have the same effect as collimation because a smaller beam area is used. However, on image intensifier systems selection of magnification reduces the gain of the image intensifier (see Ch. 6.1) and the system compensates by increasing dose rate. With older equipment, the reduction in beam area is balanced by the increase in dose rate such that the overall dose to the patient (in terms of DAP; see section 2.8.3) is unaltered. On more modern equipment, there may be some benefit in terms of dose reduction when magnification is used, but generally this is not as great as the reduction produced by simply coning down to the required field of view.

- *Supplementary shielding* may be used to protect sensitive structures within the field of view. For example, when taking a radiograph of the hips, protection of the gonads should be considered, particularly for young adults and children, provided that inaccurate positioning of the shields is not likely to result in the requirement for a repeat X-ray.

- During fluoroscopy, the image intensifier should be kept as close as possible to the patient.

- *Removal of the antiscatter grid* will reduce patient dose. This is generally possible on fluoroscopy equipment, but the loss of image quality may result in longer screening times being needed. This may be practical only for the examination of young children.

- *Increased filtration* reduces dose. Generally, the operator cannot alter the amount of filtration on the set, but some equipment is provided with additional filters (generally copper) that can be driven into place and may be automatically programmed into the system.

2.8.3 Patient doses and dose assessment

IRMER requires the practitioner to justify individual medical exposures in terms of benefit and risk. Radiation risk is directly related to effective dose, and therefore the practitioner should be aware of the magnitude of the dose for each procedure. The operator has a responsibility to ensure that doses are kept ALARP and that there is adherence to DRLs. The IRR99 requires that patient dose assessment be part of the equipment quality assurance programme. There is therefore a requirement for a programme of patient dose audit.

Patient effective dose

Typical doses from a selection of diagnostic X-ray examinations are presented in Table 2.8. These have been divided into three groups.

- *High doses* in excess of 2 mSv, i.e. doses comparable with the average annual dose from natural background radiations or above. These are associated with a moderate risk of 1 in 10 000 or greater.

- *Medium doses* between 0.02 and 2 mSv. The majority of workers who are occupationally exposed to radiation receive annual doses in this range, which includes the annual dose limit for members of the

Table 2.8 Typical effective doses in diagnostic radiology

Examination	Dose (mSv)
High dose	
CT abdomen or pelvis	10
CT chest	8
Barium enema	7
Technetium-99 m bone scan	4
Intravenous urogram	3
Barium meal	2.5
CT head	2
Medium dose	
Barium swallow	1.5
Technetium-99 m lung perfusion study	1
Lumbar spine (two films)	0.8
Pelvis anteroposterior	0.6
Head (two films)	0.04
Low dose	
Chest posteroanterior	0.015
Shoulder anteroposterior	0.005
Dental intraoral (two films)	0.004
Extremities	0.0001–0.005

CT, computed tomography.

public. The associated risks are low, in the range 1 in 1 000 000 and 1 in 10 000.

- *Low doses* below 0.02 mSv associated with trivial risk (less than 1 in 1 000 000). The doses are comparable with the average daily dose from natural background radiations (6 μSv) and from air travel (4 μSv h^{-1}). Approximately 60% of all medical X-ray examinations are included in this group.

As a rule of thumb, high-dose examinations are those involving CT or fluoroscopy with more than 1 min of screening times and several recorded images. Medium doses arise from radiographic examinations of the abdomen or pelvis with no more than two or three films, and low-dose examinations include chest radiography and examination of extremities.

Dose assessment

The standard quantities used for dose assessment in radiography and fluoroscopy are entrance surface dose (ESD) and DAP.

Entrance surface dose can be measured directly using thermoluminescent dosimeters (TLDs). Thermoluminescence is a form of luminescence (see Ch. 1.7) in which light is emitted from the phosphor only after the material has been heated. Many materials have thermoluminescence properties.

Table 2.9 Typical entrance surface doses and dose area products for X-ray examinations

Examination	Entrance surface dose (mGy)		Dose area product (Gy cm^2)	
	Typical value	*NDRL*	*Typical value*	*NDRL*
Skull AP or PA	1.9	3	–	–
Chest PA	0.12	0.2	0.09	0.12
Lumbar spine AP	4.3	6	1.3	1.6
Lumbar spine lateral	10	14	2.1	3
Pelvis AP	3.2	4	2.0	3
Intravenous urogram	–	–	12	16
Barium meal	–	–	9	13
Barium enema	–	–	22	31
Femoral angiogram	–	–	20	33
Coronary angiogram	–	–	26	36

AP, anteroposterior; PA, posteroanterior; NDRL, National Diagnostic Reference Level.
[a]NDRLs for entrance surface dose or dose area product recommended by the UK Department of Health based on surveys of X-ray doses in the UK.

The most common TLD material used at diagnostic X-ray energies is lithium fluoride. This has the advantage of an atomic number ($Z = 8.2$) similar to that of tissue so that the sensitivity, i.e. light output per unit of absorbed dose, is not strongly dependent on the X-ray spectrum. The material is supplied commonly in the form of a disk 4 mm in diameter and 1 mm thick. The TLD disk is sufficiently thin that it is not visible in the radiograph. The TLD is placed on the entrance surface, and following the examination it is placed in a reader that heats it, typically to 250°C, and measures the light output, which is proportional to the dose. The measurement uncertainty using TLD is typically ±5%.

An alternative to the direct measurement of ESD is calculation. The kV and mAs can be recorded and used to calculate air kerma from previously measured output data for the X-ray system. This will be the output at a particular distance from the focus, and air kerma at the position of the entrance skin surface is calculated using an inverse square law correction. To convert this to absorbed dose on the skin, a further correction to account for the scatter from the patient, the back scatter factor, is applied. The back scatter factor is in the range of 1.25–1.5, depending on beam area and kV. However, the accuracy of the calculation is critically dependent on the focus to skin distance, which is not generally recorded.

The use of ESD is restricted to single projections and, for auditing purposes, cannot be applied to complete examinations involving multiple projections. Typical ESDs for common radiographic examinations are shown in Table 2.9.

Dose area product meters were described in Chapter 1.6.3. They measure the product of dose and beam area in units of Gy cm^2 or submultiples. DAP display has become a standard specification on fluoroscopy equipment and on fixed radiographic installations. It is becoming the most common quantity to use for patient dose audit. Typical DAP values are shown in Table 2.9.

IRR99 has a requirement for patient dose assessment as part of the equipment quality assurance programme; however, patient dose audit is an imprecise quality assurance tool, principally because of the large patient to patient variation. An example is shown in Figure 2.6 of the spread in doses measured in a dose survey. There are a number of reasons for this variation, but it is mainly due to patient build, which may be responsible for variations by a factor of 10 or more between the maximum and minimum dose measured for a series of patients. Other factors causing this variation are pathology (particularly for examinations involving fluoroscopy) and operator competence.

IRMER requires DRLs to be set for representative examinations. DRLs are generally set taking account of the results of dose audits and require an investigation to be made if the DRL is consistently exceeded. Because of the patient to patient variation in dose, the DRL (if it is representative of standard practice and for standard-sized patients) will be exceeded for many patients, particularly for larger patients. DRLs cannot therefore be used to assess whether the dose for an individual patient is excessive. They are used, in conjunction with dose audit, to test whether the

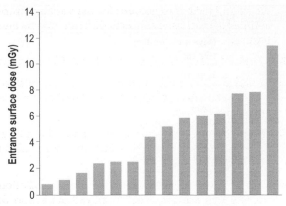

Figure 2.6 Results for a dose audit of 14 patients having an anteroposterior radiograph of the lumbar spine. The doses are given in term of the entrance surface dose.

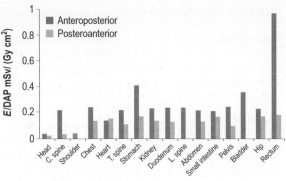

Figure 2.7 Factors to convert dose area product (DAP) to effective dose (*E*) for some common AP and PA projections used in radiography and fluoroscopy.

average dose used for a particular examination is being restricted as far as reasonably practicable.

The DRL may be considered as the boundary between good and standard practice and poor abnormal practice. Local DRLs cannot be set in isolation; there has to be some judgement as to whether they are within that boundary. IRMER requires them to be set 'having regard to European diagnostic reference levels where available'. European DRLs are not yet well established, and as an alternative national DRLs can be used. These are based on surveys of radiological practice in the UK made by the National Radiological Protection Board (NRPB).[1] National DRLs are given in Table 2.9. They represent an upper acceptable limit for DRLs set locally.

Diagnostic reference levels for CT scanning are generally set in terms of dose length product (see Ch. 7.7). For radionuclide imaging, they are based on administered activity, and some upper limits of activity are given in Chapter 8.7. Note that nuclear medicine patients are effectively radiation sources, and guidance should be given regarding this aspect when they leave the hospital, particularly with respect to air travel and airport surveillance systems, which they may activate.

Effective dose and dose area product
Dose area product is a useful quantity, because it can be easily measured. It is not directly related to risk other than that, for the same examination, a doubling

in DAP represents a doubling in risk. It is possible, however, to convert a DAP value to effective dose using theoretically derived conversion factors. The factors depend principally on the region of the body and on the projection, and to a lesser extent on kV and beam filtration. Typical conversion factors are shown for AP and posteroanterior (PA) radiographic projections in Figure 2.7.

Some observations may be made.

- The conversion factors for the skull and shoulder are very much less than in the trunk, because the organs and tissues directly irradiated are associated with lower weighting factors w_T (see Table 2.3).

- The conversion factors for PA examinations are less than for AP examinations of the same region, because generally the organs and tissues with higher weighting factors are located anteriorly and therefore receive higher doses from AP projections.

- Variations in conversion factors for examinations in the trunk are generally small. This is because the organs and tissues with the higher weighting factors are distributed fairly evenly within the trunk, and with the relatively large field sizes used in radiography the position of the beam makes relatively little difference in the result of the calculation of effective dose.

As a rule of thumb, the conversion factors for AP and PA projections in the trunk are approximately 0.2 and 0.12 mSv (Gy cm^2)$^{-1}$, respectively, for radiography. Conversion factors for projections used in barium contrast studies are more variable, because smaller fields of view are generally used. For example, the factors for the stomach are typically 0.4 and 0.17 mSv (Gy cm^2)$^{-1}$ for AP and PA views, respectively. The

[1]The NRPB became the Radiation Protection Division of the Health Protection Agency in 2005. In this text, reference to the NRPB and its reports and recommendations prior to that date are made to the NRPB.

higher conversion factor arises because, in a barium meal examination, the beam is closely collimated to the stomach, which has a high tissue weighting factor w_T (see Table 2.3). For oblique and lateral projections, the factors are generally similar to those for PA projections.

Conversion factors are also available to convert ESD to effective dose, but the validity of these factors is critically dependent on the size of the X-ray beam.

2.9 SUMMARY

- The biological effects of radiation result from ionization.

- Biological effects are dependent on radiation type, and equivalent dose is a quantity that includes a radiation weighting factor.

- Deterministic effects are associated with a threshold dose, and the severity of the effect is dependent on dose.

- Stochastic effects have no dose threshold, and the probability of incidence increases linearly with dose.

- Genetic effects arising from the irradiation of the gonads of the parent are stochastic in nature.

- Effective dose is a quantity related to the risk of developing stochastic effects and uses tissue weighting factors to account for the variable probabilities of stochastic effects in different organs and tissues.

- The risk factor for fatal cancer is 1 in 20 000 per mSv.

- Radiation protection is based on the principles of justification and optimization (ALARA) and a system of dose limits.

- UK radiation protection legislation is based on European directives, which in turn are based on the recommendations of the ICRP.

- IRR99 applies to employers who use radiation sources and are concerned with the protection of staff and the public.

- IRMER is concerned with protection of the patient.

- IRMER requires justification of individual exposures by a practitioner and optimization (keeping dose ALARP) by the operator.

- Other legislation is concerned with the use of radioactive sources, including their use in medicine and the transport and disposal of sources.

- Protection of staff in radiology is principally concerned with the minimization of exposure to scatter radiation from the patient achieved by minimization of exposure time, distance and the use of protective barriers and clothing.

Chapter 3

Imaging with X-rays

This chapter is principally concerned with the formation of X-ray transmission or projection images. It is not concerned with any specific imaging device. These are discussed in later chapters: film–screen systems in Chapter 4, digital radiographic receptors in Chapter 5 and image intensifiers in Chapter 6.

To describe the processes involved, it is necessary to introduce certain descriptors of image quality. Some general terminology used to describe image quality is introduced at the start. This terminology is common not just to imaging with X-rays but also to other imaging modalities.

3.1 IMAGE QUALITY

Radiology is concerned with the production, presentation and interpretation of images. Image production exploits a number of physical processes to provide information on both the structure and function of the human body. Images are presented in either hardcopy format, for example on film, or on a monitor display. The presentation is a two-dimensional map of structures. The interpretation of the image depends on the physical processes through which the image is created and intrinsic limits inherent in those processes and in the display system itself.

Image quality is the term used to describe the overall appearance of the image and its fitness for purpose. There are two basic descriptors:

- *Contrast* is the ability to distinguish between adjacent areas in the image
- *Spatial resolution* is the ability to detect fine detail.

3.1.1 Contrast

In most imaging modalities, the image is presented as shades of grey from black through to white. Contrast, or more strictly contrast resolution, describes the ability to distinguish between regions of the image. For example, in a chest radiograph (Fig. 3.1) the contrast between the region of the lung and the mediastinum is very marked, with the former appearing as dark grey and the latter being light. On the other hand, the contrast within the mediastinum is generally low, so that it is difficult to distinguish the spine beneath the heart. The degree of contrast between tissue types is intrinsic to the imaging technique. It depends on the properties of the tissues and the method of image formation. It may be influenced by technique and the specification of the imaging device and its display. In digital techniques, it may be enhanced using digital post-processing features.

It is one of the features of the physiology of the human eye that we are able to distinguish between neighbouring regions in an image for which the contrast is relatively low. If there is a sharp boundary between regions, the eye serves to enhance the boundary so that we are able to distinguish more clearly between the regions.

It is unfortunate that the term *contrast*, used in this context as a descriptor of image quality, is also shorthand for contrast medium, a substance introduced into the body to enhance the visualization of anatomical features.

3.1.2 Spatial resolution

Whereas contrast is the descriptor for the ability to see larger regions within the body, spatial resolution describes the ability to see fine detail. Fine detail is most clearly seen when the contrast between the feature and its background is high, for example visualization of microcalcifications that appear as white dots against a dark background in mammography, or a hairline fracture appearing as a dark line overlying a pale background of bone in radiography.

Spatial resolution may be expressed in terms of the size of the smallest visible detail. However, it is more common to quantify spatial resolution as the highest occurring frequency of lines that can be resolved in a high-contrast bar pattern. A test object used to determine spatial resolution (Fig. 3.2) consists of a number of equally spaced bars, the space between the bars being the same as the width of a bar. For X-ray imaging, the bars are strips of lead or tungsten fixed to a perspex plate. A bar and a space together make up a line pair, and the spatial frequency of the pattern is given as the number of line pairs per mm (lp mm^{-1} or lp cm^{-1}). In the test object, there are several groups of bars (generally four or five bars in each group) with progressively reduced spacing, i.e. higher frequency of line pairs. The observer determines the group with the highest spatial frequency that can be resolved, which corresponds to the limited spatial resolution in the displayed image. The smallest visible detail size is approximately half of the inverse of the resolution expressed in this way. For example, with a resolution of 10 lp mm^{-1} you might expect to be able to resolve detail as small as 0.05 mm (50 μm).

3.1.3 Noise

One of the limiting factors to contrast resolution is noise. Noise refers to the variations in the levels of

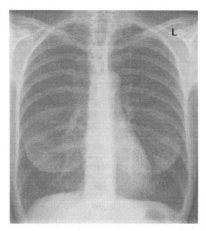

Figure 3.1 A posteroanterior chest radiograph.

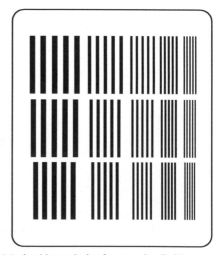

Figure 3.2 A grid test device for assessing limiting spatial resolution.

grey in the image that are distributed over its area but unrelated to the structures being imaged. The most significant source of noise in radiological imaging is *quantum noise* or *mottle*. This is generated because of the very low signal levels being detected to produce the image. For example in fluoroscopy, where low doses are employed, a relatively small number of X-ray photons are detected by the image intensifier. The detection of a photon is a randomly occurring event, and the lower the number of photons detected the greater will be the variation in the signal. Quantum mottle is seen in fluoroscopy as a graininess in the displayed image.

Only photons that are absorbed by the imaging detector convey information. Suppose that an average of M photons are absorbed in each pixel forming the image. Because of the random nature of X-ray attenuation processes, the actual number of photons absorbed varies from one pixel to another. Statistical laws dictate that the variation in the number of randomly occurring events is related to the square root of the average, $\sqrt{M}$ in this case. The variation is described by the standard deviation. Figure 3.3 shows graphically the relative number (R) of such pixels that absorb a given number (N) of photons. About two-thirds (68%) of all pixels absorb between ($M - \sqrt{M}$) and ($M + \sqrt{M}$) photons. Sixteen percent absorb more than ($M + \sqrt{M}$) and 16% absorb less than ($M - \sqrt{M}$).

This random pattern of photons, called the noise or quantum mottle, is superimposed on the signal, the pattern produced by the structures in the patient. Noise reduces the visibility of low-contrast regions within the image, particularly if they are small in area, thus reducing the visibility of finer detail in the image.

Noise, relative to the total number of photons absorbed, reduces as the number of photons increase because the relative noise is $\sqrt{M}/M$, i.e. $1/\sqrt{M}$. It is more usual to describe the significance of noise in terms of the *signal to noise ratio* that is defined as $M/\sqrt{M}$. Table 3.1 shows how the signal to noise ratio increases as the number of photons contributing to the image increases.

Quantum noise may not be the only source of noise in the image. There may be *structured noise* produced, for example in radiography using a conventional film–screen system. The screen used to convert the pattern of X-ray intensities to a pattern of light (Ch. 4.1.2) may not be completely uniform, thus it would introduce variations in intensity over the area of the film. In addition, *electronic noise* might be introduced into fluoroscopy images because of instability in the electronic circuits taking the video signal to the viewing monitor.

3.2 ATTENUATION OF X–RAYS BY THE PATIENT

In projection imaging, a fairly uniform, featureless beam of X-radiation falls on the patient and is differentially absorbed by the tissues of the body. Emerging from the patient, the X-ray beam carries a pattern of intensity that is dependent on the thickness and composition of the organs in the body. Superimposed on the absorption pattern is an overall pattern of scattered radiation.

In general, the X-rays emerging from the patient are captured on a large phosphor screen. This converts the invisible X-ray image into a visible image of light, which is then either:

- recorded as a negative image on film, to be viewed on a light box (film–screen radiography),
- recorded electronically prior to printing on a hard-copy device or display on a monitor screen (computed or direct digital radiography), or
- displayed as a positive image on a TV monitor (fluoroscopy).

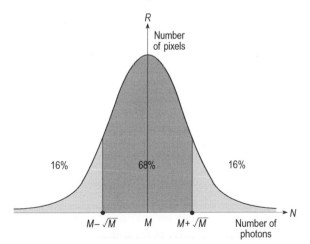

Figure 3.3 The distribution of the number of X-ray photons absorbed in each pixel of an image.

Table 3.1 The relation between the number of events, noise and signal to noise ratio

No. of events	Noise (%)	Signal to noise ratio
10	3 (30)	3:1
100	10 (10)	10:1
1000	32 (3.2)	32:1
10 000	100 (1)	100:1
100 000	320 (0.3)	320:1

Details of the image capture devices are given in Chapters 4, 5 and 6. Here, we consider the invisible X-ray image and some consequences of the properties of X-rays described in Chapter 1, namely:

● they travel in straight lines
● they are absorbed and scattered when travelling through matter.

3.2.1 Image contrast

Subject contrast
A structure in the patient is demonstrated by two things:

● the resolution, sharpness, or lack of blurring of the image of its boundary (section 3.6)
● the contrast between it and adjacent tissues caused by differences in the transmission of X-rays.

We study contrast first, with the aid of a very simple example. Figure 3.4a shows a single structure 1 (say, bone, contrast medium or gas) surrounded by another material 2 (say, soft tissue). Figure 3.4b shows the pattern of X-rays 'seen' in the image. Contrast in the pattern of X-rays leaving the subject compares E_1, the intensity or dose rate of the rays that have passed through such a structure, and E_2, the intensity of those that have passed through the adjacent tissue. All the rays suffer the same attenuation by the tissue layers lying above and below the structure. Contrast is due to the differential attenuation by the structure of thickness t and by an equal thickness of the adjacent tissues.

Accordingly, subject contrast C depends on:

● the thickness t of the structure
● the difference in linear attenuation coefficients, μ_1 and μ_2, of the tissues involved.

Thus

$$C \propto (\mu_1 - \mu_2)t.$$

So the thicker the structure the greater is the contrast. As attenuation depends on tissue density and atomic number, the more the two tissues differ in these respects the greater the contrast. The higher the kilovoltage (kV), the smaller are the attenuation coefficients and the difference between them and thus the less the contrast.

Figure 3.5 shows how the linear attenuation coefficient depends on photon energy in the case of air, fat, muscle, bone and iodine contrast medium. It will be seen that:

● the contrast C between bone (Z = 13) and muscle (Z = 7.4), which is proportional to the vertical distance between the two curves, is large at low kV because of the effect of photoelectric absorption in the higher atomic number material, and decreases noticeably as kV is increased and the relative probability of the Compton effect increases

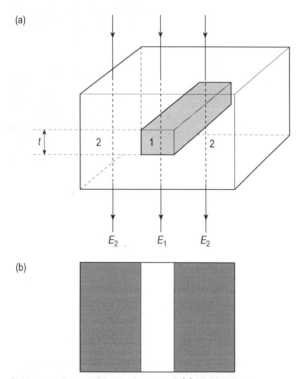

(a)

(b)

Figure 3.4 Primary contrast produced (a) on imaging a structure (1, bone) that is surrounded by a uniform block of another material (2, soft tissue), and (b) a representation of the resultant image.

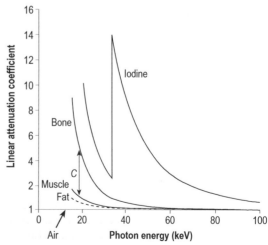

Figure 3.5 The variation of linear attenuation coefficient as a function of photon energy for fat, muscle, bone and iodine.

- the same is true of the contrast between iodine contrast media and soft tissue
- the contrast between the low atomic number tissues, fat ($Z \approx 6$) and muscle, is small and does not decrease very much when the tube kV is increased
- the contrast between air and tissue, which have similar atomic numbers, is due to the large difference in density.

Contrast media

One of the problems in radiography is the low contrast between soft tissues. One way of increasing contrast is to use a lower kV; another is to use a contrast medium. Radiopaque media are chosen to have a sufficiently high atomic number to maximize photoelectric absorption. Ideally, the absorption edge should lie just to the left of the major part of the spectrum of X-rays leaving the patient. Figure 3.5 shows that this is the case with iodine ($Z = 53$, $E_K = 33\,keV$). Barium ($Z = 56$, $E_K = 37\,keV$) also has a suitable absorption edge, and in addition a high density. Contrast media are compounds of one or other of these elements. The very low density of air or other gases make them suitable as contrast media, but their use has been superseded by computed tomography (CT) and magnetic resonance imaging and air is now used as a contrast media only in double-contrast barium enema studies.

3.2.2 Patient dose

The film–screen or any other imaging system used to convert the X-ray pattern into an image requires a specific or minimum dose to produce satisfactory image quality; about $3\,\mu Gy$ for film–screen radiography and between about 0.2 and $0.5\,\mu Gy\,s^{-1}$ for fluoroscopy.

This is the exit dose emerging from the patient and any intervening materials between the patient and the imaging device. The entrance surface dose (ESD), that is the dose to the skin proximal to the tube, has to be much higher because of the high attenuation of X-rays by the patient. ESD might be roughly 10 times greater than the exit dose for a PA chest X-ray, 100 times for an X-ray of the skull, 1000 for an AP pelvis, and 5000 times for a lateral view of the lumbar spine. The average absorbed dose within the region being imaged lies somewhere between the entrance and exit doses.

A major consideration in X-ray imaging is to restrict the dose to the patient as much as possible consistent with the primary aim of producing an image that is satisfactory for the clinical purpose. This often requires a compromise, because in general the lower the dose the poorer the image quality.

Increasing mAs, without changing any other parameter, increases both entrance and exit dose proportionately. In the case of film–screen radiography, this has the effect of producing a darker film. Changing other parameters (such as kV) generally requires a change in mAs (or milliamperage, mA) to achieve the optimum dose for the imaging system.

Effect of tube kilovoltage on patient dose

Using a higher kV makes the beam more penetrating and increases the proportion of high-energy photons that reach the film–screen. As a result, a lower entrance dose is needed for the same exit dose. Increasing the kV therefore reduces the skin dose incurred in producing a satisfactory image and, to a lesser extent, the dose to deeper tissues. This is illustrated in Figure 3.6, in which ESD is plotted against kV for an experimental arrangement in which kV is varied and mAs is adjusted to give the same degree of blackening on an X-ray film. Whereas (see Ch. 1.3) the output of the X-ray tube and the skin dose rate are roughly proportional to kV^2, the film–screen dose (at a constant mAs) is more nearly proportional to kV^4, the exponent being dependent on patient thickness and field size and in the range 3–5.

Likewise, increasing *filtration* also reduces the skin dose despite the fact that an increase in mAs is needed.

Effect of focus–film distance on patient dose

Increasing the focus–film distance (FFD) reduces the dose to the patient. This is illustrated in Figure 3.7. In delivering a specific dose to the film–screen, a sufficient number of photons need to enter through the skin. At the shorter FFD, with the focal spot at S', they are concentrated on to a surface area defined by the

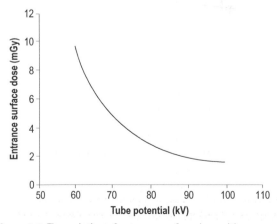

Figure 3.6 The variation of entrance surface dose with kilovoltage.

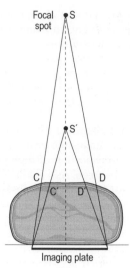

Figure 3.7 Effect of focus–film distance on patient dose.

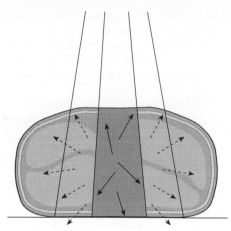

Figure 3.8 The effect of irradiated volume on amount of scatter reaching the imaging device.

points C′ and D′. At the longer FFD, with the focal spot at S, the same number of photons is required at the film to provide a satisfactory image. However, when they enter through the skin they are spread over a larger surface area represented by CD, and thus they result in a lower skin dose.

Thus, while increasing the FFD necessitates increasing the mAs needed to produce the desired number of photons at the film–screen, it nevertheless reduces the skin dose incurred in producing an acceptable image, and to a lesser extent the dose to deeper tissues.

3.3 EFFECT OF SCATTERED RADIATION

The primary radiation carries the information to be imaged, while the scattered radiation obscures it. This is similar to the way in which the ambient light in a room affects the image seen on a monitor screen. The amount (S) of scattered radiation reaching a point on the imaging device may be several times the amount (P) of primary radiation at the same position. The ratio S/P depends on the thickness of the patient's body and the area of the beam. The ratio is typically 4:1 for a PA chest (in which case only 20% of the photons recorded by the film–screen carry useful information) and 9:1 for a lateral pelvis.

Because the scattered radiation is more or less uniform over the image, it acts like a veil and reduces the contrast that would otherwise be produced by the primary rays by the factor $(1 + S/P)$, which may be anything up to 10 times.

3.3.1 Scatter reduction and contrast improvement

The amount of scatter produced in the patient may be decreased by decreasing the volume of tissue irradiated (as shown in Fig. 3.8). This may be brought about by:

- reducing the field area by the use of collimation
- compression of the patient to move overlying tissues to the side.

These two measures happily also reduce the effective dose to the patient, but use of the following three methods of scatter control requires an increase in mAs, thus carrying a penalty of increased patient dose and tube loading.

- *Kilovoltage.* As kV is reduced, the scatter produced is less in the forwards direction towards the film and relatively more to the side. At the same time, the scatter is less penetrating, so scatter produced at some distance from the film is less likely to reach it. In practice, these effects may not be very significant. Reducing the kV does increase the contrast but primarily because of the increased differential photoelectric absorption.

These first three methods reduce the amount of scatter produced and that is able to escape from the patient. The amount of scatter (relative to the primary rays) reaching the imaging device may be reduced further by interposing between it and the patient.

- *A grid.* An antiscatter grid, seen in cross-section in Figure 3.9, consists of thin strips of a heavy metal sandwiched between thicker strips of low-attenuation interspace material. The scattered photons that hit the grid obliquely are absorbed by

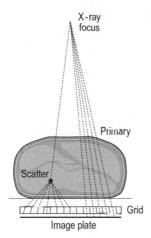

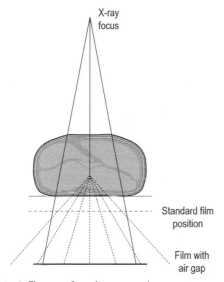

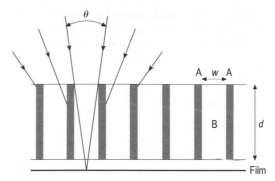

Figure 3.11 Detailed construction of a parallel antiscatter grid.

Figure 3.9 A focused antiscatter grid.

Figure 3.10 The use of an air gap to reduce scatter.

3.4 SECONDARY RADIATION GRIDS

3.4.1 Grid construction

The grid shown in Figure 3.11 is constructed using lead strips usually about 0.05–0.07 mm wide. The number of strips per cm, the *line density*, is generally in the range of 30–80, with 40 strips cm^{-1} being typical. In a grid of this specification, the repetition interval is 0.25 mm, with the gap between strips being 0.19 mm with 0.06 mm wide lead strips. The gap is filled with an interspace material that may be aluminium but is preferably a lower-attenuation material such as carbon fibre.

The *grid ratio* is the ratio of the depth of the interspace channel divided by its width (the ratio of d and w in Fig. 3.11) and is typically 8:1. In the example given above, this implies an overall grid thickness equal to $8 \times 0.19 = 1.5$ mm. The larger the grid ratio the smaller is the angle of acceptance and the more efficient is the grid at absorbing scattered radiation, thus the greater is the contrast in the image.

With very large fields, especially at a high kV, more scatter is produced, and a *high-ratio grid* (12:1 or 16:1) is preferable. A grid is generally not used with thin parts of the body such as extremities, or with children, because less scatter is generated in the patient. It is not required when the air gap technique is used.

3.4.2 Effect on scattered rays

Few of the scattered rays can pass through the channels between the strips of lead and reach the film. Because most of them are travelling obliquely and are relatively soft, they will be largely absorbed by the strips of lead. This is shown in greater detail in Figure 3.11, in which A marks the lead strips and B the interspace material. It will be seen that the grid has only a small *angle of acceptance* θ within which scattered rays can reach a point on the film.

the lead strips, while a high proportion of the primary rays pass through the gaps and reach the film. The grid is described in more detail in section 3.4.

- *An air gap.* If, as in Figure 3.10, the film–screen is moved some 20–30 cm away from the patient, much of the obliquely travelling scatter (shown dashed) misses it, and the contrast is improved. Because of the inverse square law, the increased distance causes (a) a small reduction in the intensity of the primary radiation that comes from the anode, some distance away, but (b) a larger reduction in the intensity of the scattered radiation, because that comes from points within the patient, much nearer. Use of an air gap increases contrast but necessitates an increase in the kV or mAs. It also results in a magnified image.

The *contrast improvement factor* is defined as contrast with a grid divided by contrast without a grid. It lies typically between 2 and 4, depending on the grid ratio and the various factors affecting the relative amount of scatter produced.

3.4.3 Effect on direct rays

Focused and unfocused grids

Figure 3.11 shows a small section of a grid in which the lead strips are parallel to each other and, if correctly positioned, to the central ray of the X-ray beam. This is known as an *unfocused grid*. Away from the centre of the beam, the rays strike the grid obliquely because of the divergence of the X-ray beam. They will therefore be increasingly attenuated until at an angle that is half the acceptance angle there would be complete cut-off. The effect can be reduced by using a longer FFD or a grid with a lower grid ratio. However, the use of unfocused grids is restrictive in terms of the maximum beam size that can be used.

More commonly, a *focused grid* is used in which the strips are tilted progressively from the centre to the edges of the grid so that they all point towards the tube focus. This is shown in Figure 3.9.

Grid cut-off

Within certain tolerances, the focused grid must be used at a specified distance from the anode, the tube must be accurately centred over the grid, and the grid must not be tilted about an axis parallel to the lead strips. Otherwise, cut-off of the primary rays will occur. These tolerances reduce with a higher grid ratio. The X-ray tube can be angled along the length of the lead strip (i.e. angled in the plane perpendicular to Fig. 3.9) without cutting off the primary radiation. If the tube is angled the other way, or if a focused grid is accidentally placed the wrong way round or upside down on the film, the primary beam will be absorbed, leaving perhaps only one small central area of the film exposed.

Stationary and moving grids

Grid lines are shadows of the lead strips of a stationary grid superimposed on the radiological image. If the line density is sufficiently high they may not be seen unless a magnifier is used, but they nevertheless reduce the definition of fine detail. To blur out the grid lines, the grid may be moved during the exposure. A *moving grid* (Bucky, see Box 3.1) moves for a short distance, perpendicular to the grid lines. It may move a fixed distance from side to side, with damped oscillations or in a single movement with speed reducing with exposure time. It is important that movement

begins before the exposure starts, that the speed at the start of exposure is sufficiently fast for blurring to occur at the shortest exposure times, and that it does not stop moving until after the exposure has terminated.

When a moving grid is not practical, for example for ward radiography, a stationary grid is used and this should have an increased line density. Stationary grids used with digital imaging systems such as computed radiography or direct digital radiography can produce interference patterns on the image.

Speed and selectivity

The two tasks of a grid – to transmit primary radiation and to absorb scattered radiation – may be judged by its selectivity:

$$\frac{\text{fraction of primary radiation transmitted}}{\text{fraction of scattered radiation transmitted.}}$$

An upper limit for the fraction of primary transmitted can be calculated from the geometry of the grid. It is the ratio of the width of the interspace material divided by the separation of the strips. In the example given earlier of a grid with 40 strips cm^{-1} and a strip width of 0.06 mm, this ratio is $0.19/0.25 = 0.76$. In practice, the fraction is less because of attenuation in the interspace material and the less than perfect alignment of the strips with the direction of travel of the photons. The fraction of scattered radiation transmitted depends on grid ratio and kV. Typically, the selectivity is in the range 6–12.

The use of grids necessitates increased radiographic exposure (mAs) for the same film density, because of the removal of some of the primary rays and most of the scatter. The *grid factor* is defined as:

$$\frac{\text{exposure necessary with a grid}}{\text{exposure necessary without a grid.}}$$

Typically it is in the range 3–5, and it depends principally on the grid ratio, patient thickness and kV. Using a grid therefore increases patient dose.

Scanned projection radiography

An alternative to a grid uses a slot collimator, typically 5 mm wide, to produce a narrow strip of radiation falling on the patient. There is a matching slot collimator behind the patient to allow the primary beam to reach the film. The collimators are arranged to move steadily across the field during the exposure. With only a slice of the patient being irradiated at any instant, little scatter is produced and very little of the scatter will reach the film because of the exit collimator. An increase of exposure time is necessary. Equipment for scanned projection radiography is not generally available. However, the technique is used in CT scanning to produce the scanned projection radiographs used to plan the scan series. In the CT scanner, the patient is moved through the narrow primary beam rather than vice versa.

3.5 MAGNIFICATION AND DISTORTION

Some important aspects of a radiological image arise simply from the fact that X-rays travel in straight lines. Figure 3.12a shows how the image of a structure produced by a diverging X-ray beam is larger than the structure itself.

If the diagram were redrawn with larger or smaller values for F and h, it would be seen that magnification is reduced by using a longer FFD F or by decreasing the object–film distance h. (It will be shown in section 3.6 that this also reduces the blurring B.) When positioning the patient, the film is therefore usually placed close to the structures of interest. If the tissues were compressed, this would also reduce patient dose. On the other hand, magnification may be helpful for visualizing small detail (a technique sometimes known as macroradiography), but this is generally used only in mammography (see Ch. 4.6.5).

The *magnification* M in Figure 3.12a is equal to $F/(F - h)$.

Distortion

This refers to a difference between the shape of a structure in the image and in the subject. It may be caused by foreshortening of the shadow of a tilted object (e.g. a tilted circle projects as an ellipse). It may also be caused by differential magnification of the parts of a structure nearer to and further away from the imaging device. It can be reduced by using a longer FFD.

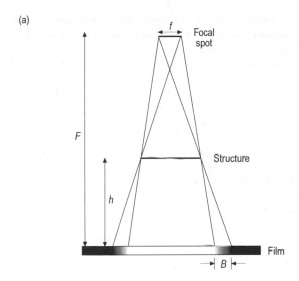

(a)

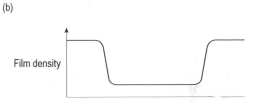

(b)

Figure 3.12 (a) Magnification of the X-ray image and geometrical unsharpness. (b) Dose profile showing the effect of geometrical unsharpness.

3.6 UNSHARPNESS AND BLURRING

Spatial resolution (section 3.1.2) is critically dependent on the visualization of a sharp edge between two regions in the imaged object. The more blurred is the edge the more difficult it is to resolve a small object in the image. Three types of unsharpness are considered below.

Geometrical unsharpness

The image of a stationary structure produced by the beam from an ideal point source would be perfectly sharp. At the edge of the shadow, the intensity of X-rays would change suddenly from a high to a low value.

Figure 3.12a shows that, in the case of an effective focal spot f mm square, the intensity changes gradually over a distance B, variously called the penumbra, blurring or unsharpness.

If the diagram were redrawn with larger or smaller values for f, F and h, it would be seen that blurring is reduced by:

- using a smaller focal spot,
- decreasing the object–film distance, or
- using a longer FFD.

From the above, it is apparent that F should be as long as possible, but for practical reasons it is generally about 1 m, possibly somewhat smaller for fluoroscopy and usually longer for chest radiography (typically 2 m).

The geometrical unsharpness can be expressed as $U_g = fh/(F - h)$. If $f = 1$ mm, $F = 1$ m and $h = 100$ mm, then $U_g = 0.11$ mm. This is shown on a plot of the profile of radiation intensity in the imaging plane (Fig. 3.12b).

Movement unsharpness

One of the problems in radiography is the imaging of moving structures. If, during an exposure of duration t seconds, the structure moves parallel to the film with an average speed v, the edge of the shadow moves a distance slightly greater than vt. This produces movement unsharpness $U_m = vt$ (approximately). If $v = 4$ mm s^{-1} and $t = 0.05$ s, then $U_m = 0.2$ mm.

Movement unsharpness may be reduced by immobilization (a technique used in mammography), by asking patients to hold their breath during exposure, and by using a short exposure time. Reduced exposure times require the use of high mA and a sensitive imaging system.

Absorption unsharpness

A gradual change in absorption near the edge of a tapered or rounded structure (e.g. a blood vessel) produces absorption blurring. This is inherent in the objects being imaged, although the effect can sometimes be reduced by careful patient positioning.

In practice, all three types of unsharpness combine to limit the resolution achievable (see Ch. 4.4.2).

3.7 LIMITATIONS OF THE X-RAY TUBE

This chapter has been concerned with the production of an optimum quality of image at the minimum level of dose to the patient. A factor with the potential to limit the achievement of these aims is the heat that inevitably accompanies the production of X-rays. This affects the design of an X-ray tube and restricts the way in which it can be used. If this heat were to be allowed to accumulate in various parts of the X-ray tube, the consequent rise of temperature might cause damage and shorten or terminate the life of the tube.

The basic components of the *stationary anode* X-ray tube were described in Chapter 1.3. A key component is the target made of tungsten. In practice, the target is typically a disk that is 10–15 mm in diameter and about 1 mm thick. It is set into a cylindrical block of copper. Most of the energy gained by the electrons as they are accelerated from cathode to anode is deposited in the tungsten as heat. This heat is transferred to the copper by conduction. The stem of the copper anode passes through the glass wall of the X-ray tube and is connected to the positive side of the high-voltage supply. The X-ray tube within its housing is surrounded with oil. The heat conducted through the copper anode passes to the oil and, through convection currents set up in the oil, passes to the tube housing and thus to the room.

In a radiographic exposure, excessive rise of target temperature, which might melt it, may be avoided by spreading the heat over sufficiently large an area of the target and during sufficiently long an exposure time. On the other hand, to minimize geometrical and movement unsharpness, the focal area should be small and the exposure time short. A compromise between these opposing requirements is affected by two aspects of the design of an X-ray tube: the focal spot size and the use of a rotating anode.

3.7.1 Focal spot size

Left to themselves, the electrons emitted by the cathode, being mutually repellent, would spread and strike the target and produce X-rays over a large focal area, thereby leading to blurred images. To obviate this, the filament coil is set in a rectangular slot in the cathode (referred to as focusing hood or cup) that is connected to one end of the filament. This arrangement acts as an electron lens. As a result, the electrons are focused on to a small elongated area on the target face (Fig. 3.13). This is the *actual focal spot*, the area over which heat is produced and which determines the tube rating (see section 3.7.3).

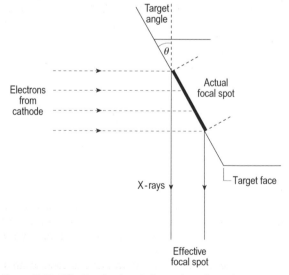

Figure 3.13 Effective focal spot size and anode angle.

Because the target is tilted, the *effective focal spot*, seen from the centre of the imaging device, is foreshortened in one direction, and appears circular or elliptical depending on the exact design of filament and focusing hood and on the target angle. A circular effective focal spot results in the same degree of geometrical unsharpness on all edges of a structure. However, the shape of the effective focal spot varies across the film. Seen from the cathode side of the film, it is elongated in the direction of the anode–cathode axis, while from the anode side it is contracted in that direction.

The *target angle* θ is the angle between the central ray of the X-ray beam and the target face. The steeper the target angle (i.e. the smaller the angle θ), the greater is the foreshortening. The target angle is generally between 7 and 20°. For a target at 18° with an effective focal spot of $1 \times 1\,mm^2$, the actual focal spot would be $3.2 \times 1\,mm^2$, whereas for a target at 12° the actual focal spot could be increased to $4.8 \times 1\,mm^2$ to produce the same effective focus spot. The tube loading in the latter tube could be increased by 50% for the same effective focal spot size. Thus the use of a steeper target serves to increase the target heat rating for a given effective focal spot or to reduce the effective focal spot size for a given target heat rating. However, as discussed in section 3.7.4, the steeper the target, the narrower the useful X-ray beam and the smaller the field covered. Thus a steep target is appropriate in mammography and in cardiac angiography where relatively small fields of view are required coupled with a requirement to image fine detail, whereas in general radiography, using large films, a shallower target angle is used.

Commonly, an X-ray tube has two filaments to provide two focal spots of different sizes that may be selected by the operator. The smaller focal spot is used for improved resolution and the larger one for thicker parts of the body where a greater intensity of X-rays is needed. Typical focal spot sizes are 0.3 mm for mammography (0.1 mm for magnification), 0.6–1.2 mm for general radiography, 0.6 mm for fluoroscopy, and 0.6–1.0 mm for CT scanning.

It is a feature of X-ray tube design that focal spot size is not constant – it depends on both mA and kV. As mA increases, the focusing of the electron beam becomes less effective. This is referred to as *blooming*, and it becomes more significant at lower settings of kV.

3.7.2 Rotating anode tube

A second method used for spreading the heat over a larger area of target is to rotate the anode during the exposure.

The basic design of a rotating anode tube is illustrated in Figure 3.14. The anode is a bevelled disk T into which is set an annulus of tungsten. It rotates during the exposure. The filament assembly is similar to that in the fixed anode tube, but it is offset from the centre of the tube. The electron stream E from the cathode is focused on the sloping edge of the disk.

The target is heated over the focal area (2, in Fig. 3.14b), but because of the rotation of the tube it is spread over a much greater area. Provided that the exposure time is greater than the period of rotation, the heat is spread over the full circumference of the disk, which is generally in the range 200–300 mm. This may be compared with the fixed anode tube in which the heat is confined to a narrow strip, with width corresponding to the focal spot size, i.e. about 1 mm.

The anode assembly, seen in cross-section in Figure 3.14a, consists of the following.

- An anode disk T, 7–10 cm or more in diameter, usually made of molybdenum because of its high melting point and (relative to tungsten) its low density. An alternative material is graphite.
- The target annulus set in the bevelled edge of the anode. The target is usually an alloy of tungsten and rhenium, which has better thermal characteristics than pure tungsten and does not roughen with use as quickly.
- A thin molybdenum stem, M.
- A blackened copper rotor, R.

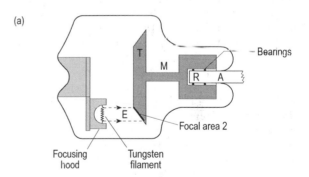

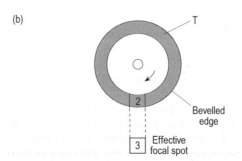

Figure 3.14 The rotating anode X-ray tube.

- Bearings lubricated with a soft metal such as silver, which enable the rotor to rotate freely around the axle within a vacuum.
- An axle A, sealed into the glass envelope, which supports the target assembly.

Rotation is effected by an induction motor. This is a device that can drive the rotating anode assembly without a direct mechanical linkage to the rotating parts. It consists of external coils (stator coils not shown in the diagram) in which alternating currents produce a varying magnetic field that induces currents within the rotor. These currents generate opposing magnetic fields that serve to drive the rotor round at up to 3000 rpm or 50 Hz, the frequency of the mains supply, i.e. a full rotation takes 20 ms. Because of the lack of direct mechanical linkage, there is a time delay before the anode comes up to its full speed of about 1 s. In a well-designed tube, the anode will continue to rotate for a long period after the stator coils are de-energized and reverse braking potentials are applied to bring the rotation to a stop. High-speed anodes are energized with three-phase mains and rotate at 9000 rpm.

Anode cooling

Heat produced on the focal track is conducted quickly into the anode disk and stored there temporarily while being transferred by radiation to the insulating oil. The molybdenum stem is sufficiently long and narrow to control the amount of heat that is conducted to the rotor, so that it is not in danger of overheating and seizing up. Heat radiation is promoted by blackening the anode assembly. The rate of heat radiation increases as the anode gets hotter, being *proportional to the fourth power of the temperature* expressed in K (the kelvin scale is the absolute temperature scale starting at 0 K, equal to $-273.15°C$). Thus a 40% increase in the output of X-rays and accompanying heat involves a rise of rather less than 10% in the temperature. Because heat loss is so dependent on temperature, the anode disk temperature rapidly rises when the tube is energized up to a level at which the rate of heat loss matches the heat input. Thus there is the requirement for the disk and its stem to have good thermal properties with a high melting point and relatively low conduction rate in its stem.

Heat is taken up by the oil and transferred by convection to the housing, from which it is lost by radiation and, in some designs, by fan-assisted convection through the surrounding air. High-powered tubes used in CT and angiography may pump the oil through an external heat exchanger.

The oil in the tube housing expands as its temperature rises. The housing is therefore designed with a bellows system that allows for this expansion. The oil serves not just to transfer heat from the tube to the housing – it is also electrically insulating. The housing itself is lead-lined so as to prevent radiation being emitted in directions other than that of the useful beam.

Choice of tube type

The rotating anode tube is the choice of tube for the majority of X-ray applications. However, it is very much more expensive than the stationary anode tube and there are applications for which the simpler tube is preferred. The principal exception is dental radiology, in which, for both intraoral and panoramic radiography, a stationary anode tube is invariably used.

A stationary anode can sustain long periods of running at a low mA so that continuous fluoroscopy is possible. Because of their restricted use, mobile fluoroscopy units used, for example, in orthopaedic theatres and for guiding temporary pacemaker insertions commonly have a stationary anode tube. Similarly, if the system is to be used for a limited number of radiographic exposures at a higher mA, such as is the case for ward radiography, a rotating anode tube is not required.

3.7.3 Heat rating

The heat loading of an X-ray tube may be calculated in joules and is equal to kV × mAs for a constant potential or three-phase system. For single-phase generators, the heat loading is $0.7 × kV_p × mAs$. Heat loading may also be expressed in terms of heat units (see Box 3.2).

Single radiographic exposure

In order to 'freeze' and display a moving structure, individual exposures should be as short as possible

---

Box 3.2 Heat unit

The heat unit is the original unit of energy input to the target. It was defined in the days when single-phase generators were standard (Ch. 1.3). The number of heat units is simply kVp × mAs. Because single-phase generators have a sinusoidal voltage variation, the energy in J is less, and there is the relationship that 1.4 HU = 1 J. In some manufacturers' data sheets, tube ratings are still given in terms of the heat unit. The same abbreviation (HU) is also used for the Hounsfield unit in computed tomography. The two should not be confused.

and may be limited by the heating of the X-ray tube. A combination of kV, mA and exposure time used should be such that, at the end of the exposure, the temperature of the anode does not exceed its safe value, i.e. there should be no risk of the target melting, vaporizing, emitting gas or prematurely roughening. The *allowable mAs* at a particular kV increases as the exposure time is lengthened. Conversely, if the mAs needed to produce a satisfactory radiograph can be reduced, the exposure time can be made shorter.

The rating is usually stated as the *allowable mA*, and this:

- decreases as the exposure time is lengthened
- decreases (in inverse proportion) as the kV is increased
- increases with the effective focal spot size and, for a given effective focal spot, is greater for smaller target angles
- is greater for a rotating than a stationary anode
- increases, in a rotating anode tube, with disk diameter
- is greater for a high-speed anode because the heat is spread more evenly along the focal track
- for exposures shorter than 1 s, is greater for a constant potential than for a single-phase pulsating potential, because the former produces heat more evenly throughout the exposure.

The control system for the equipment should be designed so as to prevent exposures being made that exceed the tube rating.

Repeated radiographic exposures

Certain investigations, such as angiography, require a rapid series of exposures. Each exposure is sufficiently short to freeze movement, and each must be within the rating of the focal area. As a result of the repeated exposures, heat accumulates in the anode assembly and the oil. Neither of these can be allowed to exceed its maximum safe temperature. The rapidity with which a series of such exposures can be made depends on the maximum amount of heat that can be temporarily stored in the tube housing as a whole and the anode in particular, and on the rate at which they lose that heat by cooling processes.

Whereas for standard radiography an anode heat capacity in the region of 250 kJ may be sufficient, for angiography it may be in excess of 1 MJ and up to 5 MJ for an X-ray tube in a CT scanner. The generator control system should not allow the operator to select sequences in which the total exposure time would result in this heat capacity being exceeded at the required levels of kV and mA. There may also be a requirement built in the system to prevent repeated examination sequences causing the overall heat capacity of the X-ray tube assembly (typically 1 MJ) to be exceeded. When the intensity of use of the tube approaches these limits, it may take a significant time for the anode and for the complete assembly to cool down before further exposures are allowed by the control system.

Continuous operation: fluoroscopy

If heat is produced on the focus continuously over a long period, it must be removed at the same rate from the housing if it is not to cause overheating of the oil. The rating depends only on the cooling rate of the tube housing and not at all on the focal spot size or the type of generator. Typically, tubes can be run continuously at $350\,\mathrm{J\,s^{-1}}$ (watts), corresponding to approximately 4 mA at 90 kV, but much greater cooling rates can be achieved when cooling systems are incorporated into the design.

Other ratings

There is a maximum kV that may be applied, depending on the insulation of the tube, cables, etc. There is a maximum mA that can be drawn without having to heat the filament to too high a temperature. The maximum mA is smaller at a low kV than at a high kV (because of what is called the space charge effect). In general, X-ray tubes for diagnostic radiology do not operate above 150 kV, and the maximum mA for radiography is no greater than about 700 mA. Generators used to produce the high-voltage supply have a rating given in kW, and typically this is in the range 40–60 kW. This limits the mA at a particular setting; for example, a 50-kW generator could not be operated above 500 mA at 100 kV but could be operated at 625 mA at 80 kV.

3.7.4 Uniformity of the X-ray beam

An X-ray tube emits some X-rays in every direction, necessitating lead shielding inside the tube housing to protect the patient and staff from unnecessary exposure. A collimator system is used to adjust the beam to the required size (Box 3.3).

The useful beam is taken off where it is most intense, in a direction perpendicular to the electron stream. The central ray (B in Fig. 3.15) emerges at right angles to the tube axis from the centre of the focal spot. It is usually pointed towards the centre of the area of interest in the body.

Towards the anode edge A of the field, the beam would be cut off by the face of the target. The beam could extend further in the cathode direction but is deliberately cut off at C by the edge of a circular

Box 3.3 Collimation

X-ray sets have a collimator system so that the beam can be adjusted to the required size by the operator. In radiographic equipment, this comprises two sets of parallel blades made of high-attenuation material that can be driven into the beam to define the required (rectangular) area. The collimator incorporates a light source to the side of the X-ray beam and a mirror in the beam. The position of the light bulb and the angle of the mirror are adjusted so that the divergent light beam appears to emanate from the X-ray focus. This allows the radiographer to see the position of the X-ray beam projected on to the patient. The collimator assembly is referred to as the *light beam diaphragm*.

For fluoroscopy, the detector (image intensifier) is circular and, to prevent unnecessary irradiation of the patient, circular collimation should be used. The equipment may incorporate fixed circular collimators that are automatically moved into the beam at each magnification setting of the intensifier to restrict the beam to the maximum size that can be seen on the TV monitor. These will be used with variable collimators that will either be rectangular or have iris diaphragms to produce near circular collimation (in fact they commonly have eight blades mechanically linked to produce an octagonal beam).

Some radiologists, when talking about adjustment of the X-ray beam size, talk about bringing in the cones or coning down. The origin of the term *cone* goes back to the time that fixed, interchangeable collimators were used that had to be manually fitted to the X-ray tube. These could be either rectangular (generally to match the standard film cassette sizes) or circular. A collimator designed for a circular beam would have been conical in shape, the origin of this terminology.

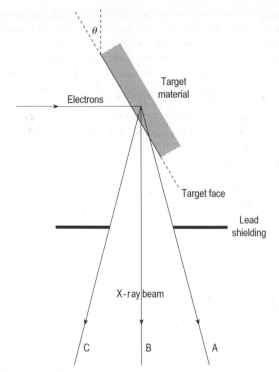

Figure 3.15 The anode heel effect.

travelling towards the cathode edge (C). The intensity of the beam decreases across the field, and this is most apparent from B to A. Less importantly, the half-value layer increases because of the filtration effect and, as was noted in section 3.7.1, the effective focal spot decreases. The steeper the target, the greater is the heel effect. At longer FFD, the heel effect is reduced for a given film size.

The heel effect, being gradual, is generally not noticeable even on the largest film. Where the patient's thickness varies considerably across the field, advantage may be taken of the heel effect by positioning the patient with the thicker or denser part towards the cathode of the tube where the exit beam is more intense (see, for example, mammography, Ch. 4.6.3).

The target surface roughens progressively during the life of an X-ray tube because of bombardment by the electrons. As a result, X-rays produced in the 'valleys' have to penetrate the 'hills' of tungsten, and this both reduces the output of X-rays and increases the heel effect. Overloading of the tube accelerates roughening and its adverse effects.

The intensity of the beam decreases somewhat either side of the central ray, in a direction perpendicular to AC (i.e. parallel to the tube axis), because of the inverse square law, the X-rays at the edges having further to travel.

aperture in the lead shield. Thus the X-ray field is made symmetrical around the central ray B, and A and C are the limits of the useful beam.

The maximum size of the useful beam is determined by the angle θ of the anode. In practice, it is narrower than suggested because of the *heel effect*. As indicated in Figure 3.15, most of the electrons penetrate a few micrometres into the target before being stopped by a nucleus. On their way out, the X-rays are attenuated and filtered by the target material. It will be seen that X-rays travelling towards the anode edge of the field (A) have more target material to cross and so are attenuated more than those

Box 3.4 Performance tests on the X-ray tube and generator

Light beam diaphragm alignment and Bucky centring

Regular checks should be made to ensure that the light beam and the X-ray beam match, and that the centre of the field lies at the centre of the film when the cassette is positioned in the Bucky assembly behind the patient. Any misalignment would lead to repeat examinations or the use of unnecessarily large field sizes. For the test, the X-ray tube is centred over the Bucky. A test object incorporating a metal frame (generally 150 mm square) is placed on the tabletop and the light beam is adjusted so as just to cover the metal frame. A film is taken. Alignment of the X-ray beam and the image of the metal frame and the centring of the beam on the film are assessed. Generally discrepancies of up to 10 mm are acceptable.

Kilovoltage and output

The kV is generally measured indirectly using a penetrameter. The instrument usually has two radiation detectors placed behind metal filters of different thickness. The ratio of the response of the two detectors is dependent on the penetrating ability of the beam and thus on kV. The instrument can sample the signal from the detectors at a sufficiently high frequency to enable it to display the kV waveform, normally by interfacing the instrument to a computer. For standard use, this interface is not required – the instrument will display a single kV value corresponding either to the peak kV or to an average value. The kV meter has to be calibrated against a standard.

The output of the tube can be measured using a dosimeter, often an ionization chamber (Ch. 1.6.3). For a constant mAs, the output is a function of kV^x,

where x is about 2, as noted in Chapter 1.6.4. For a constant kV, the output is a linear function of mA and exposure time and, if the time is measured using an appropriate instrument, any discrepancy in the output curves can be attributed to malfunctions in either kV, mA or exposure time.

Step wedge

A simple alternative to the use of a kV meter and ionization chamber is to use a step wedge. This is a block of material, generally aluminium, which is machined so as to have successive steps of differing thickness. Typically, there might be 15 steps from 1 to 15 mm thick. A radiograph is taken of the wedge, and the optical density of one or more of these steps is measured using a densitometer (see Ch. 4.1.1). The measured densities are compared with baseline values. A change in optical density may be due to kV, output or processor performance. This is a constancy test in which a consistent result demonstrates that the imaging system is performing satisfactorily at the chosen settings used for the test. A deviation from the baseline does not identify the problem; rather, it identifies a requirement for further investigation.

Further tests

The tests described above are those that might be incorporated into a regular quality assurance programme for the X-ray tube and generator. Other tests that could be carried out at the time of acceptance or to investigate particular performance problems could include:

- total filtration assessed by measurement of the half-value layer
- focal spot size measured using a pinhole camera or a star test tool.

We have seen that two of the limiting factors in X-ray imaging are the amount of heat that is acceptable to the X-ray tube and the dose of radiation that is acceptable to the patient. A third limiting factor, the sensitivity and performance of the film–screen or other recording media, will be the subject of the following chapters.

3.7.5 Quality assurance of exposure parameters

The principles of quality assurance were discussed in Chapter 2.5.4. In regard to the X-ray tube and generator, there are certain tests that may be carried out periodically by radiography staff to determine whether parameters have changed that could affect image quality or patient dose. These are described briefly in Box 3.4.

3.8 SUMMARY

- Contrast in the image depends on the thickness, density and atomic number of structures within the body.
- Contrast media use high atomic number materials with suitable K-edge energy.

- For a particular imaging device, patient dose is affected by kV, FFD and filtration.
- Scattered radiation reduces image contrast.
- The amount of scatter depends on the size of the X-ray beam and the thickness of the body part.
- Scattered radiation may be reduced using a grid or an air gap.
- The grid is generally focused to minimize cut-off and may be moved during exposure to blur out the grid lines.
- Image unsharpness may be caused by large focal spot size and movement.
- Target angle influences the heat loading on the target and can be used to minimize the effective focal spot size.

- The anode heel effect causes reduction in beam intensity at the anode side of the tube.
- Small target angles limit the maximum useful beam size.
- Rotating anode tubes are used to increase the tube rating.
- The rotating anode tube is cooled by radiation heat transfer from the anode disk to the surrounding oil.
- Heat rating of an X-ray tube indicates the maximum allowable mA for the specified kV and exposure time and the maximum sustainable continuous mA without damage to the tube.
- The X-ray system should be subject to a quality assurance programme.

Chapter 4

Film–screen radiography

In the previous chapter, we showed how the X-ray transmission image is produced by the differential attenuation of X-rays by the organs and tissues within the body. It was seen how the subject contrast is influenced by the atomic number and density of the overlying tissues and by the kilovoltage (kV) and spectrum of the X-ray beam. Spatial resolution was shown to be a function of focal spot size. It was demonstrated how contrast is reduced by scatter and unsharpness is influenced by the focal spot size and the distance between the object and imaging plain.

This chapter is concerned with image capture on film; that is, film–screen or analogue radiography. Digital radiographic systems are considered separately in Chapter 5.

4.1 FILM–SCREEN RADIOGRAPHY: IMAGE FORMATION

4.1.1 Film

The radiographic image is recorded on a sheet of X-ray film. The film consists of a polyester base (typically 0.2 mm thick) on which is coated (usually on both sides) a thin photographic emulsion (about 5–10 μm thick). The emulsion is a suspension in gelatine of silver halide crystals, generally silver iodobromide with 90% bromide and 10% iodide. Each crystal is about 1 μm in size and contains a million or more silver atoms. Both films and screens have a very thin transparent antistatic supercoat to protect against abrasion and are designed not to curl. A photographic emulsion is sensitive to ultraviolet and visible light and, much less so, to X-rays. It is affected by mechanical pressure and creasing, by static electricity, and by chemical liquids and vapours, all of which have implications for storage and handling.

Exposure to light

Two features of the silver iodobromide crystal account for the photographic process: the small proportion of iodide relative to bromide ions distort the lattice, which allows some of the silver ions to move through the lattice; and the silver halide crystals are manufactured to possess sensitivity specks on their surfaces.

When a crystal absorbs a light photon, an electron may be liberated that migrates to the sensitivity speck, where its potential energy will be lowest. When a hundred or so photons have been absorbed by a crystal, enough electrons have accumulated at the sensitivity speck to attract mobile silver ions from within the crystal to join them and be neutralized. They form a submicroscopic speck of silver metal on the surface of the crystal. The distribution of the specks of silver within the emulsion forms a latent image in the film that is awaiting development.

Processing

The invisible pattern of latent images is made visible by processing. The film is processed in three stages:

1. The film is first *developed* by immersion in an alkaline solution of a reducing agent (an electron donor), which is able to enter the crystal at the site of the latent image. It proceeds to reduce the positive silver ions to silver atoms, and the latent image grows into a grain of metallic silver.

   The unexposed crystals, which carry no latent images, are unaffected by the developer. The layer of bromine ions forming the surface of the crystal repel electron donor (developer) molecules and allow their entry only at the latent images where the ion barrier is breached.

   However, given sufficient time, the developer would penetrate the unexposed crystals. The amount of background fog produced by the development of unexposed crystals is a function not only of development time but also of developer strength and temperature.

2. The film is now *fixed* by an acid solution of thiosulfate ('hypo'), which dissolves out the unaffected silver ions so that the image is stable and unaffected further by light.

3. After each of stages 1 and 2, the film is *washed* in water, and finally it is dried by hot air. The result of inadequate washing would be for any retained hypo to turn the film brown/yellow in time, causing the stored films to have a familiar vinegary smell.

Automatic processors use a roller feed system to transport the film through different solutions. Processor performance is maintained through a comprehensive quality assurance programme (see section 4.2).

Optical density

The film now carries a pattern of silver grains corresponding to the pattern of X-rays leaving the patient. The image is viewed by transmitted light on an illuminator or light box of uniform brightness. It is a negative image: where the X-rays have been most intense, the film is darkest, and vice versa.

The grains of silver scatter and absorb the light as it passes through the processed emulsion. The optical density (D) or blackening of an area of the film depends on the number of silver grains per unit area. It is defined as the log of the ratio of the intensities of the incident and transmitted light:

$$D = \log_{10}(\text{incident light}/\text{transmitted light}).$$

The log is used because the eye responds logarithmically to the brightness of light. Optical density is measured by an instrument known as a *densitometer*, which incorporates a small light source, generally 1–2 mm in diameter, and a light detector.

From the definition, it can be deduced that if 1% of the light is transmitted then the density of the film is 2.0, and if 10% is transmitted the density is 1.0. The density of a completely transparent film in which there is no light absorption is zero.

Densities are additive: if the front and rear emulsions each have a density of 1.0, the film has a total density of 2.0. The density of the area of interest on a properly exposed film averages about 1.0, although in the lung field of a chest film it may be about 2.0. Areas with density above 3 are too dark to be viewed on a standard light box and require a bright lamp if any detail is to be seen.

4.1.2 Intensifying screens

X-ray film is relatively insensitive to X-rays and, if used in isolation, would require unacceptably high levels of radiation to produce a satisfactory image. With the exception of intraoral dental radiography, film is used for clinical radiography only in association with intensifying screens that convert the pattern of X-ray intensities to light.

An intensifying screen is a sheet of material that is the same size as the sheet of film. The screen has a polyester base (typically 0.25 mm thick) on which is coated a dense layer (0.1–0.5 mm thick) of fine phosphor crystals (3–10 μm in size) bound by a transparent resin. The crystals absorb X-rays and emit light of intensity proportional to the intensity of the X-rays (see Ch. 1.7 for an explanation of luminescence).

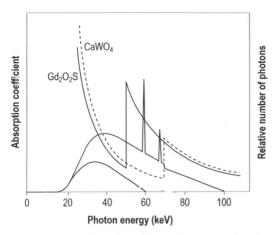

Figure 4.1 Relative absorption of X-ray photons as a function of photon energy for two screen materials. The spectra for 60 and 100 kV X-rays are superimposed.

The screen converts the pattern of X-ray intensities emerging from the patient into one of light that is then recorded by the film.

Photon absorption in the screen is determined by the absorption coefficient of the phosphor material. The traditional phosphor used for radiography was calcium tungstate ($CaWO_4$), a material that emits blue light when irradiated with X-rays. The variation of mass–energy absorption coefficient for calcium tungstate with photon energy is shown in Figure 4.1. The coefficient is predominantly influenced by tungsten (W) with $Z = 74$ and its K-edge at 70 keV. Superimposition of the spectra of 60 and 100 kV X-rays demonstrates that the absorption coefficient is not optimally matched to the typical spectra used in radiography, with relatively low attenuation at the peak of the X-ray spectrum and poor detection of the characteristic radiation.

The use of calcium tungstate has been superseded by the use of rare earth materials. The rare earths are those elements with atomic numbers in the range 57–70 and K-edges between 39 and 61 keV. The phosphors most commonly used for intensifying screens are lanthanum oxybromide, lanthanum oxysulphide and gadolinium oxysulphide (Gd_2O_2S). The absorption coefficient for gadolinium oxysulphide is also shown in Figure 4.1. The phosphors incorporate impurities (or activators) that form the energy traps referred to in Chapter 1.7. The combination of phosphor and activator produces a spectrum of light that is specific to that material. The sensitivity of the film should match the spectrum of the emitted light. This is discussed further in Box 4.1.

Rare earth screens are chosen not just on the basis of atomic number. They are also more efficient than calcium tungstate in converting absorbed X-ray energy into emitted light. The two factors together make rare earth screens more sensitive ('faster') than calcium tungstate screens. They require a smaller exposure, resulting in a patient dose that is 2–3 times lower while producing images of the same quality.

X-ray film is usually double-coated with an emulsion on each side of the base, and it is used with a pair of screens. Each emulsion is in contact with the phosphor coating of an intensifying screen. About a third of the X-radiation falling on the front screen (nearer the patient) is absorbed, and about half the light so produced travels forwards and exposes the nearer (front) emulsion. The rear screen absorbs about a half of the X-radiation transmitted by the front screen, i.e. about two-thirds of the total fluence is absorbed by the two screens in combination. Light from the back screen exposes the rear-facing emulsion.

Screen materials are chosen that do not emit delayed fluorescence (phosphorescence; see Ch. 1.7), because these would retain a 'memory' of the previous exposure. On reloading the cassette, the previous image would be recorded on the new film and superimposed on the image of a subsequent exposure.

4.1.3 The film cassette

An *X-ray cassette* is a flat, light-tight box with internal pressure pads designed to keep its contents (a film) in close and uniform contact with the two intensifying screens. The front of the cassette, nearer to the tube, is made of a low atomic number material, possibly carbon fibre (Z = 6), in order to minimize the attenuation of the beam and so reduce the patient exposure required. The use of low atomic number materials between the patient and the intensifying screens in the cassette is particularly important at lower kV such as those used for mammography and extremity radiography. The cassette back usually incorporates a thin lead sheet to minimize any backscattered radiation arising from interactions between the radiation transmitted through the film–screen combination with the materials behind the cassette.

4.2 CHARACTERISTIC CURVE

The response of a film and screen combination to X-rays is described by its characteristic curve. This is a graph of optical density as a function of exposure plotted on a logarithmic scale (Fig. 4.2). The term *exposure* is used loosely here; more correctly, it is air kerma. However, in practice the characteristic curve is not measured using an X-ray beam to irradiate the film–screen combination to varying levels of air kerma; it is measured from a film exposed to light of varying intensity using an instrument known as a *sensitometer* (see Box 4.2).

The characteristic curve shown in Figure 4.2 has three distinct regions:

● The *region of correct exposure* is the (nearly) straight line portion, where the slope or gradient is

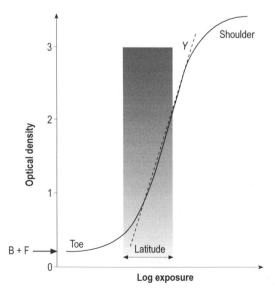

Figure 4.2 The characteristic curve of a photographic film.

steepest. The densities within the area of diagnostic interest should lie within this range.
● The *toe* is the low-density region in which the slope of the curve is shallow.
● The *shoulder* is at higher densities and also has a shallow slope.

At higher doses beyond the shoulder region, the curve flattens off at a density of about 3.5, representing saturation, in which all the silver bromide crystals have been converted to silver. At extremely high levels of exposure, the density will begin to fall because of an effect called solarization, but this is not relevant for the radiographic image.

Certain properties may be derived from the characteristic curve:

● *Base plus fog* level (B + F) is the density of processed but unexposed film. The film has an intrinsic base

Box 4.2 Sensitometry

A *sensitometer* is an instrument that can be used to derive the characteristic curve shown in Figure 4.2. It is a small portable instrument that is generally battery-operated. It has a light source with an array of filters that enable a film to be exposed to a series of exposure steps. Each step produces an area of blackening on the film and, in a common design, there are 21 steps set in a line with the light intensity increasing by $\sqrt{2}$ at each successive step in the series. Thus the light intensity of the 21st step is $2^{10} = 1024$ times greater than that of the first. Measurement of the optical density of each step (using a densitometer) and plotting this against step number gives the characteristic curve shown in Figure 4.2.

For performance testing, it is not necessary to measure the full characteristic curve. It is simpler to measure density on just three steps: the least exposed step to measure base plus fog, a step with net density just above 1 to give an index of speed, and a third step with net density just above 2. The difference in densities between these last two steps gives an index of contrast. Plotting the three indices against time will show trends. Variations greater than 10–15% from the baseline value indicate that remedial action may be required.

This simple test (known as sensitometry) gives information on the performance of the processor, which is a key element in maintaining good image quality in film–screen radiography. It also serves to indicate any changes in performance between batches of film.

density due, about equally, to some of the silver bromide crystals having acquired latent images during manufacture and the film base absorbing light when viewed. Additional fog may arise during storage (particularly if the temperature and humidity are too high or if the film is old) and from accidental exposure to X-rays. It may be increased by the processing conditions (over-strength developer, high developer temperature, long development time). Fog reduces the contrast of the image and should be as low as possible. Generally, the density of base plus fog is in the range 0.15–0.2.

- *Speed* is loosely defined here as the reciprocal of the exposure required to produce a net density of 1.0; that is, the density with the base plus fog subtracted. A net density of 1 is the approximate average density of a correctly exposed radiograph. In Figure 4.3, film A has higher (or faster) speed than film B. The speed of the film increases with the average size of the crystals in the film emulsion, because the smaller crystals require a higher level of light exposure to form the latent image. Speed of the film and screen in combination is also dependent on the properties of the screen and of the X-ray beam. This is discussed further in section 4.3.1.

- *Film gamma* (γ) is the average slope of the characteristic curve. It influences the amount of contrast displayed in the radiographic image. In Figure 4.3, film A has a higher γ (a steeper slope), and it therefore displays more contrast than B because greater differences in density are produced for the same difference in exposure. The slope of the curve increases as exposure and density are increased, and γ generally refers to the average slope between net densities of 0.25 and 2.0. Typically, γ is in the range 2–3.

   The value of γ depends on the *range* of crystal sizes (not their average size). If all the crystals in an emulsion were of the same size, they would all acquire latent images at the same level of exposure, and the characteristic curve would theoretically be vertical, i.e. with a very high value of γ. The bigger the crystal, the smaller is the light exposure required to form a latent image. Therefore the wider is the range of sizes, the greater is the range of exposure required to produce the latent images and the shallower the slope of the curve.

- *Film latitude*. This is shown in Figure 4.2. It is the range of exposures that produce net densities lying in the *useful density range* between 0.25, below which the gradient is too low, and 2.0, above which

the film is too dark for details to be seen using a normal illuminator. For $\gamma = 2.5$, the log of the difference in the doses to give net densities of 0.25 and 2.0 is equal to $1.75/2.5 = 0.7$. This represents a dose ratio of 5.

Figure 4.3 shows that γ and latitude are inversely related. It compares the characteristic curves of two film–screen combinations, A and B. A has the steeper slope and higher γ. It also has the narrower latitude, $L(A)$. B, with lower γ, has the wider latitude, $L(B)$. A wide latitude is needed in chest radiography (in which the range of radiation intensities between the lung and mediastinal regions is great), whereas in mammography there is a requirement for a high γ because of the low subject contrast.

Effect of developing conditions
Increasing the developer temperature will increase the rate of chemical reaction and so cause an increase of speed but also of fog level. It also causes γ to increase initially, but above the temperature recommended by the manufacturer of the film the increase in fog level will *reduce* the average γ. Increasing developer concentration or developing time will have similar effects.

Developing conditions are optimized to give maximum γ and minimal fog. In an automatic processor, the *temperature* is controlled thermostatically and the *time* by roller speed. *Concentration* is controlled by automatic replenishment of the developer that depends on the throughput of film.

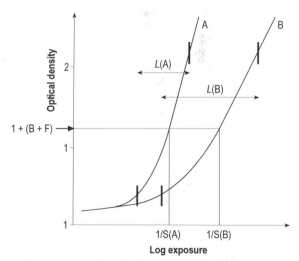

Figure 4.3 Characteristic curves for two film–screen combinations.

Quality assurance

The control of processing conditions is critical to the production of optimum image quality in film–screen radiography. There is therefore a requirement for a quality assurance programme to assess performance on a regular, preferably daily, basis. The most effective measurement method is sensitometry (see Box 4.2). A successful quality assurance programme should serve to reduce the incidence of repeat films and the consequent unnecessary dose to the patient and waste of materials.

4.3 FILM–SCREEN SENSITIVITY

4.3.1 Intensification factor

Film exposed on its own to X-rays is relatively insensitive. Only about 2% of X-ray photons incident on the film will interact within the emulsion, and in each interaction a single latent image is produced. The phosphor in the intensifying screens has a higher atomic number than silver bromide, and the screen itself can be made thicker. Consequently, the probability of interaction in the two screens on either side of the film is greater than with film alone and is generally in the region of 30%. In the interaction, the X-ray photon generates up to 1000 light photons (the intensification process). Just under half of these reach the film.

It may require up to 100 light photons to produce a single latent image, but the combination of increased detection efficiency and intensification leads to an overall reduction in dose required to produce a particular density on the film. This is described as the intensification factor (IF), defined as the ratio of air kerma required to produce $D = 1$ for film alone to the air kerma required with the film plus screen. IF is typically in the range 30–100. For a particular phosphor, IF can be increased by increasing the efficiency of light capture by adding a reflective layer to the base of the phosphor to reflect those light photons that initially travel away from the film back towards the film.

4.3.2 Speed class

Intensification factor is not generally used to express the sensitivity of a particular film–screen combination. The more common descriptor is the speed class. It is defined as:

$$speed = 1000/K,$$

in which K is the air kerma (in µGy) required to give a film density of 1 above base plus fog. The definition applies to a specific radiation geometry and X-ray beam quality.

Speed class depends on a number of factors, including phosphor type, thickness of phosphor and type of film. Typical rare earth screen–film systems have a speed classification of 400, indicating that the dose to the film cassette is in the region of 2.5 µGy for a satisfactorily exposed radiograph.

4.4 RADIOGRAPHIC IMAGE QUALITY

4.4.1 Contrast

In Chapter 3.2.1, it was shown that subject contrast depends on the attenuation coefficient of adjacent regions in the patient, and in Chapter 3.3.1 that this is reduced because of the influence of scattered radiation. The contrast seen in the film is due both to the subject contrast and to film γ.

In film–screen radiography, contrast is defined as the difference in optical density between adjacent areas on the film. In Figure 4.4a, the radiographic contrast between two areas having exposure E_2 and E_1 would be the difference between the corresponding densities, i.e. $D_2 - D_1$. Because γ represents the slope of the curve, it follows that the radiographic contrast is the product of γ and the difference in exposure $(E_2 - E_1)$, the subject contrast. Thus γ (generally in the range 2–3) amplifies contrast, and the contrast seen with the film in Figure 4.4a will be significantly greater than that for the film represented in Figure 4.4b. However, the downside is that the more contrasty film has a lower latitude, so that image detail is more likely to be lost in the darker or lighter areas of the image. In Figure 4.4b, although the contrast is much less, the latitude of exposure is greater, as shown by the displacement of the dashed lines.

Contrast is described here as an objective measure of density differences. However, a film is evaluated and reported by the radiologist subjectively, and the viewing conditions can significantly affect the limits of contrast that can be seen in the film. In particular, higher levels of ambient light prevent the eye seeing the full range of contrast in the beam. That may be high levels of room lighting or the glare from unmasked areas of the viewing box surrounding the film. The viewing box itself needs to have an adequate and uniform brightness in order to ensure that the full range of contrast can be perceived by the eye.

4.4.2 Screen unsharpness

In Chapter 3.6, the influence of focal spot size, movement and absorption on image unsharpness was discussed. Here, we will consider the influence of the imaging device, i.e. the film–screen system.

(a)

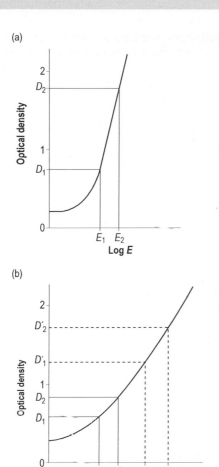

(b)

Figure 4.4 A comparison of exposure latitude for two films with (a) high and (b) low γ.

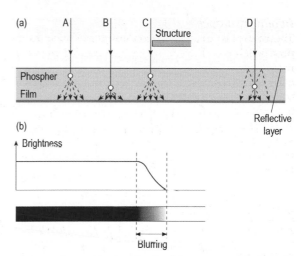

(a)

(b)

Figure 4.5 Screen blurring showing (a) a cross-section through the screen and film emulsion, and (b) the profile of film blackening caused by an edge in the imaged structure.

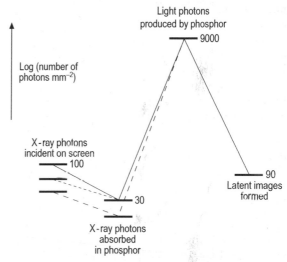

Figure 4.6 The numbers of photons transmitting information at various stages of imaging with a film–screen system. The solid line represents screen A, the dotted line in a thicker screen with the same phosphor as screen A, and the dashed line a more efficient phosphor than screen A.

For a film exposed to X-rays without a screen, a single X-ray interacting in the emulsion would produce a single latent image in an iodobromide crystal, i.e. a near point image in the film. The size of the point is limited only by the size of the film crystals. However, when screens are used light is given out in all directions from the point of interaction in the screen, as shown in Figure 4.5a. In effect, photon A in the diagram produces a blurred disk of light on the phosphor. The extent of the blurring is determined by the distance of the phosphor crystal from the film. Photon B interacts with a phosphor crystal closer to the film and therefore produces a smaller disk of blackening on the film.

We can now consider what happens to the image of a sharp-edged, highly attenuating structure lying above the film. Photons falling on the structure will be attenuated and will form no image in the film below the structure, whereas photons well away from the edge will produce uniform blackening in the film. However, a photon falling just outside the structure, photon C in the diagram, causes some blackening within the film behind the structure because of the blurring effect. The image of the edge is therefore unsharp, as seen in Figure 4.5b. The degree of unsharpness increases with phosphor thickness. However, as phosphor thickness is increased so does the likelihood that the photon will interact in it. Thus the thicker the phosphor, the greater is the sensitivity or speed of the screen. Figure 4.6 illustrates this, as described in Box 4.3.

Box 4.3 Quantum noise and film–screen speed

If a film without a screen is exposed to X-rays, the probability of an X-ray photon being absorbed in the emulsion is low (about 2%). However, because of the large number of secondary electrons produced following the interaction, each photon that is absorbed will produce a single latent image. In a film–screen system, there are a series of events taking place, illustrated in Figure 4.6. For the purpose of this illustration, it is assumed (solid line) that we start with 100 photons per mm^2. Approximately 30% of these may be absorbed within the screen. There follows an amplification process in which each X-ray photon generates some 600 light photons, half of which may reach the film, i.e. 9000 in total. Light photons are less efficient than X-rays in the production of a latent image and, assuming 1% efficiency, 90 latent images will be formed per mm^2. The noise in the final image is related to the point in the process at which the fewest number of photons is carrying the signal. This point may be referred to as the *quantum sink*. Any amplification of the signal after this stage will amplify the noise to the same extent. In this situation, the quantum sink is the number of X-ray photons absorbed in the screen.

We can now consider the influence of screen speed on noise. There are two principal ways in which speed of the system might be increased. The first is to increase the detection efficiency of the phosphor by making it thicker.

This is illustrated by the dotted line in the figure. It is important to note that the aim is to produce the same density in the film, i.e. the same number of latent images, for a reduced dose. There are therefore fewer incident photons, but because the phosphor material is the same the degree of amplification of the signal remains the same. The net effect is therefore to make no change in the noise despite the fact that the dose to the screen has been reduced.

The second method of increasing film–screen speed is to use a more efficient phosphor. This may have a higher absorption efficiency but, more importantly, it is likely to produce a greater signal amplification. This is illustrated by the dashed line in the figure. It can be seen that to produce the same number of latent images, the number of photons absorbed in the phosphor is reduced and thus the noise is increased.

Returning to film exposed without a screen, the number of incident photons needed to produce 90 latent images would be 4500, showing that the intensification factor of the screens is 45. However, despite the very much higher dose required, the noise is reduced by very much less than this would suggest. The number of X-ray photons absorbed is only 3 times greater than in the film–screen example.

It is a common feature of X-ray imaging that a compromise has to be struck between the sensitivity or speed of the system and image quality. Increased speed, and therefore lower patient dose, can be achieved by using a thicker phosphor, but at a cost of greater unsharpness. In film–screen radiography, it is common practice to use different speed class systems for different applications. A standard 400-speed class system, having a relatively thick phosphor, may be used for radiographs of the thicker sections of the body (e.g. abdomen or pelvis), and a thin phosphor system may be used for extremities. The latter screens, sometimes referred to as definition screens, may have a speed class in the region of 100–150 and thus require about 3 times the dose for the same optical density. However, their use is appropriate for those situations in which fine structures are to be imaged and for which the radiation dose to the patient is relatively low.

There are a number of other features in the design of screens that may affect both sensitivity and unsharpness. Two of these are mentioned here. To increase sensitivity, a *reflective layer* may be added to the screen

base at the outer surface of the phosphor. Light travelling away from the film is reflected back to the film (see photon D in Fig. 4.5a), thus increasing both the blackening of the film and unsharpness. To reduce unsharpness, *coloured dyes* may be incorporated in the phosphor layer to absorb some of the light as it passes through the phosphor. Light photons emitted at a wider angle are more likely to be attenuated, thus reducing unsharpness. However, this is at the cost of reducing the overall sensitivity of the system.

An additional cause of blurring is *crossover*. A small proportion of light from the front screen may pass through the emulsion and be detected on the rear emulsion of the film, and vice versa. Because of the divergence of the light from a point in the screen, the diameter of the disk of light will be increased. Crossover can account for as much as 25% of the blackening on the film and is a major contributor to the overall unsharpness in a film–screen system.

A smaller effect contributing to unsharpness in double-emulsion systems is *parallax*. The film essentially has two images, the one on the rear emulsion being slightly larger because of the divergence of the X-ray beam. In practice, this difference is insignificant when the film is viewed straight on, but it may make a small contribution to overall unsharpness should the film be viewed obliquely.

The sharpness of the image on the film depends critically on *film–screen contact*. If the screen and film are not in contact, the light has further to travel and the probability of the disk blackening from a single-photon interaction in the phosphor increases. Poor film–screen contact can occur because of damage to the cassette and can be seen as a region of blurring in the processed image.

Combination of unsharpness

In Chapter 3.6, it was shown that edges may be blurred by the focal spot size and geometry and by movement. These effects are described as geometrical and movement unsharpness, and their magnitudes can be expressed as U_g and U_m, respectively. In this section, screen unsharpness (U_s) has been discussed. The total unsharpness (U_t) can be derived from the three components:

$$U_t = \sqrt{(U_g^2 + U_m^2 + U_s^2)}$$

For example, should the unsharpness from each component be 0.2 mm, then the total unsharpness would be 0.35 mm and not 0.6 mm, the sum of the three components.

4.4.3 Noise

Noise was discussed in Chapter 3.1.3. In film–screen radiography, the number of photons contributing to the image is of the order of 100 000 photons per mm², so that signal to noise is high, approximately 300:1. The influence of the factors affecting film–screen speed on noise is considered in more detail in Box 4.3.

4.5 FILM–SCREEN RADIOGRAPHY IN PRACTICE

The amount of radiation reaching the film is controlled by the tube potential (kV), the tube current (milliamperage, mA) and the exposure time. In general, the X-ray control unit allows each of these parameters to be selected separately. However, more commonly the product of mA and exposure time, referred to as *mAs*, can be selected as a single parameter and the control unit will automatically adjust the mA to the maximum permitted for the kV selected, thus giving an exposure in the shortest possible time consistent with the generator power and the tube rating (Ch. 3.7.3).

Kilovoltage

The choice of kV has a significant influence on image quality and patient dose. Patient dose decreases with increasing kV, because the more penetrating beam at the higher kV requires less radiation to produce a satisfactorily exposed film (see Ch. 3.2.2). The advantages of high kV are:

- increased penetration, leading to reduced patient dose
- increased exposure latitude of exposure, resulting in a larger range of tissues displayed
- reduction in mAs, allowing shorter exposure times.

However, the disadvantage is reduced subject contrast, as discussed in Chapter 3.1.1.

Milliampere seconds

The choice of kV is the key parameter determining image quality and patient dose. The correct mAs must then be selected to ensure the correct blackening of the film. Selection of mAs cannot be determined from a simple equation. It depends principally on:

- the quality of the radiation beam, not only kV but also filtration and waveform
- the focus–film distance
- attenuation in the tabletop, grid, etc.
- the speed of the film–screen combination
- the region of the patient being examined
- patient thickness.

The first four of these are equipment-related, so that for any examination room standard exposure factors, i.e. kV and mAs, can be established for each examination to be performed in that room. The biggest variable is the last: patient size. Larger, fatter patients may require the use of very high values of mAs, resulting in unacceptable levels of tube loading or extended exposure times. In those circumstances, an increased kV might be used.

Reciprocity law

In radiography, it is generally assumed that the film density depends only on the total quantity of radiation (mAs) and not on the particular combination of mA and exposure time. This is known as the reciprocity law. This assumption is true for films exposed to X-rays, i.e. without screens. However, it is not strictly true when film is exposed to light, as in films used with screens. The blackening produced, by the same mAs, in very short or very long exposures is less than with a 1-s exposure. This effect, which is a consequence of the involved way in which latent images are formed, can usually be ignored in clinical practice, except perhaps with the longer exposures associated with mammography.

Automatic exposure control

Because of the limited latitude of film–screen systems, selection of the correct mAs for patients of widely ranging thickness requires considerable skill and experience. As an alternative, the exposure can be terminated automatically when the right amount of radiation has reached the film.

This is achieved using a thin radiation detector positioned in front of the cassette and behind the grid. The detector is generally a flat parallel plate ionization chamber (see Ch. 1.6.3). There are usually three separate chambers covering different areas of the film. One is positioned so that it is over the middle of the cassette but displaced towards the patient's feet, while the other two are to the right and left of midline and displaced towards the head. When a preset amount of radiation has been detected, the system will terminate the exposure. The system is referred to as automatic exposure control (AEC). It is important that the detector does not itself cause a significant amount of attenuation and that it does not itself produce an image on the film.

Depending on the examination type, the operator can select which detector or combination of detectors is used. For example, for a chest radiograph the two outer detectors covering the lung fields might be used, whereas for an anteroposterior view of the lumbar spine the central detector alone may be selected. In addition, there is a density control that increases or decreases the cut-off point at which the AEC system terminates the exposure, allowing the production of darker or lighter films.

The use of an AEC system is limited to those films taken in the Bucky. Its use is also compromised because the detectors have a fixed geometry that may not be ideal for all beam sizes. For example, for small cassettes ($18 \times 24\,\text{cm}^2$) the detectors would extend beyond the area of the film. AEC systems therefore may have limited use in situations such as paediatrics.

4.6 MAMMOGRAPHY

Mammography aims to demonstrate both microcalcifications, features with high inherent contrast that may be $100\,\mu\text{m}$ or less in size, and larger areas of tissue having much lower intrinsic contrast than would be imaged in general radiography. It is therefore being taken as a separate subject within this chapter.

4.6.1 Target and filter materials

The breast is composed of a mixture of glandular and adipose tissues that are similar in atomic number

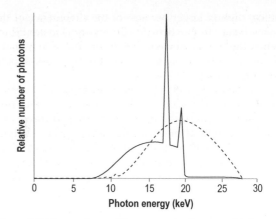

Figure 4.7 The spectrum of X-ray energies from a molybdenum target using a molybdenum filter, with the spectrum from a tungsten target with aluminium filter superimposed (dashed line).

(approximately 7.4 and 6.5, respectively). To differentiate between the two – that is, to maximize subject contrast – it is necessary to use a low tube potential. The breast, when compressed, is generally no more than 60–80 mm thick and on average between 40 and 50 mm. This allows for the use of low-energy X-rays that would ideally be monoenergetic in the range 16–22 keV. For this imaging situation, the use of a broad bremsstrahlung spectrum from a tungsten target is far from ideal, and it is now standard practice to make use of the characteristic radiation from a lower atomic number material. Two target materials used for mammography are molybdenum ($Z = 42$) and rhodium ($Z = 45$), the former being the most common.

Molybdenum has a K-edge at 20 keV and produces characteristic radiations at 17.4 and 19.6 keV. The spectrum emitted from the X-ray tube, which incorporates a beryllium exit window to minimize attenuation, is shown in Figure 4.7 for a tube potential of 28 kV. In order to achieve a more nearly monoenergetic beam, the emerging spectrum is filtered by the same material (molybdenum, about 0.03 mm thick). This provides the highest attenuation both for the low-energy photons and for higher energies above the K-edge with relatively low attenuation of the characteristic radiation, as shown in the figure. The use of alternative target–filter combinations is discussed in Box 4.4.

4.6.2 Film–screen systems for mammography

The detection of microcalcifications necessitates better spatial resolution than is achieved in standard radiography. The screens used in mammography are rare earth screens in which the principal interaction is

The most common target–filter combination is molybdenum with molybdenum (Mo–Mo). However, this is less suitable for thicker breast thicknesses. As an alternative, tubes may be designed with dual Mo and rhodium (Rh) targets. Rh produces characteristic radiation at 20.2 and 22.8 keV that can be filtered by Rh to produce an X-ray spectrum suitable for thicker breast thicknesses.

A more common approach is to have a single target material (Mo) with selectable filters (Mo and Rh). The Rh filter is automatically selected for the larger patients. The Rh filter has its K-edge at 23.2 keV. Use of a Mo–Rh target–filter combination increases the mean energy of the spectrum, because it will transmit bremsstrahlung photons in the energy range just below 23.2 keV, thus increasing the beam penetration.

For progressively increasing breast thickness, Mo–Mo, Mo–Rh and Rh–Rh may be used. The materials used are selected not simply on the basis of atomic number, and thus K-edge energy, but also on their physical characteristics (high melting point, manufacturing qualities). The combination Rh–Mo is not used, because the effect of the filter would be to attenuate the Rh characteristic radiation with energy that is just greater than the K-edge of Mo.

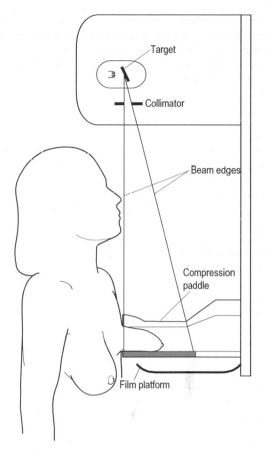

Figure 4.8 Key components in a mammography X-ray set.

the photoelectric effect with the L-shell electrons (the K-edge for rare earth materials is in the region of 50 keV). Because of the low X-ray energy, the screens are thinner than for routine radiography, thus reducing unsharpness (see section 4.4.2). More significantly, a single screen is used to eliminate parallax and cross-over. A single screen is used with a single-sided emulsion. The screen (and emulsion) is on the distal side of the film, furthest from the X-ray tube and patient. This arrangement is used because the highest proportion of the photon interactions, and thus light production, will be on the side of the screen closest to the film. This serves to minimize further the screen unsharpness. The film–screen systems used for mammography are able to produce a limiting resolution of 15 lp mm^{-1} or better.

Although not the subject of this chapter, it may be noted that computed radiography and direct digital radiography systems are available for mammography. Computed radiography plates and readers are available with pixel sizes down to 50 μm, giving a limiting resolution of about 10 lp mm^{-1}.

4.6.3 The mammography unit

A diagram of a mammography set is shown in Figure 4.8. The cathode–anode axis of the X-ray tube is perpendicular to the chest wall, with the cathode on the chest wall side of the patient. The reason for this orientation is that the anode heel effect reduces tube output on the anode side (i.e. on the nipple side of the breast). Although compression is used to even out the breast thickness over the whole field of view, this cannot be fully achieved, with the thickness invariably being greater on the chest wall side.

The target focus is located directly above the chest wall edge of the platform in order to minimize beam divergence into the patient. Dual focal spot sizes are used, with the large size being in the region of 0.4 mm and the small size, used for magnification views, being about 0.1–0.15 mm. Because of focal spot size, tube currents are generally limited to about 100 mA (40 mA for the small focal spot). Operating potentials are generally in the range of about 24–35 kV, although the lower half of the range is used for most patients.

For radiography, the breast is positioned on the support platform and held in place by the compression paddle. Compression reduces the breast thickness by spreading the tissues over a wider area, and it helps to equalize tissue thickness, which is essential for the production of a radiograph with a reasonably homogeneous density across the whole breast. In addition, dose is reduced because of reduced thickness, and by bringing the structures closer to the film, the geometrical unsharpness is reduced. It also serves to immobilize the patient. Exposure times for mammography are long (up to 2 s or more in some cases), and it is essential to minimize the risk of movement that would introduce an additional source of unsharpness.

Although the amount of scatter is small at these low energies, it is still important that the effects are minimized so that a moving grid is used. The AEC detectors are positioned behind the film cassette, because they would cause additional attenuation of the beam, thus increasing dose, but more importantly an image of the structure of the system would be superimposed on the mammogram.

4.6.4 Dose

Patient dose is a particularly significant issue in mammography, because the majority of mammograms are taken in the context of screening healthy women for breast cancer. Because the majority of women examined will gain no direct health benefit, it is especially important to adhere to the principle of restricting dose as far as reasonably practicable. The design of the equipment ensures that the only part of the woman exposed to a significant radiation dose is the breast. For this reason, the quantity effective dose is not used, and it is more useful to consider the average absorbed dose to the glandular tissue in terms of the mean glandular dose. Typically, it is in the range of 1.5–3 mGy per film. At a dose of 2 mGy, the fatal cancer risk is approximately 1 in 50 000 for women in the age range 50–65.

Quality assurance in mammography is particularly important. In part, this is due to the issues involved in screening healthy individuals, but it is also required because optimization of image quality for low-kV radiography is more dependent on, for example, small changes in kV and processor conditions.

4.6.5 Magnification films

Magnification radiography is sometimes referred to as macroradiography. It is only in mammography that magnification views are still routinely performed. For magnification views, a raised platform to support the breast is placed above the film holder approximately halfway between the focus and cassette. The image is therefore magnified by a factor of two. However, the net effect of this is to greatly increase unsharpness (see Ch. 3.6) so that, in order to be able to view the same small detail in the magnified view, the smaller focal spot must be used. This has the effect of increasing exposure time because of the lower mA (see Ch. 3.8.3). However, this can be offset by removing the grid, because scatter is reduced by the introduction of an air gap. Inevitably the patient dose will be increased, so this procedure is justified only for symptomatic patients.

4.7 LINEAR TOMOGRAPHY

So far, we have considered conventional projection radiography, in which the shadows of structures further from the film are superimposed on those closer to the film. This leads to an inability to determine the depth of an object in the body, a limited ability to resolve the shape of an object, and an overall reduction in contrast between objects of similar composition. The first of these can be overcome through orthogonal projections (e.g. anterior–posterior and lateral views). In certain specific situations, conventional or mechanical tomography may assist in overcoming the other limitations.

In tomography, only structures in a selected slice of the patient, parallel to the film, are imaged sharply. Those above and below are deliberately blurred so as to be unrecognizable. This blurring is produced by simultaneous movement, during the exposure, of two of the three following: tube, film and patient.

In *linear tomography*, depicted in Figure 4.9, the tube and film/cassette carrier are linked by an extensible rod that is hinged about a fulcrum or pivot, which in turn is attached via a vertical arm to the tabletop. During the exposure, the cassette tray moves horizontally, for example from right to left, along rails under the couch top, while the tube is driven in the other direction, from left to right. While moving, the tube head is rotated such that the central ray of the X-ray beam is always directed towards the pivot point.

Figure 4.9 depicts the start and finish positions of the tube and its focal spot (T_1 and T_2) and the corresponding positions of the film. It shows that the shadow of a structure, P, at the level of the pivot moves from P_1 to P_2 at the same speed as the cassette so that it remains at the same position on the film, producing a sharp image. The shadow of a second structure, X, at the same height above the film (described as being in the focal plane) moves from X_1 to X_2, retaining the same

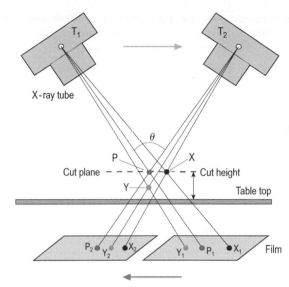

Figure 4.9 The principles of image formation in linear tomography.

off-focus anatomy are spread over the film, contrast is low and a reasonably low kV must be used, consistent with penetrating the patient. The technique has been most useful when imaging structures of high inherent contrast (e.g. bony structures in the inner ear and iodine-filled vessels in urography). Because for much of the exposure the beam is passing obliquely through the patient, attenuation is higher and patient dose is greater than in conventional radiography.

Linear tomography is less effective at blurring out linear structures lying in the plane of movement of the tube and film. It is possible to devise alternative movements (e.g. circular or elliptical) to blur out such structures. However, equipment of this type is generally no longer available because of the preponderance of computed tomography.

The equipment described here for linear tomography relies on mechanical linkage between tube and film. More recently, equipment with electronically controlled linear movements of tube and film and of tube angulation has been introduced.

position relative to the shadow of P and therefore also produces a sharp image. However, the shadow of a structure Y below the pivot moves from Y_1 to Y_2. This is a shorter distance than the distance moved by the film, and therefore the shadow of Y sweeps across the film and is blurred out. Structures above the pivot are similarly blurred.

The further the structure is from the pivot plane, the greater the movement blurring. Structures lying within a slice of thickness t are sufficiently sharp to be recognizable, whereas those lying outside that slice are too blurred and of too low contrast (see below).

The level of cut or *cut height* is adjusted by raising or lowering the pivot. The *thickness of cut* is controlled by adjusting the tomographic angle, angle θ. As the angle is reduced, the degree of blurring (represented by the distance between Y_1 and Y_2 in Fig. 4.9 relative to the distance between P_1 and P_2) is decreased, thus increasing the thickness of the structures appearing to be in focus. At the limit, when θ is reduced to zero, a conventional radiograph would result in which all structures appear sharp. The thickness of cut also becomes smaller as the fulcrum (level of cut) is raised, as this increases the movement of the cassette and the tomographic effect. Decreasing the focus–film distance has a similar effect.

Typically, in tomography θ is 40°, resulting in a cut thickness of about 3 mm. Because such a thin slice of each structure is being imaged, and the shadows of

4.8 SUMMARY

- Intensifying screens convert the X-ray image into a light image.

- The light image is captured on film.

- The most commonly used screens have rare earth phosphors with a K-edge near the peak in the diagnostic X-ray spectrum.

- Film–screen systems for general radiography commonly are 400-speed class, speed class being defined as 1000 divided by the dose (in μGy) required to produce a net optical density of 1.

- Optical density is defined as the log to the base 10 of the incident light intensity divided by the transmitted intensity.

- The characteristic curve of the film is a plot of optical density against the log of dose to the film.

- Film gamma (γ) is defined as the slope of the characteristic curve between net optical densities 0.25 and 2.

- Contrast is directly related to γ.

- Film latitude is the range of film exposures that produce optical densities in the useful range of the film.

- Both γ and speed are affected by processor performance.

- Increasing thickness of the phosphor in the screen increases sensitivity at the cost of increased screen unsharpness.

- Mammography uses special equipment that generally has a tube with a molybdenum target with a molybdenum filter.

- A rhodium filter may also be used with a molybdenum target for mammography.

- Films used for mammography have a single-sided emulsion and are used with a single intensifying screen.

- Compression helps to produce a more uniform image of the breast, reduces breast dose and helps to minimize movement unsharpness.

- Linear tomography utilizes a technique in which the X-ray tube is rotated about a pivot point at the height of the cut plane at the same time as the film is moved behind the patient.

Chapter 5

Digital radiography

CHAPTER CONTENTS

The previous chapter was concerned with the recording of an analogue radiographic image on film. This method of radiography is being rapidly superseded by digital radiographic systems. There are many advantages to producing images in a digital format, i.e. in a format that can be stored and processed in a computer and displayed on a monitor. Indeed, certain medical imaging modalities, in particular computed tomography (CT) and magnetic resonance imaging (MRI), could not have been realized without the computer. One of the key drivers in switching to digital radiographic technologies is the introduction of picture archiving and communication systems (PACSs).

In this chapter, it is the intention to introduce digital radiography (DR) by considering general principles and terminology that is common to other imaging modalities.

5.1 DIGITAL IMAGING

5.1.1 Image structure and size

In digital imaging, the image is divided into a matrix of individual cells or *pixels*. Each pixel has an assigned value that is related to the intensity of signal in the corresponding part of the image. In film–screen radiography, the image is presented as a negative, with white representing low dose and black high. This convention is retained in DR, with pixels having high values being displayed dark and those with low values light, although the reverse, or positive images, might equally well be displayed. The matrix size (i.e. number of pixels), pixel size and field of view are clearly interrelated. For example, a 512×512 matrix is commonly used in CT scanning to cover a field of view that may be 350 mm. The pixel size in that situation is 350/512, i.e. approximately 0.7 mm. Clearly, pixel size is related to spatial resolution, because objects smaller than the dimensions of a pixel will not be seen unless there is a very high degree of subject contrast, in which case the partial volume effect may make it visible (see Ch. 7.1.1).

The value stored in each pixel is stored in binary format, and the maximum value that is stored is related to the bit depth of the pixel (see Box 5.1). The greater the bit depth, the greater is the potential to display contrast. A single bit would store images only as either black or white, whereas a 12-bit pixel has 4096 (2^{12}) levels of grey. Computer memory size is expressed in terms of the number of bytes of information. A byte can carry up to 8 bits, i.e. a number up to a value of $2^8 - 1 = 255$ (1 less than 2^8, because zero is included as a possible value). For a pixel with a bit depth that is greater than 8, the number of bytes used per pixel is increased proportionately. Thus a typical single-slice CT image consisting of 512×512 pixels with 4096 levels of grey and a bit depth of 12 requires $512 \times 512 \times 12/8 = 0.375$ Mbytes (MB) of memory.

Image storage size is important because of potential limitations in computer memory and archive capacity, in processing time, and in transmission times (e.g. the time to transfer an image from archive to the reporting workstation in a PACS). The maximum matrix size is largely determined by the imaging modality. For example, in CT scanning, although matrix size per se defines the limit to spatial resolution, there are also limitations imposed by detector size and sampling frequency (see Ch. 7.5.1) that mean that matrix sizes greater than 512×512 would not significantly improve spatial resolution. Radiography has an intrinsic spatial resolution that is high, and film–screen radiography has the potential to take full advantage, with resolution up to 10 lp mm^{-1}. DR systems therefore need large matrix sizes (see section 5.3.3).

The required bit depth for image storage is influenced by noise and by the dynamic range of the imaging device. With an image associated with high levels of noise, such as radionuclide images, bit depth may need to be no greater than 8. In DR, detectors have a very wide dynamic range, so that for data acquisition bit depths of 16 may be used. However, the full range of data may not be needed in the final image, and 12- or 14-bit depth may be sufficient for storage.

Compression

To reduce storage requirements and to increase transmission times, the image can be stored in a compressed format. There are a number of ways in which this may be achieved. For example, if consecutive pixel values in the matrix array are identical, it is possible to store the value and the number of successive pixels sharing that value.

Compression techniques can be divided into those that are *lossless* or *reversible* and those that are *lossy* or *irreversible*. In the former case, the image can be restored into an identical version of the original, whereas lossy compression will result in a displayed image that does not perfectly reproduce the original. The extent to which lossless compression can reduce image storage size depends on the image modality, but lossless reduction in file sizes by factors of 2 to 3 are generally possible. Lossy compression allows reduction of image storage size by much greater factors, up to about 40, without immediately apparent loss in image detail when redisplayed. However, this may not be acceptable if the image is to be used for primary diagnosis.

5.1.2 Image processing

Many imaging processing techniques are available to assist in the visualization of detail in the displayed image. Particular techniques are considered in the sections on the different imaging modalities, but certain generally applicable methods may be considered here.

Noise limits the ability to see low-contrast detail. In a real-time acquisition system, such as fluoroscopy,

---

Box 5.1 Binary system of numbers

Our numerical system is decimal; that is, a system in which there are 10 base numbers (including zero). We count in powers of 10, i.e. 10^1 is written as 10, 10^2 as 100, 10^3 as 1000, etc. In the binary system, there are only two base numbers. In the smallest memory location, the computer holds a voltage signal that may either be zero or a single discrete value representing 1. This is a single memory bit. If there were 4 bits of memory, then, with the zero value included, there would be just 16 possible values, represented as 0, 1, 10, 11, 100, 101, etc. to 1111). The maximum value, represented by 1111, is $15 = 2^4 - 1$. Likewise, 8 bits corresponds to a maximum of 256 (2^8) discrete values. Unlike the decimal system, the binary system has no equivalent of the decimal point. In our standard notation, we are able to use negative powers, for example $10^{-1} = 0.1$. There is no equivalent in binary, i.e. there cannot be any value between, for example, binary 100 and binary 101.

Computer memory is expressed in terms of the number of bytes (B), with each byte consisting of 8 bits.

noise can be reduced by adding the signal from successive frames to give a time-averaged image. This is equivalent to increasing exposure time in radiography. Frame averaging is a useful technique provided that there is no movement between frames, otherwise the image will be blurred.

Noise may also be reduced by low-pass spatial filtering. This is a technique in which the greyscale value stored in each pixel has added into it a proportion of the value of the neighbouring pixels and the resultant value averaged. The effect is to smooth the final image, but it will blur small details or edges.

Edge enhancement or high-pass filtering has the opposite effect. Rather than display a weighted average value of neighbouring pixels, a high-pass filter adds in a proportion of the difference between the greyscale value of the pixel and that of its neighbours. The effect is to exaggerate the contrast at the boundary between structures, thus making the structures more visible. However, the process also serves to increase noise. It may generate false structures in the image when a high level of filtering is applied.

5.1.3 Image display

A key component of the digital imaging system is the display. Two types of display are available: the cathode ray tube and flat panel monitors. The cathode ray tube monitor utilizes a scanning electron beam whose intensity is modulated in accordance with the stored pixel values. Typically, there are up to 1250 scan lines, limiting the resolution in the perpendicular direction, with the resolution parallel to the scan lines being limited by the frequency of the modulating signal. There are several types of flat panel monitor, the most common in use in medical imaging being the liquid crystal display. The screen is composed of individual pixels with matrix sizes up to about 2000 by 2500 in rectangular arrays.

An important feature of the image display is its calibration. The image produced by the imaging system is a matrix of pixel values that may have 12-bit or greater depth, as described above. To maximize the visibility of detail in the image, these values are matched to a display curve that is optimized to the imaging task (see section 5.3.2). It is then essential that this optimized pattern of values is consistently displayed on any display monitor (and, it should be emphasized, printed to film if that is done). There is a standard for display calibration in the Digital Imaging and Communications in Medicine standard (DICOM; see section 5.5). The standard takes account of the perceptivity of the human eye. Image displays that are used for primary diagnosis should be subject to a quality assurance programme to ensure that any changes in calibration with time are detected and rectified.

5.2 IMAGING TERMINOLOGY

5.2.1 Fourier analysis, sampling and aliasing

An image is composed of a pattern of signal levels on a two-dimensional map, for example the pattern of X-ray intensities that are transmitted through the patient in radiography. In recording and displaying the image, the ability of the imaging system to transfer that information accurately is an important feature in determining the performance of the system. Some basic descriptive terms for image quality were given in Chapter 3.1, i.e. contrast, spatial resolution and noise. In this section, some additional imaging terminology is introduced that is more closely associated with digital systems.

A mathematical approach to understanding the performance of the imaging system is *Fourier analysis*, in which the image signal may be broken down into a series of sine waves that vary in terms of spatial frequency and amplitude. To give a brief insight into Fourier analysis, a simple example is given in Box 5.2. This form of analysis demonstrates that to image small, sharp structures the system has to be able to handle high spatial frequencies without loss of signal or contrast. How well it does so is measured by its modulation transfer function (MTF), described below in section 5.2.2.

Sampling is a feature of imaging. A TV image is sampled by the raster of scan lines. A digital image is presented as a matrix of samples, i.e. pixels. A video signal is sampled before digitization. If there are too few TV scan lines or if there are too few pixels in the matrix, fine detail will obviously be lost. It is perhaps not so obvious why fine image detail is also lost if too few samples are taken of a video signal.

A complex analogue video signal is composed of Fourier sine wave components of many frequencies. When it is sampled for digitization, some information is inevitably lost. At too low a sampling frequency, the high-frequency components carrying information about small structures with sharp edges will be lost. The *Nyquist* criterion states that the signal must be sampled *at least twice in every cycle or period*, i.e. the sampling frequency must be at least twice the highest frequency present in the signal. Otherwise, high-frequency signals will erroneously be recorded as low, referred to as *aliasing*. The maximum signal frequency that can be accurately sampled is called the Nyquist frequency and is equal to half of the sampling frequency.

Box 5.2 One-dimensional Fourier analysis

The square wave (A) in Figure 5.1 represents the pattern of X-rays that would be produced in an ideal imaging system by scanning across the resolution grid in Figure 3.2. The peak value represents black on the radiograph, i.e. the gap between the lead bars, and the trough is white, i.e. behind the lead bars. In an ideal system, there is no blurring of the edges and the transition from black to white is represented by a vertical line. Spatial frequency is defined as the number of peaks in a given distance, commonly expressed as line pairs (lp) per mm, as discussed in Chapter 3.1.2.

A sine wave (B) with the same spatial frequency is drawn on to the graph. The amplitude, or peak to peak height, has been adjusted so that the area below the sine wave is equal to that below the square wave. The sine wave is a poor representation of the original. A closer fit may be achieved by adding a second sine wave with 3 times the spatial frequency and one-third the amplitude (profile C). Successive additions of sine wave with 5, 7 and 9 times the frequency and one-fifth, one-seventh and one-ninth of the amplitude and so on will provide an increasingly close fit to the square wave. Profile D in the figure goes up to the sine wave with 15 times the spatial frequency and one-fifteenth of the amplitude. Note that only odd numbers are used in this mathematical technique. Continuing up to an infinite series would produce a perfect reproduction of the original.

The signal produced by scanning across a single narrow strip of lead can similarly be analysed into a spectrum of sine waves, but now the spectrum contains a wider range of frequencies and the higher frequencies have more amplitude. The narrower the strip, the wider the band of sine wave frequencies involved and the more important the high frequencies.

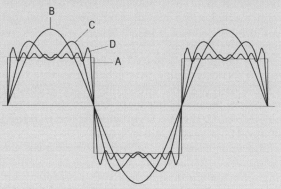

Figure 5.1 One-dimensional Fourier analysis of A, a square waveform that can be represented by: B, a single sine wave; C, the sum of two sine waves; and D, a function with eight sine wave components.

This is what is meant by saying that a fine structure with a sharp edge is composed of or corresponds to high spatial frequencies, whereas a large diffuse structure is composed of or corresponds only to low frequencies. In order to reproduce small, sharp structures in the image, the system has to be able to handle high spatial frequencies without loss of signal or contrast. How well it does so is measured by its modulation transfer function, described in section 5.2.2.

The technique of converting from the spatial to frequency domain is possible in two dimensions as well as in one dimension as illustrated here. The process is known as the Fourier transform and is a powerful mathematical tool used in the reconstruction of images, particularly in computed tomography, magnetic resonance imaging and ultrasound.

Figure 5.2a shows a sine wave (solid curve) that is sampled four times in three cycles. The samples, shown by the squares, are interpreted by the imaging system as a wave (dashed curve) of much lower frequency. Sampling six times in the same period, as in Figure 5.2b, preserves the correct frequency.

Aliasing artefacts caused by such under-sampling can take various forms.

- In CT, the body section is sampled by a fan beam containing a limited number of X-ray pencil beams, coming from a limited number of directions. If

these are too few, the system does not have the information to reproduce sharp high-contrast boundaries, instead producing the 'low frequency' streak artefacts.

- In MRI (see Ch. 10.8), failure to sample the whole of the field of view causes wrap-round, translocation of anatomy from one side of the image to the other.

- In pulsed Doppler imaging (see Ch. 9.13.2), the flow of blood corpuscles is sampled by a series of ultrasound pulses. If these pulses are not repeated

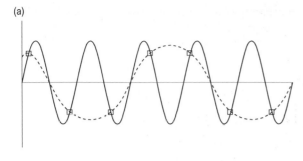

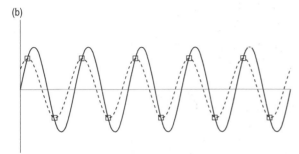

Figure 5.2 (a) Aliasing produced by under-sampling and (b) sampling that satisfies the Nyquist criterion.

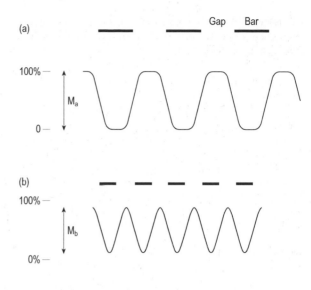

Figure 5.3 The output signal behind a grid pattern, showing reduction in modulation caused by blurring as spatial frequency increases.

sufficiently rapidly, fast flow in one direction will be interpreted as a slower flow in the opposite direction.

5.2.2 Modulation transfer function

The ability to visualize detail in an image was described in Chapter 3.1 in terms of the limiting spatial resolution that could be seen of the system for a high-contrast test pattern. Limits to resolution are intrinsic to the imaging modality and equipment. In particular, sharp edges are not perfectly represented but suffer a certain degree of blurring, for example caused by focal spot size or light spread in the phosphor of a film–screen system. This is illustrated in Figure 5.3, in which the profile of the grid pattern produced by a test object such as that described in Chapter 3.1 is shown. Figure 5.3a represents a low spatial frequency (i.e. widely spaced detail) in which blurring is not sufficient to prevent the modulation of the output signal profile from matching the modulation present in the object, modulation being defined here as the difference between the maximum and minimum amplitude as a proportion of the average signal. As the spatial frequency is progressively increased in Figure 5.3b and c, the blurring reduces the output modulation such that with the addition of noise it would become impossible to visualize detail at the higher spatial frequencies.

The ratio of the output and input modulation is known as the modulation transfer function. MTF varies with spatial frequency, generally reducing progressively from 100% at low spatial frequencies towards zero at higher frequencies. MTF as a function of spatial frequency is shown in Figure 5.4 for various imaging systems.

There are mathematical techniques for assessing MTF using Fourier analysis of the image of a sharp edge. Data produced in this way provide an objective method for comparing the imaging performance of different systems. It is a common way to compare two systems by quoting a single figure such as the spatial frequency at which the MTF is 10%.

5.3 COMPUTED RADIOGRAPHY

5.3.1 Imaging plates and readers

Computed radiography (CR) is the most common method of producing digital radiographic images and

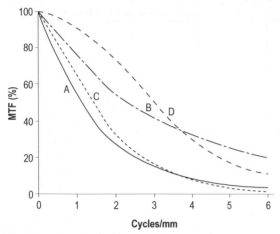

Figure 5.4 Modulation transfer function (MTF) as a function of spatial frequency for various radiographic systems: A, 400-speed film–screen system; B, detail film–screen system used for extremity imaging; C, computed radiography; and D, direct digital radiography.

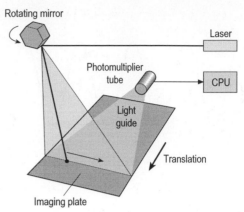

Figure 5.5 Formation of the computed radiography image using a scanned laser beam. CPU, central processing unit.

the first technology that was commercially available. CR uses a storage phosphor that requires light input to release the trapped energy in the form of light that is proportional to the X-ray intensity. It is referred to as a *photostimulable phosphor*. The material is commonly barium fluorohalide doped with europium (BaFX:Eu), in which the halide (X) is a combination of bromide and iodide, typically 85% and 15%, respectively. The phosphor in a powdered form is mixed with a binder or adhesive material and laid down on a base with a thickness of about 0.3 mm. A surface coat protects the phosphor from physical damage. The imaging plate thus formed is similar in appearance to the intensifying screen used in conventional radiography. The plate is inserted into a light-tight cassette, also similar in appearance and with the same dimensions as that used for film–screen radiography. For this reason, X-ray equipment used for conventional radiography can be used for CR, making the transition from analogue to digital radiography straightforward.

The signal from the imaging plate is read in a CR reader. In the reader, the plate is removed from the cassette and scanned by a laser beam (see Fig. 5.5). Scanning is achieved using a rotating mirror. Above the plate, there is an array of optical fibres to direct the emitted light to one or more photomultiplier tubes to measure its intensity. The position of the light-emitting centre is determined from the time at which the light is received. While there is repeated scanning across the plate, it is progressively moved through the scanning beam so that the complete pattern of light intensities

can be extracted. Most phosphors used for CR emit light at the blue end of the spectrum and need a scanning laser emitting red light for simulation.

Following the read cycle, the residual signal from the plate is erased by exposing it to a bright light source. The time for a CR reader to extract the image from the plate is generally between about 30 and 45 s, and the faster readers are capable of reading 100 or more plates per hour. To achieve the fastest throughput, stacking readers are available in which several cassettes (at least four) may be placed in a queue for automatic feed into the reader. Stacking readers are particularly useful for readers serving more than one X-ray room.

5.3.2 Computed radiography image processing

Photostimulable phosphors have a very wide dynamic range, being able to record photon intensities varying by a factor of about 10000:1. This is illustrated in Figure 5.6, in which the log of the light intensity from the screen is plotted against the log of the X-ray dose. This is a linear relationship. Superimposed on the plot is the characteristic curve of a film–screen system. It can be seen how the latitude of the CR system, i.e. range of doses that can be imaged, is very much greater than for conventional radiography. If the light signal were directly converted to greyscale on an image monitor such that, for example, black was assigned to a signal level of 10000 in the figure and white was set at level 1, as shown by the bar above the graph, the image seen would be very flat and display minimal contrast. This is in contrast to the film, for which the greyscale is compressed into a narrower range. Effectively, the raw CR image would be equivalent to a film–screen image with a film γ (Ch. 4.2) of about 0.4 compared with 2 to 3.

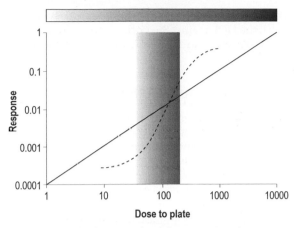

Figure 5.6 Relation between signal from a computed radiography plate and dose to the plate. For comparison, the characteristic curve of a film–screen system is shown (dashed line).

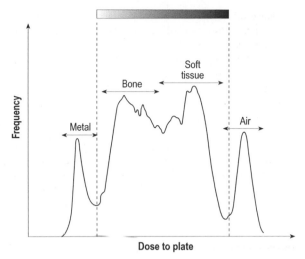

Figure 5.7 Distribution of signals from the computed radiography plate as a function of dose.

To display a useful image, it is necessary to process the data from the reader. The first part of the process is to detect the collimated edges of the X-ray beam. The signal outside the collimated area is then ignored. The second stage (histogram analysis) involves an analysis of the distribution of the light intensities within the collimated area. Very high and low signals are rejected. These may correspond to areas outside the body (high pixel values) or low pixel values in the region of, for example, a metal implant (Fig. 5.7). The third stage is to map the intensity values identified as being useful to a gradation curve that is similar in shape to the characteristic curve of a film–screen system. However, unlike film–screen radiography, in which one curve has to be used for all radiographic projections, the shape of the curve can be optimized for the particular projection.

Post-processing may also include edge enhancement and noise reduction (see section 5.1.2). Because the parameters used in the histogram analysis and the choice of gradation curve are dependent on the projection, it is important that these are selected correctly before the image is printed or archived to the PACS.

5.3.3 Computed radiography image quality

Spatial resolution with CR images is less than with conventional film–screen radiography. One factor limiting spatial resolution is pixel size. Pixel size generally varies with plate size. For the smaller plates (18 × 24 cm²) pixel sizes are generally approximately 90 μm, implying a matrix size of 2000 × 2670 pixels (5.3 Mpixels) and limiting resolution of 5.5 lp mm⁻¹,

whereas for the largest plates (35 × 43 cm²) they are generally about 140 μm, giving a 2500 × 3070 matrix (7.7 Mpixels) with limiting resolution of about 3.5 lp mm⁻¹. The increased size for the larger plates is not a physical limitation. It is introduced by the manufacturer, because fine detail is not generally required for the projections for which these plates are used, such as chest and abdominal radiography. The larger pixel size helps to reduce scanning time and image file size. The values of limiting resolution may be compared with those for film–screen radiography, which are typically 8 lp mm⁻¹ but may be increased to 12 lp mm⁻¹ with detail screens.

There are intrinsic limits to resolution in CR other than those imposed by the choice of matrix size. The most important of these is scattering of the laser light in the phosphor layer that spreads the area over which the detected light signal is emitted. This effect increases with the thickness of the phosphor. CR phosphors are being developed that have a crystalline structure that acts as a light guide in the same way as is used in the image intensifier input screen (see Ch. 6.1). However, such screens are more fragile and may be suitable only for use in fixed plates built into the X-ray equipment. Additional influences on spatial resolution are the size of the phosphor grains and the diameter of the scanning laser beam. High-resolution screens are available for mammography. These have a thinner phosphor layer and permit a reduced pixel size of 50 μm.

The ability to detect finer detail in the CR image may be enhanced by the partial volume effect (Ch. 7.1.1) and by the use of edge enhancement algorithms.

Contrast in the CR image is determined by the processing techniques outlined in the previous section. Through the selection of gradation curves that have been optimized for the radiographic projection, the CR image should display more contrast than can be seen in film–screen radiography.

5.3.4 Detector dose indicators

The restricted latitude of the film–screen system results in a clear indication of film dose. A dark film indicates excessive exposure and a light film underexposure. The film serves as its own quality control device. For CR and other DR systems, the detector has a very wide latitude, and processing of the data from the imaging plate ensures that the image provided to the viewer is optimized in terms of its greyscale presentation. There is therefore no obvious indication as to whether the imaging plate has received the 'correct' dose; superficially, the image would look the same whether the plate had received 5 times too much or 5 times too little dose, although in the latter case quantum mottle would be apparent and could lead to unacceptable levels of low-contrast resolution.

To provide assurance that the dose to the patient is being kept as low as reasonably practicable, CR manufacturers have introduced detector dose indicators (DDIs). DDIs are analogous to optical density of film. In film–screen radiography, it would be possible to measure optical density to determine whether it was over- or underexposed, but it would be the average value determined over a broad area of the image in the region of clinical interest. In the case of film, the human eye is sufficiently accurate to assess whether the film has an acceptable range of optical densities. In CR, DDI is determined from the signal from the plate averaged over a broad region of the plate but restricted to signal values that lie within the region of the histogram used for mapping the signal to the gradation curve (Fig. 5.7).

Unfortunately, the definition of DDI is manufacturer-dependent. Some systems use a definition in which the DDI is inversely proportional to dose, thus high DDI values indicate underexposure and vice versa. Other manufacturers have DDIs that are functions of the log of the dose. The latter case may be more intuitive, but it is important to recognize that, although high values indicate overexposure, a doubling of the dose does not double the DDI; the increase may be no more than 15%.

Manufacturers provide normal ranges for DDIs that may be examination-dependent. However, it is important that radiology departments validate these in terms of their diagnostic reference levels (see

Ch. 2.6.3). The person making a CR exposure should check the DDI against the normal range to ensure that the doses given to the patient are being adequately controlled.

5.4 DIGITAL RADIOGRAPHY

Computed radiography, like film–screen radiography, has the disadvantage that the production of the final image involves removing the cassette from the X-ray set, taking the plate to a reader, and waiting for a period of about 1 min while the film is processed or the CR plate is scanned. Although the delay time is not great and the distance between X-ray equipment and CR reader may be short, this may be inconvenient and may limit patient throughput. DR systems use imaging devices that remain in situ and produce an image with a delay that is generally no more than about 10 s.

The distinction between computed and digital radiography is somewhat artificial, because both are digital technologies employing computers for their implementation. There are CR systems (i.e. systems that use photostimulable phosphors) that incorporate the plate reader into the X-ray equipment so that for the operator there is little difference between the two. DR itself is divided into two main classes: indirect DR and direct DR (often referred to as DDR).

The most common DR detectors are based on amorphous silicon thin-film transistor (TFT) arrays, the dimensions of the array being the size of the area to be imaged. A transistor is a device that amplifies an electrical signal, and in the TFT array the amplified signal is stored as an electrical charge. The charge can be released by applying a high potential. In the TFT array, which is essentially a large integrated circuit, each row of detectors is connected to the activating potential and each column to a charge-measuring device. The potential is applied row by row, so that the timing of the detected signal determines the position of the pixel from which it originated.

In a TFT array, there are as many transistors as there are pixels, and the size of each transistor, or pixel, is in the range 100–200 μm. The electronics and detectors are deposited in several layers on a glass substrate (Fig. 5.8).

Deposited above the charge collection device on the plate is an X-ray or light detector. Two types of detector are considered here.

Indirect conversion

One of the most common classes of flat plate detectors is that which uses indirect conversion of the X-ray pattern into an electronic signal. A phosphor is

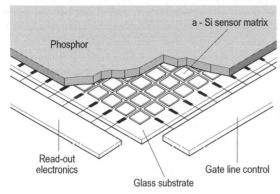

Figure 5.8 The structure of a flat plate detector used for indirect digital radiography. a–Si, amorphous silicon.

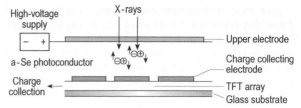

Figure 5.9 Cross-section of an amorphous selenium (a–Se) detector for direct digital radiography. TFT, thin-film transistor.

used to convert the X-ray photons to light. The light is then detected by photodiodes incorporated into the amorphous silicon TFT array. A common phosphor is caesium iodide laid down as a crystalline structure above the photodiode array. The elongated crystals (with diameters very much smaller than the pixel size) are grown so that they are perpendicular to the surface of the detector. Light produced by an interaction in the crystal is internally reflected so that it is directed towards the photodiode element that is directly below the point of interaction. Because of this method of reducing the spread of light, a relatively thick layer of scintillator may be used, thus increasing the detection efficiency. This is the same principle that is used for caesium iodide input screens on image intensifiers (see Ch. 6.1).

An alternative is gadolinium oxysulphide, a phosphor commonly used for film–screen radiography. It gives greater light spread so that a thinner layer is used, thus reducing detection efficiency. However, it is cheaper to produce and more robust, and is therefore more suitable for, for example, ward radiography using mobile X-ray equipment.

The flat plate detector described here may be produced as a single detector to cover the full field of view (up to $45 \times 45\,\text{cm}^2$). However, in practice there are manufacturing problems with this size of detector, and the full field detector may comprise four separate detectors. These are described as tiled detectors. Abutting detectors require some image processing and interpolation to ensure that the join between them is not visible in the displayed image.

Direct conversion: amorphous selenium detector

Amorphous selenium is a photoconductor, which is a material that will pass an electrical charge on

irradiation. It is deposited on the amorphous silicon TFT array as a single layer of material (Fig. 5.9). The upper surface is bonded to an electrode connected to a high positive potential. An X-ray photon interacting in the photoconductor material causes ionization, i.e. produces positive and negative charges. The positive charges are drawn to the charge collectors in the TFT array, with minimal lateral diffusion.

The efficiency of an X-ray detector system can be described by its *detective quantum efficiency* (DQE). This is a parameter that reflects the efficiency of photon detection and the noise added to the detected signal. If every X-ray photon is recorded in the image with no additional noise, then DQE would be 100%. In practice, DQEs are lower because of less than 100% absorption of X-rays in the device and internal sources of noise. DQE for DR systems may be as high as 65%, whereas for CR and film–screen systems it is closer to 30%. Thus DR systems can be used at lower doses without any increase in quantum noise.

The disadvantages of DR in comparison with CR (or film–screen radiography) are cost and versatility. A radiographic room generally has two Bucky positions: in the table and in the chest stand. For DR, two separate (very expensive) detectors would be required, whereas a single CR reader will serve not only both Buckys but also additional X-ray rooms. In addition, for angled projections of extremities, for example, and for ward radiography, a DR plate does not have the same flexibility in positioning as a CR plate. However, there are new approaches to X-ray equipment design that provide greater versatility in positioning the DR imaging plate than in the conventional X-ray room with a table and an erect Bucky.

CCD detector

An alternative detector that can be used for DR is based on CCD detectors. These are light-sensitive detectors of the type that are used in video and digital cameras. The problem with CCD detectors is that they cannot be manufactured in a size that is very much greater than $5\,\text{cm}^2$. They are used in conjunction with a phosphor to detect the X-rays, and the light emitted from the phosphor is focused on to the CCD. This leads to a deeper detector than the flat plate, TFT systems described above. To cover the full field required in radiography, systems are built with tiled array of CCDs. CCD-based digital detectors have been used in mammography for stereotactic films used for biopsy localization. For this application small fields are sufficient, so that detectors with a single CCD are sufficient.

5.5 PICTURE ARCHIVING AND COMMUNICATION SYSTEMS

The benefits of PACS are self-evident, but some may be summarized briefly here.

- The facility to have images available almost instantaneously in any location, not only within the hospital but elsewhere (such as peripheral clinics).
- The facility for images to be viewed simultaneously in different locations.
- Security of image storage.
- Elimination of film stores.
- Integration of imaging with other electronic patient records.
- The facility to build teaching files of images.

The disadvantages are few, but it should be borne in mind that filmless radiology is not necessarily cheaper. Although the costs associated with film and film storage are eliminated, there are additional costs associated with the management of a sophisticated computer network and the costs of upgrades to both software and hardware. These will almost inevitably be greater than the costs saved.

In a PACS configuration, the various imaging devices and associated workstations are linked to the *PACS workflow manager*, the computer and associated software at the heart of PACSs that control the flow of images and information.

A key feature in the design of the PACS is that the image data sent from the modalities and stored in the archive are in a format that can be recognized and used within the complete system. The image file contains the basic digital data that allow it to be displayed, but it also contains essential information including the imaging modality, annotations, display preferences, the patient's name and other identifying data. The presentation of these data must be in a standard format, and the standard used is DICOM. The standard is complex. There are a number of services that can be provided, and these are considered briefly in Box 5.3.

The PACS workflow manager can send or retrieve images from the archive. The archive may be split into

---

Box 5.3   Digital Imaging and Communications in Medicine services

There are two classes of DICOM service: service class user and service class provider. The service class user role is to invoke an operation, and the service class provider role is to perform the operation. For example, the computed tomography scanner is a user of the storage function of the picture archiving and communication system (PACS), whereas the PACS archive is the provider of storage.

When purchasing an item of radiology equipment, the purchaser needs to identify the specific Digital Imaging and Communications in Medicine (DICOM) compliances that are required. The software for these services may be provided with the imaging device. However, the purchaser has to buy the software licences to enable the services to be used. Examples of some common DICOM definitions are given here of service class user functions that might be required on imaging modalities.

- *Modality worklist* permits retrieval of scheduling information for that modality and patient

demographics from the radiology information system. This saves the operator from having to input these data for every imaging request and eliminates the risk of input errors.

- *Modality push* allows the system to store images to PACS.
- *Modality pull* uses the query and retrieve service that allows the modality to query PACS to find out about previous images for the patient and to fetch those images from archive to the workstation. This is clearly essential for viewing workstations but not necessarily so for all imaging modalities.
- *Print service* allows the modality to print to a network printer. This may not be needed in a filmless environment.
- *Modality performed procedure step* provides information on whether the examination in the worklist is in progress or completed. This can be used, for example, to show that the examination is ready for reporting.

two parts. One of these is a short-term archive for current cases, i.e. for inpatients or those about to attend an outpatient clinic. The short-term archive is designed for rapid access on demand. The larger the archive the more difficult is rapid access, so there is a need for a longer-term archive for those images that are unlikely to be of immediate interest and for which access time is slower. There will be automatic systems in place to transfer images from the long-term into the short-term archive prior, for example, to a patient attending an outpatient clinic. For security, the archive is usually backed up to a second archive in a separate location often at some distance from the hospital.

A PACS is ineffective if it is not connected to other information systems within the hospital. In particular, the *hospital information system*, more commonly referred to as the *patient administrative system*, must be fully integrated, as must be the *radiology information system*. These systems hold information such as patient demographics and appointment dates that is then available to the radiology user. Other standards apply to these systems: HL7, a standard for the interchange of text data, and Integrating the Healthcare Environment. A *PACS broker* provides an interface between these systems and the workflow manager. The function of the PACS broker is to ensure that the various information systems can communicate and that their simultaneous use is transparent to the user.

The images are accessed by workstations for reporting or review. There are various types of workstation. These include modality workstations that are supplied with the imaging equipment. These incorporate imaging software provided by the manufacturer of, for example, the CT scanner that are specific to the images produced on that scanner, for example proprietary software for CT angiography. If provided with the appropriate DICOM licences, the modality workstation can display images from the archive, for example to display MRI images together with the CT images on the CT workstation.

Reporting workstations are generally those used by radiologists. They have high-quality image display monitors (normally two for each workstation) and a wide range of software tools for image manipulation and measurement. It is essential that the display monitor is calibrated to the DICOM standard to ensure optimum display conditions (see Box 5.4). It is also essential that the display environment is suitable: that

---

Box 5.4 Quality assurance of display monitors

A display monitor is calibrated so that the greyscale rendering of the image is optimized to the performance of the human eye. This can be checked using standard test images. One example of a tool used for display quality assurance was developed by the Society of Motion Picture and Television Engineers and is known as the SMPTE test pattern (Fig. 5.10). It incorporates areas of varying brightness from zero (black) to 100% (white) in 10% steps. Measurement of the luminance of these squares provides a check against the DICOM standard. It can also be used as a visual check. There are smaller 5% contrast squares within the zero and 100% squares that should both be visible on a well-adjusted monitor. Failure to see these low-contrast details is an indicator to show that the monitor may be out of calibration. The appearance of the image on the monitor can be adjusted using contrast and brightness controls. However, these will not bring an out of calibration monitor back into calibration, and it is generally recommended that these controls are disabled. If the user wishes to change the appearance of the image on the monitor, the software windowing tools provided within picture archiving and communication systems should be used in preference.

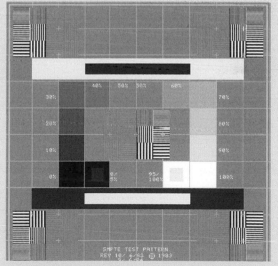

Figure 5.10 SMPTE test pattern used for calibration of display monitor.

the background lighting is kept low and that there are no extraneous light sources to produce reflections from the screen.

Elsewhere, such as in clinics, there may be review workstations with lower specification monitors and limited imaging software. Primary reporting from review workstations should be done with caution, because the image display is not as good.

Access to the archive is more generally available through web browsers installed on standard PCs. These do not have image manipulation tools. Access to images can then be made more generally available (with appropriate password protection) to any PC linked into the hospital network. Users need to be made aware of the limitations of such systems and the inherent risks in using them for diagnosis. The displays are unlikely to conform to the DICOM standard, and they may have limited resolution and are almost invariably used in locations in which the lighting levels are high and in which there are many sources of light causing reflections off the screen.

5.6 SUMMARY

- The digital image is stored as a matrix of pixels having values in binary notation.
- The image size (in bytes) depends on the size of the matrix and the number of binary digits (bit depth).
- Image storage size may be reduced by compression, which is either lossless or lossy.
- Image processing may be used for noise reduction (low-pass filtering) or edge enhancement (high-pass filtering).

- The image data are mapped to greyscale for display.
- Fourier analysis is a technique of representing an image by a series of sine waves.
- Aliasing may be produced when there is insufficient sampling of the imaging data.
- MTF describes the ability of the system to represent the image as a function of the spatial frequency of the information presented.
- CR is a method of image capture based on photostimulable phosphor plates.
- The phosphor is a barium fluorohalide that emits light following irradiation when it is scanned by a laser beam.
- The image data are fitted to a gradation curve that is designed for the particular image task or radiographic projection.
- DDIs provide information on dose to the imaging plate.
- DR based on amorphous silicon TFT arrays may use either a light-emitting phosphor with photodiode light detectors or an amorphous selenium photoconductor for direct digital imaging.
- PACS are used for archive and distribution of digital images.
- Imaging devices with a PACS must comply with DICOM standards.
- The quality of the image displayed depends on the specification and calibration of the monitor and on the viewing environment.

Chapter 6

Fluoroscopy

Radiography is concerned with the recording of an image produced by the transmission of X-rays through the body, using either a film–screen system or a digital recording device as discussed in Chapters 4 and 5. Fluoroscopy is also concerned with X-ray transmission images, but instead of recording a single frame a sequence of images is viewed in real time.

Fluoroscopy has existed as an imaging technique for almost as long as radiography. Direct viewing fluoroscopy involved the use of zinc sulphide fluorescent screens. The phosphor was backed by lead glass, and the radiologist viewed the image from behind the screen while being shielded from the radiation transmitted through the patient and the phosphor. There were many limitations to such a system, the main one being the brightness of the image; it was so dim that fluoroscopy had to be carried out in a dark room so that the radiologist's vision would be sufficiently adapted to be able to see an acceptable level of contrast in the image. Even then, the level of contrast that could be displayed was very poor in comparison with today's systems.

The development of the image intensifier dates back to the 1950s and 1960s, and it has become the device at the heart of all fluoroscopic systems. However, in the future it is likely that flat plate detectors will be used predominantly for real-time imaging. These have gradually become available since about 2000, initially for cardiology systems because of the more limited requirement in terms of field of view, but more recently with larger detectors that can be used for other applications, particularly angiography.

6.1 THE IMAGE INTENSIFIER

A schematic diagram of the image intensifier is shown in Figure 6.1. The device is contained within

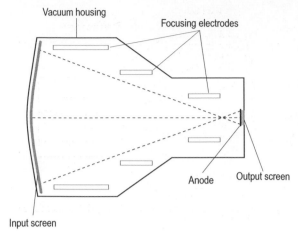

Figure 6.1 Cross-section of an image intensifier.

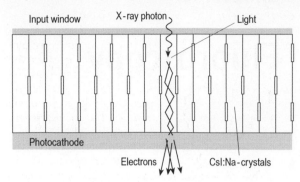

Figure 6.2 Detailed view of the input screen of an image intensifier, demonstrating internal light reflection in the caesium iodide crystals.

an evacuated glass or ceramic envelope that is itself surrounded by a metal housing that has the function of preventing light from getting into the tube and of shielding the device from the effects of magnetic fields.

Within the tube itself, there are three main components:

- the input screen
- the electron-focusing electrodes
- the output screen.

Input screen

The input screen is curved, with the radius of curvature being approximately equal to the distance from the screen to the focal point of the electron beam (see below). The screen has two components (Fig. 6.2). On the outer (X-ray beam) side is the input phosphor layer laid down on a thin metal layer. On the inner side of the screen, there is a thin coating of a material that acts as a photocathode, a material that emits electrons when irradiated by light. A common photocathode material is antimony caesium $SbCs_3$. The intensity of light produced in the phosphor and the number of electrons produced in the photocathode are directly proportional to the intensity of X-ray photons.

In modern image intensifier systems, the phosphor is invariably caesium iodide. Caesium iodide is chosen partly because of its absorption efficiency. It has its K-edges at 36 keV (caesium) and 33 keV (iodine), which fall just below the peak of the bremsstrahlung spectrum used for most clinical situations (Fig. 6.3). In practice, about 60% of the incoming X-ray photons are detected by a phosphor layer that is 0.1–0.4 mm thick. In addition, caesium iodide has a crystalline structure, and the input phosphor can be manufactured so that

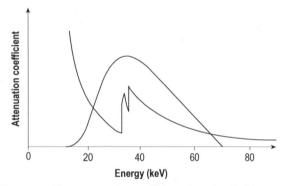

Figure 6.3 Mass attenuation coefficient of caesium iodide superimposed on a 70 kV X-ray spectrum.

the narrow needle-like crystals (approximately 5 μm in diameter) are laid down perpendicular to the screen. Light produced in the crystals is internally reflected. This minimizes the spread of light in the phosphor layer (Fig. 6.2) and thus minimizes the unsharpness caused by having a thicker phosphor layer.

The input screen is maintained at a high negative voltage with respect to the anode shown on the right side of the intensifier in Figure 6.1, the potential difference being about 25 kV. The effect of the voltage is that the electrons generated in the photocathode are accelerated within the vacuum towards the anode and the output screen.

The input screen size may be between about 150 and 400 mm in diameter, its size being selected on the basis of clinical application. The smallest sizes may be used for applications such as fracture fixation in orthopaedics, whereas the largest sizes are suitable for angiography and interventional radiology. For applications such as barium contrast studies of the gastrointestinal tract, an input diameter of 350 mm is typical.

Output screen

The output screen is between about 25 and 35 mm in diameter. It comprises a thin phosphor layer, usually zinc cadmium sulphide (ZnCdS:Ag), to convert the pattern of electron intensities into light. It needs to be no more than a few micrometres in thickness, because of the very limited range of the electrons; because it is so thin, there is very little light spread in the screen. Because the screen gives out light in all directions, including backwards, the inner part of the screen has to be covered. If it were not, light from the screen would be detected by the photocathode, causing a cascade of electron emission that would completely white-out the image. The screen is covered with an extremely thin coating of aluminium (about 0.5 μm) to prevent this happening. This aluminium coat also acts as the anode.

It is worth noting that there is a direct relationship between the brightness displayed on the output screen and the intensity of X-ray photons falling on the input phosphor – doubling X-ray exposure doubles the light output; effectively, the system has γ = 1. This is in contrast to the situation in film-screen radiography (Ch. 4.2).

Electron focusing

The anode is the aluminium coating on the output screen. Without additional focusing electrodes, the electrons would cross the tube to the anode in a more or less disorganized fashion and no image would be formed. The focusing electrodes are metal rings within the tube that are held at positive voltages with respect to the photocathode. The voltages are set so that the electrons are constrained to travel along paths that lead them directly to the output screen, such that the pattern of electron intensities falling on the screen are an exact (but minified) replica of the pattern of intensities on the input screen. The electrodes are effectively acting as an electron lens.

Gain

Gain is the descriptive term used to indicate the extent to which the image intensifier has intensified the light emitted from the output screen in comparison with that from the input screen; that is, it is the ratio of the brightness of the output phosphor to that of the input phosphor. Two factors are responsible for the gain.

- Generally, a single light photon produced in the input phosphor causes a single electron to be emitted from the photocathode. Following acceleration to about 25 keV by the focusing field in the intensifier, each electron causes many light photons to be emitted from the output phosphor.

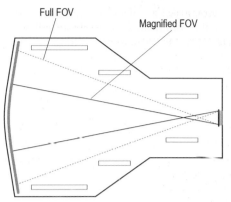

Figure 6.4 Electron beam path in the image intensifier for a magnified field of view (FOV).

This is described as *flux gain* and is typically about 50.

- *Minification gain* is the term used to describe the intensification caused by reducing the image size from the input to output screen. It is equal to the ratio of the areas of the two screens. For a 300 mm intensifier with a 30 mm output screen, the minification gain would be $(300/30)^2 = 100$.

The overall brightness gain is the product of the two, which in this case is approximately 5000.

Gain is not a measurable quantity. It is more common to describe the performance of an image intensifier in terms of the *conversion factor* (G_X). G_X is defined as the ratio of the brightness (luminance) of the output phosphor (in units of candela m^{-2}) and the dose rate at the input surface of the image intensifier (μGy s^{-1}). Typical values are in the range 25–30 Cd m^{-2} (μGy s^{-1})$^{-1}$. One of the features of image intensifiers is that the gain, and therefore the conversion factor, deteriorates in time and with equipment usage because of loss in the detection efficiency of the phosphor.

Magnification

In Figure 6.1, it was seen that the image in the output phosphor is a minified version of the image from the full area of the input screen. By changing the voltages of the intermediate electrodes, the electron crossover point (or focus) can be moved nearer to the input screen so that the intensifier operates in a magnification mode. The central part of the input image then fills the whole of the output phosphor (Fig. 6.4). This effectively magnifies the image seen on the output screen. Because the TV system that is viewing the output phosphor is one of the major limits to spatial resolution, the resultant image will display better resolution than is displayed with the full field of view. However, because magnification effectively reduces the minification gain, there will be reduced brightness on the output screen. To restore brightness requires an increase in exposure factors, thus increasing the patient's skin dose. This is discussed further in section 6.3.

Generally, all image intensifier systems offer at least one magnified field of view. With the larger intensifier, sizes up to four magnified fields may be provided down to a minimum size of about 150 mm.

6.2 TV SYSTEM

The image from the output screen is displayed on a monitor using a TV imaging system. It is not the intention in this text to give a full description of the TV system. It is sufficient to consider the various elements in the TV chain and their development over time.

The original TV image intensifier systems used a lens system between the output screen of the image intensifier and the camera tube to focus the image from the output screen on to the input screen of the camera. The camera was a vacuum device that incorporated a scanning electron beam that produced a voltage on the signal plate incorporated into the input screen of the camera. This voltage (the video signal) is proportional to the intensity of light falling on the area of the plate being scanned. The signal is then fed into the TV monitor to display the image in real time.

There have been several subsequent developments that have led to significant improvements.

Digital fluoroscopy

Modern image intensifier systems have digital functionality. The signal from the video camera is converted to digital format that is input into a computer before being displayed. The computer has a number of functions. One is to provide an image storage facility (see section 6.5). Second, having created images in digital format it is then possible to carry out a number of image-processing functions such as noise reduction or edge enhancement, as discussed in Chapter 5.1.2. Additional functions include black and white reversal (i.e. display of positive or negative images), geometrical inversion (left to right or top to bottom), and mapping to display look-up tables to maximize contrast (see Ch. 5.1.2). The processing can be done in real time so that these techniques can be applied to the fluoroscopic image as well as to recorded images.

CCD camera

The TV camera described briefly above is a vacuum device producing an analogue video signal. It is more effective to use a camera that produces a signal that is in a digital format. The input screen of a CCD camera is a thin layer of amorphous silicon that is divided into individual pixels (generally 1024×1024). Each element acts as a small capacitor, with the charge collected being proportional to the intensity of light falling on it. The collected charge on each pixel is measured sequentially from a single row of the matrix and then from row to row. The read-out is extremely rapid, sufficient for image sequences at 30 frames s^{-1} or faster.

CCDs are used widely in the domestic market for video recorder and digital cameras. They are now the standard for image intensifier–based fluoroscopy systems. One significant advantage is the increased dynamic range, because CCD cameras generally have 12-bit image depth.

Optics

Good optical connection between the output face of the intensifier and the camera input is essential. Lens systems have traditionally been used, but these are now being replaced by fibre-optic coupling. This provides more efficient light collection and improved geometrical integrity.

6.3 AUTOMATIC BRIGHTNESS CONTROL

In radiography, the amount of radiation reaching the image receptor is controlled either manually by the radiographer (kilovoltage, kV, and mAs setting) based on standard exposure factors and experience, or by using an automatic exposure control system that terminates exposure when the correct quantity of radiation has been detected at the film or imaging plate (see Ch. 4.5). In fluoroscopy, the manual option is not practical, because the region of patient being imaged may change throughout the course of the examination and the radiological thickness may change rapidly with the administration of contrast. An *automatic brightness control* (*ABC*) system is essential.

Automatic brightness control systems may take as input signal either a measurement of the light intensity of the output screen or a measurement of the signal from the camera. In older systems, with optical coupling, it was common to incorporate a partially reflecting mirror in the optics (this means that only a small fraction of the light would be reflected – most would pass through the mirror to the camera). The light intensity of the output screen of the image would be measured, and changes would be fed back to the generator for the automatic adjustment of kV and/or milliamperage (mA) to restore the output light intensity to the required level. In modern equipment, it is

Box 6.1 Dose control curves

The purpose of the automatic brightness control system is to maintain the brightness at an acceptable level on the output screen. This is achieved by a feedback mechanism using a measurement of brightness either taken directly from the output screen or taken from the signal from the TV camera. The measured signal is fed back into the generator to allow for automatic adjustment of kilovoltage (kV) and/or milliamperage (mA) designed to maintain the signal at the appropriate level. The kV and mA adjustment follows brightness curves programmed into the system by the manufacturer. Most generators have several dose control programmes to allow the user to select the curve that is most appropriate for the particular clinical task.

In general, as radiological thickness increases it is necessary to increase kV to provide better penetration through the patient. Most commonly, mA is also increased with radiological thickness, as shown in curve A in Figure 6.5. This type of control curve is referred to as an *anti-isowatt* curve. Curve A has a higher mA at each kV setting, so the input power increases with patient thickness as necessary to the maximum of about 400 W.

Two common variants on the anti–isowatt curve are shown in Figure 6.5. Curve B might be used to maximize image quality for iodine contrast studies (e.g. for angiography). Rather than having a continuous increase in kV with increasing thickness, the system holds the tube potential at between 60 and 65 kV to provide the optimum spectrum for imaging iodine that has a K-edge at 33 keV. With increasing radiological thickness, mA is increased with the kV being held at this value. However, the tube can sustain continuous fluoroscopy only up to

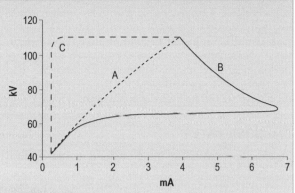

Figure 6.5 Relationship between kilovoltage (kV) and milliamperage used for automatic brightness control. Curve A is an anti-isowatt curve, curve B is optimized for iodine contrast imaging, and curve C is for low-dose high-kV fluoroscopy.

a particular level of input power, typically about 400 W. At 62 kV (a typical value), this level is reached when the tube current is equal to $400/62 = 6.5\,mA$. Therefore for radiological thicknesses that would need higher tube currents, the system is programmed to increase kV while reducing mA to ensure that the maximum power rating is not exceeded.

Curve B is designed to maximize image quality, but at a cost of increased dose because of the use of a low kV. In contrast, curve C in Figure 6.5 minimizes dose at the cost of image quality by increasing kV rapidly as radiological thickness increases, up to the maximum kV that can be sustained by the tube. As thickness is increased further, the maximum kV is used with increasing mA. A high-kV curve might be suitable for paediatrics, for which dose minimization is particularly important.

more usual to take the camera signal to provide this information.

Adjustment of brightness is made by increasing either kV or mA or both. This is discussed further in Box 6.1. The area of the output screen used by the ABC system is not the full screen. In general, the brightness in the central area of the screen is selected because the user will have centred the imaging system to the area of radiological interest; it is the brightness in this central region that should be optimized without the influence of changes in brightness in peripheral areas that may be influenced by, for example, collimation or the presence of lungs. Some systems allow the operator to select the region of the image to be used with the ABC system, although a default

region may be programmed into the system on selection of a particular clinical programme.

Automatic gain control

It would be equally possible to adjust the brightness of the image seen on the TV monitor by adjusting the sensitivity (or gain) of the TV system itself (*automatic gain control*). This is, after all, what is done with TV images to compensate for the varying light levels in scenes that are being filmed. However, in fluoroscopy this would be at the cost of either increased image noise or of unnecessary dose. For large radiological thicknesses (e.g. oblique views in the pelvis), the kV and mA factors need to be relatively high to give sufficient transmission to produce an image in which noise does not obscure image contrast. If the kV and mA factors were not altered as radiological thickness was reduced, a brighter and less noisy image would be produced on the output screen and the TV system gain could be adjusted to give an acceptable brightness level on the TV monitor. However, for thinner radiological sections in which the kV and mA had been selected to be sufficient for thicker sections, the dose rates would be unnecessarily high.

6.4 DOSE RATES

Fluoroscopy screening times depend on the clinical task and the expertise of the operator. They may be as short as a few seconds in orthopaedic theatres for fracture fixations; for barium contrast studies, the screening times are typically in the range 1–3 min, and for complex interventional techniques the time may be 15 min or more. As a result, there is the potential for delivering high doses to the patient during fluoroscopy and a proportionately high dose to the operator (see Ch. 2.8.1).

Fluoroscopy dose rates depend to some extent on the detective quantum efficiency (see Ch. 5.4) of the image intensifier. For intensifiers with caesium iodide input screens, this is generally high, about 65%. However, the critical factor in determining dose rate is the level of noise that can be accepted in clinical practice. The gain that can be applied to the TV system means that very low levels of brightness on the output screen on the intensifier can be displayed at an acceptable brightness level on the monitor display. However, at these low-output brightness levels the image noise may be unacceptable. Because output brightness is directly proportional to the input dose rate at the image intensifier face, this parameter is frequently used to define the dose efficiency of the system. For standard settings and for the maximum field of view, manufacturers generally set the input dose rate of image intensifier systems to be in the range 0.1–$0.5\,\mu Gy\,s^{-1}$, most commonly between about 0.2 and $0.3\,\mu Gy\,s^{-1}$. As radiological thickness changes, kV and mA are adjusted as described in section 6.3 to keep the output brightness or camera signal at a nearly constant level with relatively small variations in input dose rate. As a general rule, the lower the input dose rate to the intensifier, the greater is the noise in the displayed image.

On magnification, the gain of the intensifier reduces (see section 6.1); that is, the brightness in the output image is decreased in proportion to the reduction in area of the field of view. If the gain of the TV system is not adjusted, then the input dose rate must be increased in inverse proportion to area in order to retain the same level of image brightness on the output screen. Because the increase in dose is inversely proportional to the reduction in area, the dose area product should be the same when a magnified field is used. However, in practice some increase in camera gain is applied so that the increase in input dose rate for magnified fields of view is less than would otherwise be required. Dose area product is therefore reduced to some extent on magnification.

The patient entrance surface dose (ESD) rate in fluoroscopy depends on the sensitivity of the detector (image intensifier), and systems with low input dose rates will generally have lower ESD rates. One internationally accepted design feature of fluoroscopy systems is that, for standard fluoroscopy settings, the ESD rate cannot exceed $100\,mGy\,min^{-1}$ for any field of view, and that for the largest field size it cannot exceed $50\,mGy\,min^{-1}$. Reference to Table 2.8 shows that screening for 1 min at this latter dose rate would be equivalent to approximately 15 radiographs of the pelvis. In practice, for an average size patient and using well-adjusted, modern equipment, ESD rates in the range 10–$30\,mGy\,min^{-1}$ are typical.

Pulsed fluoroscopy

Fluoroscopy systems can commonly be used in pulsed mode. The X-ray generator supplying voltage to the tube is switched on and off at regular intervals to give pulses of X-rays from the tube. Indeed, most fluoroscopy systems provide pulsed radiation as standard, with what is described as 'continuous' fluoroscopy being pulsed at either 25 or 30 pulses s^{-1}. At these rates, the eye is not able to detect the difference between pulsed and continuous images. Pulse rates may then be reduced, generally by successive halving of the standard rates, for example from 30 to 15, 7.5 and 3.75 pulses s^{-1} and so on down to about 1 pulse s^{-1}, the pulse width being generally in the range 2–20 ms. Dose rate falls approximately, but not necessarily exactly, in proportion to pulse rate; the precise relationship between pulse and dose rates depends on equipment design. Each successive image is retained on the display monitor until the following image is displayed. Therefore with a static scene, no flickering is seen on the screen even at the lowest pulse rates. However, with movement in the field of view, the lower pulse rates will display blurring or lag that may be unacceptable for particular examinations.

As an alternative to switching the X-ray beam at the generator, it is possible to use the tube itself to switch the beam on and off. In a *grid-controlled tube*, an additional electrode is built into the tube between the cathode and anode. This is a circular electrode through which the electrons pass as they are accelerated from the filament (cathode) to the target (anode). When a negative voltage (approximately 2 kV) relative to the cathode is applied to the grid electrode, then the electrons emitted from the target will be repelled and effectively be pushed back into the filament. Therefore by switching a negative voltage to the grid, the electron flow and thus X-ray production can be switched off. Pulsing the X-ray beam using this technique is called *grid-controlled fluoroscopy*. It has the advantage that switching is more precise, giving greater control over the intensity of the X-ray beam in each pulse.

6.5 RECORDED IMAGES

Fluoroscopy is used almost exclusively for positioning, whether of the tube, the patient, contrast or inserted devices such as catheters or biopsy needles. The live fluoroscopy image is rarely used for diagnosis, both because of the difficulty in analysing the content of an image in real time and because of the relatively poor image quality. It is therefore important to have a facility to record images. Older, non-digital systems required sophisticated mechanical or optical systems to be able to record diagnostically acceptable images (see Box 6.2). The current generation of image intensifier systems record images in digital format using the signal from the TV camera. Recording images produced by an image intensifier can be described by the term *fluorography*.

In the simplest case, the computer stores the last frame of a fluoroscopy sequence and that frame continues to be displayed on the TV monitor after the X-ray beam has been switched off (*last image hold*). This allows the operator to inspect the image without additional radiation. In certain circumstances, this image may be sufficient for the clinical purpose and it may stored permanently as a record or for subsequent reporting. This feature may be referred to as *fluoro grab*. More commonly, a higher-quality image is required for diagnosis. *Digital spot images* are single-shot images taken with a single pulse of radiation at a high mA to produce a low-noise image. Digital spot images generally require an image intensifier dose in the range of 0.1–5 μGy to provide adequate image quality, the exact value depending on the amount of magnification and the clinical requirements for image quality. An acquisition requiring 0.5 μGy gives a dose that is equivalent to 2 s of screening at a typical image intensifier dose rate of 0.25 μGy s^{-1}. Digital spot images are stored in the computer for subsequent transfer to a picture archiving and communication system or to be printed on film.

Systems may have the facility to record sequences of images. These may either be diagnostic quality

Box 6.2 Image recording in non-digital fluoroscopy

For analogue image intensifier systems, image recording was principally done by film–screen radiography. The equipment incorporated a cassette holder that could be introduced between the grid and image intensifier. During fluoroscopy, the holder, with film cassette in place, was parked outside the radiation beam. On pressing the radiographic exposure switch, the cassette with film in place was automatically driven into position in front of the intensifier and the exposure made, the time delay between initiation and exposure being generally not much greater than 1 s. The equipment commonly incorporated mechanisms for positioning the film and cassette linked with selectable collimator settings so that multiple exposures could be made on a single film. This was particularly useful for rapid image sequences such as for barium swallows, for which there was insufficient time to change film cassette between exposures. These films were commonly referred to as spot films.

An alternative method of taking spot films was to use a camera attached to the image intensifier, which, using a mirror introduced between the output screen and TV camera and a separate lens system, could take a picture of the image on the output screen of the intensifier. The film size was typically 105 mm, giving an image that was about 30% of the size of what would be seen on the conventional spot film. These films were sometimes referred to as photospot images, and the term *fluorography* was introduced to describe recorded images produced by fluoroscopy equipment. To take a photospot image, a short exposure time with an increased milliamperage was used in order to minimize noise. As an extension to this method, the static camera could be replaced by a cine camera. By using pulsed exposures from the X-ray tube and synchronizing the pulse rate with the frame rate of the camera, cine recordings could be made. Such systems were standard in cardiac studies prior to the introduction of digital systems.

sequences such as in angiography or recording of fluoroscopy sequences. The total number of images that may be stored from a single run depends on the size of the computer memory (RAM), because they have to be stored in memory in real time before transfer to disk. A few hundred sequential images may be stored in this way.

6.6 IMAGE QUALITY

Spatial resolution

Spatial resolution and its measurement were introduced in Chapter 3.1.2. In the image intensifier itself, it is principally limited by blurring caused by the spread of light in the output phosphor. At this stage, resolution is generally in the range 4–5 lp mm^{-1} and somewhat better for magnified fields of view. Here, the resolution is defined in terms of the image size at the input face of the image intensifier, not at the position of the patient. The resolution that is seen on the monitor display is more limited, because it is degraded in the TV system. The CCD camera used to view the output screen may have 1024 × 1024 pixels. Thus for a 350-mm field of view, the pixel size is about 290 µm, giving a theoretical resolution of 1.7 lp mm^{-1}. However, the spatial resolution in the fluoroscopic image as viewed on the display monitor is somewhat less than this and is generally no better than about 1.2 lp mm^{-1}, improving to about 3 lp mm^{-1} in the magnified image. Similar spatial resolution may be produced with the older vacuum tube camera. In that case, the resolution is limited by the number of scan lines used to form the image and the band width (or frequency) of the signal carrying the TV signal.

Noise

Noise is a significant feature of fluoroscopy that influences the contrast resolution in the displayed image. In Chapter 4.4.3, the quantum sink was discussed with respect to film–screen radiography and defined as that part in the imaging chain in which the fewest number of photons is carrying the image signal. For an image intensifier, the quantum sink corresponds to the photons absorbed in the input screen. No increase in image intensifier or camera gain will improve the signal to noise ratio from that point forwards.

Noise may be reduced by increasing the input dose rate by increasing fluoroscopy mA, but this is undesirable because of the increase in patient dose (see section 6.4). It is possible to reduce noise by frame averaging. In this technique, successive images are added together pixel by pixel and the average value is then displayed. The level of smoothing depends on the number of frames that are added. This technique is useful provided that there is no significant movement between frames, in which case the image would be blurred. In effect, it is no different from using pulsed fluoroscopy at an increased mA per pulse.

Veiling glare

Veiling glare is produced by scattering effects in the image intensifier. It is mainly from light scattering in the output window of the intensifier but is also caused by X-ray and light scattering in the input phosphor and electron scattering in the tube itself. Its overall effect is to reduce image contrast, because dark regions of the images appear lighter because of the surrounding light areas. This not only affects contrast, it is also one of the causes of the central area of the image being brighter than the periphery; this latter effect is known as *vignetting*. In general, the larger the image intensifier the greater is the veiling glare.

Geometrical distortion

The image from an image intensifier is subject to geometrical distortion. There are two main types. Pin cushion distortion, in which there is a magnification towards the edges of the image, is produced by the curvature of the input screen. S-type distortion imposes curvature on straight line features and is caused by ambient magnetic fields influencing the path of the electrons from input to output screens of the intensifier. Generally, neither of these is significant, or noticeable, when imaging the complex shapes within the body.

Testing image quality

Spatial resolution is tested using a grid test object as described in Chapter 3.1.2. Generally, the test is carried out without any attenuating material in the beam. A low kV is used to minimize scatter. When testing, it is usual to angle the test grid (generally at 45°) with respect to the matrix of the TV system in order to avoid interference artefacts on the displayed image. It is a useful test, because it will detect any deterioration in the focusing of the image intensifier.

Contrast resolution may be tested with a low-contrast test object. There are a number of such test objects commercially available. These include those originally developed at the University of Leeds and referred to as Leeds test objects. In appearance, these are flat disks approximately 6 mm thick and 200–300 mm in diameter. They contain circular inserts of higher atomic number material that produce varying levels of contrast in the final image. To test image quality, the test object is imaged under standard fluoroscopy conditions. The observer is required to count the number of details that can be seen in the displayed image. Use of one of the standard Leeds test objects (TO.10) is described in Box 6.3.

6.7 DIGITAL SUBTRACTION ANGIOGRAPHY

The object of digital subtraction angiography (DSA) is to produce images of contrast-filled vessels in isolation from other tissues. This provides improved

Box 6.3 A test object for assessment of low–contrast resolution

The layout of details in Leeds test object TO.10, which is used for assessing low-contrast resolution, is shown in Figure 6.6. It incorporates 12 groups of circular details, with the diameter of each group varying from 0.25 to 11.1 mm. Each group comprises nine disks with thickness (and thus contrast) varying progressively. The system is generally used to test fluoroscopy images using 1–2 mm of copper filtration to drive the kilovoltage (kV) up to about 70 kV. Under these conditions, it is generally not possible to see more than about six details in each group, and possibly no more than one detail in the group with the smallest detail diameter. The test object is provided with calibrated contrast data enabling the user to determine the minimum visible or threshold contrast (C_T) for each detail size. From this, the threshold detection index $H_T(A)$ can be derived:

$$H_T(A) = [C_T(A) \times A^{1/2}]^{-1}.$$

Plotting $H_T(A)$ against $A^{1/2}$ provides a good indication of imaging performance and allows comparison with previous tests or with a standard as is shown in Figure 6.7.

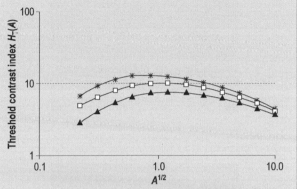

Figure 6.7 Contrast detail diagram derived from Leeds test object TO.10.

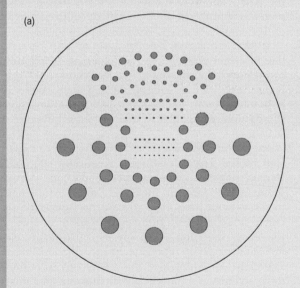

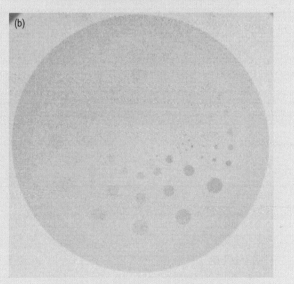

Figure 6.6 Details in Leeds test object TO.10: **(a)** the layout of the 12 sets of details, and **(b)** a simulated fluorography to show the varying levels of contrast.

clarity in the image of the vessels and permits the use of a lower dose of contrast medium. Images of the same region are taken before and after injection of the contrast medium. Between imaging sequences, it is important to avoid any movement of the patient or equipment, and therefore in general the images should be acquired in rapid succession.

The process is illustrated schematically in Figure 6.8.

- The non-contrast image (a) is taken before the contrast medium has reached the target area. It shows normal anatomy only. Commonly, two frames are acquired; the first is used by the system to stabilize

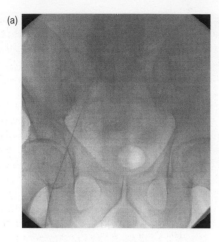

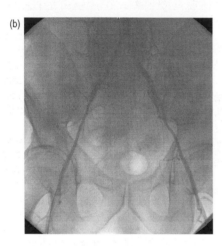

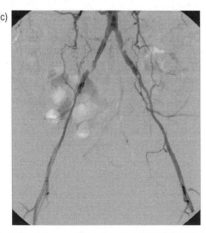

Figure 6.8 Digital subtraction angiography (DSA) showing
(a) the precontrast mask image, (b) the unsubtracted image
following contrast injection, and (c) the subtracted DSA image.

the X-ray factors and the second is stored in the computer memory (the *mask* image).

- The contrast image (b) is taken when the vessels have filled with contrast medium. It shows the filled vessels superimposed on normal anatomy and is stored as a second frame.

- The first stored image (the mask) is then subtracted from the second on a pixel by pixel basis. The resulting subtraction image (c) is stored as a third frame. This shows the filled vessels only.

- Recording can continue to provide a sequence of subtracted images based on the initial mask.

In general, the subtracted images may be viewed in real time. Inevitably, there will be some misregistration of images caused by movement between frames. This can be seen particularly at the boundaries between high-contrast details (e.g. at bone edges). This effect may be minimized retrospectively by adjustment or movement of the mask (pixel shifting). However, this can be done only over the full area of the image and does not allow for differential movements within the field of view. Pixel shifting may be done manually or using automated techniques.

It may be noted that because of the exponential nature of attenuation, the signals in the contrast images and the mask are first converted into their logarithms prior to subtraction and then converted back into intensity values for display. Additional algorithms may be applied to minimize the influence of scatter.

In section 6.6, it was noted that the effect of quantum mottle may be reduced by adding successive frames. Effectively, the number of photons contributing to each pixel is increased, and because noise increases with the square root of the signal, the signal to noise ratio is improved by this technique. In the same way subtracting images causes a decrease in signal to noise ratio, the image appears noisier. Therefore to counteract this effect, DSA requires increased mA in comparison with unsubtracted image acquisition.

In the description given above, it has been assumed that the image sequence is concerned with a single static field of view. This is not always the case. For example, in femoral angiography the length of anatomy to be imaged is very much greater than the field of view of the intensifier. To acquire views of the full length of the legs might have to be done as three or four separate sequences. This would require separate contrast administrations for each region that was to be imaged. Most DSA systems include software that allows acquisition of several mask images, in this case down the full leg length, and the contrast images can then be acquired along the full leg length with the table longitudinal movement being used to track the progress of the contrast. The table's position is recorded for each contrast image, and the appropriate mask image for that position is used in the subtraction. The advantage of such techniques is to reduce the amount of contrast medium needed and to minimize the time taken for the examination. A potential disadvantage is the increased likelihood of movement between the mask and contrast images.

Digital subtraction angiography may be used for more complex techniques such as rotational angiography. Mask images are taken at several angles for a 90° rotation of the X-ray tube and intensifier about the patient. This is followed by a post-contrast rotation during which images of the filled vessels are acquired at the same angles. DSA images are then produced at each angle. Subsequently, these images may be used for three-dimensional reconstruction of the vasculature that can then be viewed from any angle. This permits identification of the optimum imaging angle to view vessels that might otherwise be hidden behind other vessels at standard viewing angles.

Dual energy subtraction

Another subtraction technique involves taking images in rapid succession at low and high kV. At low kV, the image will display high contrast between bone and soft tissue, whereas at high kV the contrast of bone is significantly reduced, image contrast being primarily influenced by tissue density rather than atomic number. Subtracting the low-kV image from the high-kV image therefore minimizes the visualization of bone and improves soft tissue contrast. This might be of value in chest radiography, because the ribs overlying the lung region are effectively removed. Conversely, subtracting the high-kV from the low-kV image displays the bony structure in greater detail.

6.8 FLAT PLATE DETECTORS

The detectors used for fluoroscopy are essentially the same as those used for digital radiography. Most commonly, they use amorphous silicon detectors with caesium iodide scintillators (see Ch. 5.4). The detective quantum efficiency for these detectors is comparable with that of an image intensifier (i.e. about 65%). The principal advantages are increased dynamic range and improved spatial resolution. Image intensifier systems have a limited contrast ratio, no better than about 30:1, because of the high background signal and veiling glare. Even though good contrast resolution may

be displayed within this range when a 12-bit CCD camera is used, the overall image contrast that can be displayed is limited. For a flat plate detector, the range of signals that can be detected is very much greater and makes full use of the 14-bit depth that is typically available.

The pixel size for flat plate detectors is typically about 150 μm, giving high-contrast resolution of about 3 lp mm^{-1}. This may be compared with the displayed spatial resolution of an image intensifier, which is generally no better than 1–1.2 lp mm^{-1} for the largest intensifier at the largest field of view (about 40 cm). This is equivalent to a pixel size of about 400 μm. The spatial resolution when using a flat plate detector does not, however, improve with magnification other than through the display of a magnified image, because the pixel size remains the same. In contrast, the resolution of the image intensifier–based system improves with magnification to the extent that for the smallest fields of view the resolution of the two systems is comparable.

With the flat plate system, there is no distortion in the displayed image as described in section 6.6 for image intensifier–based systems. In that section, it was noted that distortion was generally not of clinical significance.

One of the facilities that may be provided on angiography systems with flat plate detectors is computed tomography (CT). The flat plate detector with 1024 ×1024 pixels may be thought of as a multislice scanner with 1024 rows of 1024 detectors. Using a single 180° rotation of the C-arm about the patient, a CT scan can be produced covering the collimated length of the patient. Image quality is less good than with a standard CT scanner because of the effect of beam divergence, which is very much greater than for the standard multislice CT scanner (see Ch. 7.4.2 regarding the cone beam effect), and because of the greater proportion of scatter radiation reaching the detectors. In principle, an image intensifier could be used in the same way. However, its use is limited because it has a circular field of view, because of geometrical distortion, and because of the limited dynamic range.

6.9 SUMMARY

- The image intensifier is a device that converts an X-ray image to a minified light image displayed on its output screen.

- The output image from the image intensifier is viewed by a TV camera (generally CCD) and input to a computer.

- Following image processing, the image may be displayed in real time (fluoroscopy) or be stored (fluorography).

- The gain of the image intensifier depends on the relative size of the input and output screens and the accelerating potential applied to the output screen.

- Magnified images are produced by altering electron focusing in the II tube so as to use a smaller area of the input screen.

- The output brightness is controlled by automatic adjustment of kV and mA to maintain near constant brightness.

- The kV and mA adjustment programme is generally selectable depending on clinical application.

- Pulsed fluoroscopy may be used to reduce patient (and staff) dose.

- Spatial resolution is principally limited by the TV system and is generally no better than 1.2 lp mm^{-1} for the largest available fields of view.

- Image contrast in fluoroscopy is limited by quantum noise.

- Test objects may be used for the subjective assessment of changes in image contrast.

- Fluoroscopy systems may be used for DSA, in which a mask image taken before administration of a contrast medium is subtracted from a post-contrast image to display the vasculature without any other structures.

- Other subtraction techniques include dual energy subtraction imaging.

- Flat plate detectors may be used in place of image intensifiers to provide superior image quality.

Chapter 7

Computed tomography

CHAPTER CONTENTS

7.1 INTRODUCTION

Tomography literally means a slice view of the patient, although the term *sectional imaging* is now preferred. Linear tomography was described in Chapter 4.7. As described in that section, tomography is an X-ray imaging technique that produces sectional views of the patient in a plane parallel to the tabletop on which the patient is lying. The contrast demonstrated by this technique is poor because of the influence of overlying tissues. Computed tomography (CT) generates images in transaxial sections, i.e. perpendicular to the axis of rotation of the X-ray tube about the body and generally perpendicular to the cranocaudal axis of the patient's body. Unlike linear tomography, CT images are not influenced by the properties of neighbouring regions of the body. They are therefore able to display levels of contrast that truly represent the subject contrast within the imaged section, with the only limitations being imposed by the width, i.e. thickness, of the section (Fig. 7.1).

Computed tomography was introduced in the early 1970s. It is worth noting that it was originally described as computed axial tomography, known popularly as CAT scanning. The term *axial* was used to distinguish it from the conventional tomography techniques, and the word *computed* was included in the description indicating the key role of the computer in the development of this technology. Methods of image reconstruction that could be used for CT had been formulated many decades before its introduction but only as a branch of abstract mathematics. The employment of such methods required such intensive arithmetic application that they were of no practical use. It was with the advent of the digital computer that theory could become practice, and it is in large

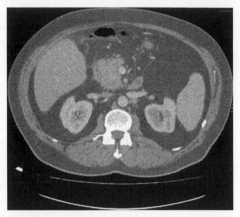

Figure 7.1 A computed tomography scan of the abdomen.

Table 7.1 Approximate range of CT numbers for various tissues

Tissue	Range of CT numbers
Bone	500–1500
Muscle	40–60
Brain (grey matter)	35–45
Brain (white matter)	20–30
Fat	−60 to −150
Lung	−300 to −800

part because of the developments in computer technology over the succeeding years that the technique has been transformed from basic transaxial imaging to true three-dimensional representation of the body.

7.1.1 The computed tomography image

The CT image is most commonly calculated on a 512 × 512 pixel matrix, although 256 × 256 and 1024 × 1024 matrices may also be used. It should be recognized that each pixel should more correctly be described as a *voxel*, i.e. it is a volume element having three dimensions with a depth that is equal to the thickness of the section. The value stored in each pixel, the *CT number* (*CTn*) represents the average linear attenuation coefficient, μ_t, of the tissues within the voxel and is given by:

$$CTn = 1000 \times \frac{\mu_t - \mu_w}{\mu_w},$$

in which μ_w is the linear attenuation coefficient of water. By definition, water has a CT number equal to zero, and air, because of its very low density giving it effectively an attenuation coefficient of zero, has a CT number equal to −1000.

It should be noted that in several texts the term *Hounsfield unit*, named in honour of Sir Godfrey Hounsfield, the pioneer of CT scanning, is used in place of CT number. However, the latter terminology is now the more common and will be used in this chapter.

Air and water are used for the calibration of the CT number scale of the scanner. The CT numbers of body tissues themselves are variable because of the heterogeneity of the tissues themselves, and the variation in the attenuation coefficient of each tissue relative to water, being dependent on kilovoltage (kV) and filtration of the X-ray beam. Representative values of

some tissues are presented in Table 7.1. It can be seen that the CT number of cortical bone (the tissue with the highest attenuation coefficient) may be as high as 1500, although higher values may be displayed. The range of CT number values is most commonly from −1024 to +3071 (4096 levels of grey corresponding to 12-bit storage), although wider ranges may be used by some manufacturers.

Partial volume effect

The CT number stored in each voxel represents the average attenuation coefficient in that voxel. A high-contrast object that is smaller than the voxel may therefore be seen even though its dimensions in the transaxial plane may be less than the displayed pixel size. More significantly in CT scanning, a thin high-contrast structure, such as a vessel filled with contrast or the skull, that crosses the transaxial plane at an oblique angle will be visualized in several adjacent pixels, giving an appearance of a much larger structure in the displayed image. The extent to which the partial volume affects the image depends on the thickness of the transaxial slice, thinner slices providing better resolution. Partial volume effect may also reduce the visibility of low-contrast detail. If the detail only partially fills the voxel, then the CT number will lie between the CT number of the detail and the surrounding structure. There may then be insufficient difference in CT number to visualize the low-contrast detail.

7.1.2 Image display

It was seen above that the CT image is represented by pixels having CT number in the approximate range −1000 to +3000, i.e. 4000 levels of grey. However, the human eye does not have the capacity to distinguish between so many levels of grey and is limited to a range that is not much greater than 50. A CT scan displayed with CT number −1000 represented as black and +3000 as white, with all shades of grey displayed between, would appear very flat with little differentiation being apparent between the various tissues. Windowing is a common technique in digital imaging

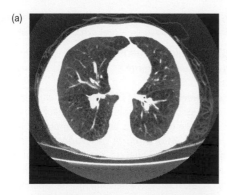

(a)

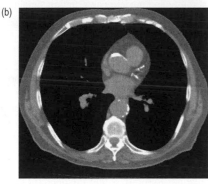

(b)

Figure 7.2 Computed tomography scan of the chest to demonstrate the effect of window width and level. Window levels in (a) have been set to display structure in the lung and in (b) the soft tissue structures.

to bring out the hidden detail in the image. Figure 7.2a is a transaxial scan of the thorax. Window range has been set to -900 to -400 to display the detailed structure in the lungs. All pixels with CT number of 100 and greater are displayed as white, and therefore little detail can be seen in the mediastinum or in the chest wall. Figure 7.2b is the same scan but in this instance the window level has been set from -240 to 300, providing no information in the lungs but good structural detail outside.

Generally, the viewing window is set automatically depending on the imaging protocol. However, the viewer has the opportunity to alter this manually.

7.2 EQUIPMENT FOR COMPUTED TOMOGRAPHY SCANNING

There have been many significant developments in CT technology since the earliest scanners were installed up to the present generation of multislice scanners that are based on *third-generation scanner* geometry. It is not the intention of this text to describe scanner development in detail, but some further information is given in Box 7.1. In this and the following section, a description will be given of the components of a typical single-slice scanner and an outline of the methods used to reconstruct images from the measured transmission data. It is recognized that the single-slice scanner is becoming a rarity; however, the principles of scanning are best understood by using this as a starting point. In section 7.4, two of the principal developments in equipment, helical scanning and multislice detectors, will be described in further detail.

The principal components of the scanner are shown in Figure 7.4. X-ray tube, collimator and detector array are mounted on a rotating gantry. By convention, the rotation axis is referred to as the z-axis. The X-ray beam is collimated as a wide fan beam sufficient to cover the patient cross-section at its widest. It has a narrow width parallel to the z-axis that, for a single-slice scanner, generally defines the imaged slice thickness.

Behind the patient is an arc of detectors, with the radius of the arc being equal to the focal distance so that each detector is the same distance from the source. The total number of the detectors is in the range 500–1000.

Although not shown in the figure, it is now a general design feature to mount the high-voltage generator alongside the X-ray tube on the gantry. On a helical scanner (section 7.4), the gantry can rotate around the patient in 1 s or faster, the minimum time on the newest scanners being about 0.3 s for a full 360° rotation. It is worth noting that the rotating gantry weighs about 500 kg. In discussing the developments in CT technology, it is easy to forget the improvements in the mechanical design and construction of this equipment. It is an impressive sight to have the covers of a CT unit opened up and to see such a heavy structure being rotated so smoothly and quietly about the table at a rate of 2 revolutions s^{-1} or faster.

The patient lies on a couch that has a tabletop that can be moved longitudinally through the gantry aperture. Normally, the plane of gantry rotation is perpendicular to the long axis of the tabletop. However, it is possible to tilt the gantry usually by up to 30° about the vertical. This allows the transaxial scans to be produced at an angle in the body, remembering that transaxial was defined as being perpendicular to the axis of rotation. The main application is in scanning the head, for which the scan planes may be made parallel to the base of the skull.

7.2.1 X–ray tube

The X-ray tube is mounted with its anode–cathode axis parallel to the axis of rotation of the scanner. This

Box 7.1   Scanner generations

The earliest clinical computed tomography scanner had an X-ray source and a single detector (Fig. 7.3a). Data acquisition involved moving both tube and detector across the scanning plane to acquire a series of transmission measurements. Detector and tube were then rotated by 1° and the process repeated. In all, data were collected through a 180° rotation. This scanner may be referred to as the *rotate–translate* type. To reduce scan times, the next generation of scanner had, instead of a single detector, a bank of up to 30 detectors that could measure data simultaneously but that were still insufficient to cover the full cross-section of the patient (Fig. 7.3b). Therefore the rotate–translate procedure was still needed, but it became possible to reduce scan times from just under 5 min for the earliest scanner to less than 20 s. Note that these are the data acquisition times for a single slice. Inevitably, these two early designs became known as *first* and *second generation*.

The inevitable next step in scanner technology was of the type described in this chapter; that is, a scanner with a large number of small detectors arranged in an arc to cover the complete cross-section of the patient. This eliminated the requirement for the linear translation of tube and detectors and allowed for continuous data collection through a full 360° rotation. This may be described as a *rotate–rotate* or *third-generation scanner* (Fig. 7.3c).

One of the technological problems with early scanners was detector stability, and this was made worse by the movement of the gantry. This and other problems led to the development of a *fourth-generation* or *rotate-stationary scanner*, in which the detectors were arranged in a stationary ring outside the path of the rotating tube (Fig. 7.3d). This overcame some of the problems of detector stability and made reconstruction simpler. An additional advantage was that the outer part of the fan beam would always pass outside the patient, and during each rotation every detector would be able to measure unattenuated radiation. This measurement could be used to adjust the calibration of each detector throughout the scanning cycle. However, the downside to the design is that the total number of detectors is increased by a factor of about 6, and this becomes prohibitive, particularly with multislice scanners. In addition, higher doses are required because of the increased distance between the patient and the detectors due to the fact that the tube has to rotate within the detector ring.

A so-called *fifth-generation scanner*, more correctly referred to as an electron beam scanner, was introduced in the early 1980s. It employed an electron source that produced an electron beam that could be focused on to and swept round a high-voltage target ring that covered a 210° arc below the patient. X-rays would be produced and following collimation detected above the patient on an offset 216° ring of detectors. Because there were no mechanical parts, the electron beam could be swept across the full arc in no more than 50 ms. This rapid imaging time permits imaging of the heart, for which the system was designed.

The *generation* terminology for describing scanners is now largely redundant. With the advent of multislice scanners, the rotate–rotate geometry of the third-generation scanner has become an industry standard. These scanners, with up to 64 submillimetre detector rows and scan times of 0.4 s or less, linked with gated data acquisition techniques and improved reconstruction algorithms, provide devices that produce genuine three-dimensional images even of the beating heart.

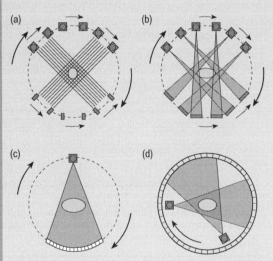

Figure 7.3 The development of the computed tomography scanner from **(a)** first to **(d)** fourth generation.

is so as to minimize the influence of the anode heel effect, because the size of the beam parallel to the axis of rotation (the z-axis) is no more than a few centimetres even with a multislice scanner.

Tubes for CT scanning have to be capable of prolonged exposure times at high milliamperage (mA). Typically, tubes have two focal spot sizes, the smallest being about 0.6 mm. Many are designed to run

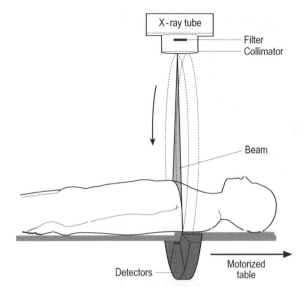

X-ray tube

Filter
Collimator

Beam

Detectors

Motorized
table

Figure 7.4 Basic components of a computed tomography scanner.

continuously for periods of 90 s or greater at 120 kV and 200 mA. To achieve this performance, they have heat capacities of 4 MJ or more. In order to reach this standard, they incorporate heat exchangers to cool the oil, and the air within the gantry enclosure is maintained at a low temperature.

Typically scanners are operated at 120 kV, but a range of kV is usually available, with three or four fixed settings between about 80 and 140 kV.

7.2.2 Collimation and filtration

Ideally, a monoenergetic photon beam would be used for CT, but this cannot be achieved with an X-ray source (see section 7.6 on beam-hardening artefacts). Earlier scanners used additional copper filters to remove low-energy photons, but because of improvements in reconstruction algorithms this is no longer necessary, and generally scanners have a total tube filtration of about 6 mm aluminium.

The collimator is mounted on the X-ray tube. The beam is collimated to a fixed width that is generally about 50 cm at the axis of rotation, sufficient to cover the full cross-section of the patient. On the z-axis, the size is variable and, in the case of the single-slice scanner, defines the imaged slice thickness; typically, there are fixed width settings between 1 and 10 mm. For single-slice scanners, there may also be a post-patient collimator. This is mounted in front of the detectors. Its purpose is to reduce scatter radiation from reaching the detectors when the slice thickness is less than the width of the detector. Some manufacturers have

also used post-patient collimation to get accurate thickness selection for the smallest slice widths.

For multislice scanners, post-patient collimation is neither necessary nor possible because the full width of the detectors in each row is used to form the image, and shielding from scatter radiation would also shield from direct radiation.

The cross-section of the patient is generally elliptical, so that at the edges of the patient the ray path from focus to detector passes through a relatively low tissue thickness. This has the effect that noise levels are poorly matched over the area of the transaxial section, being highest at the centre where doses are low, and also that the dose at the periphery and on the skin is unnecessarily high. To minimize this effect, some manufacturers introduce additional shaped filters that are thin at the centre and progressively thicker towards the edges of the fan beam. These serve to equalize the transmitted intensities emerging from the patient. They also even out the beam-hardening effect across the projected fan beam. Because of their shape, such filters are sometimes referred to as *bow tie filters*. Generally, different sizes of filter are used for head and body scanning.

7.2.3 Detectors

The requirements for scanner detectors are as follow.

- To be small in order to allow good spatial resolution. For the single-slice scanner with 600–900 individual detectors in the detector bank, the width of each detector is no more than about 1.5 mm.

- To have a high detection efficiency.

- To have a fast response with negligible afterglow so as to keep up with fast scanning times and rapid changes in radiation intensity.

- To have a wide dynamic range. The X-ray intensity may vary over a range of 5000 to 1 between the situation in which the beam passes by the side of the patient with no attenuation to that in which it passes through the lateral projection of a heavy patient.

- To have a stable, noise-free response.

Prior to the development of multislice scanners, the detector of choice for most manufacturers was the ionization chamber. It fulfilled most of the criteria above. To have a reasonably high detection efficiency linked with a small size, the chambers had to be relatively deep, i.e. elongated in the direction parallel to the X-ray beam. They used xenon gas because of its high atomic number ($Z = 54$) and K-shell binding energy (35 keV), and the gas was kept at high pressure (about 20 atm, 2 MPa). These detectors have a detection efficiency of about 60%. Ionization chamber detectors are not suitable for multislice scanners, and greater detection efficiency can now be achieved with solid state devices so that scanners with ionization detectors are no longer manufactured.

Solid state detectors incorporate a scintillant with an embedded silicon photodiode to detect the light output. The scintillant may be cadmium tungstate, bismuth germinate or a rare earth ceramic. The detection efficiency is very high (up to 98%), although it is effectively less than this because the detectors have to be separated to prevent light crossover. If this geometrical factor is included, the overall efficiency is closer to 80%. Solid state detectors can be made very small (down to about $1 \times 0.5\,mm^2$), they have negligible afterglow (i.e. signal lag), and they have a stable response.

7.3 IMAGE RECONSTRUCTION

The tube and detectors described above rotate smoothly around the patient. In the modern scanner, X-rays are produced continuously and the detectors are sampled (i.e. measurements are taken) approximately 1000 times during the course of a 360° rotation.

Figure 7.5 represents a matrix of tissue voxels traversed by the fan beam of X-rays that are then incident on the array of detectors. For simplicity, the figure is drawn with a straight detector array and with the pencil beams of photons labelled A to E parallel to each other. The signal measured by each detector depends on the attenuation coefficients of the overlying voxels that are traversed by the pencil beam as it passes through the patient. In the calculation process, account is taken of the fraction of the volume of the voxel through which the pencil beam passes, as shown by the shaded area in the figure, and of the fan beam divergence.

Figure 7.5 represents one position of the fan beam. Each individual voxel is traversed by one or more X-ray pencil beams for every measurement taken during the full 360° rotation of the gantry. The attenuation of each voxel therefore contributes to the measured transmission for a large number of the ray sums.

The logarithm of the ratio of the intensity of the unattenuated pencil beam to that measured by each detector after transmission through the patient is equal to the sum of the linear attenuation coefficients multiplied by the average path length of the pencil beam in each voxel through which the pencil beam has passed before reaching the detector. The number of measurements taken in scanning a single section of the patient depends on the number of detectors and

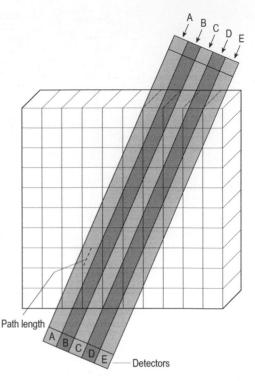

Figure 7.5 Pencil beams crossing a matrix of tissue voxels.

on the number of measurements that are taken in the full rotation. With 800 detectors and with measurements taken at 0.5° intervals, this amounts to some 576 000 individual measurements. That is more than the total number of voxels for which the attenuation coefficient is to be calculated, approximately 260 000 for a 512×512 matrix, and in theory CT numbers for each voxel could be calculated from a series of simultaneous equations. In practice, this would not work for many reasons, including the influence of individual measurement uncertainty on the final result. For the purpose of reconstruction, complex mathematical techniques referred to as *algorithms* are required.

Back projection

Most algorithms are based on the method of backprojection. The simplest illustration of this is to consider a cylindrical uniform body incorporating a hole down the centre filled with air (Fig. 7.6a). A beam passing through this body from one direction will have a transmitted profile in its central region, as shown in Figure 7.6b. This single measurement cannot determine the position of the hole other than identifying that it is in the line of the pencil beam passing through the centre of the body. Pixel values along this line are decreased by the amount calculated from the

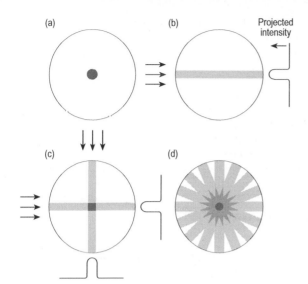

Figure 7.6 The back-projection reconstruction technique: (a) a cylindrical body with a hole running through its centre, (b) the back-projected image for a single beam, (c) the image combined with a second orthogonal beam, and (d) the reconstructed image for eight beams.

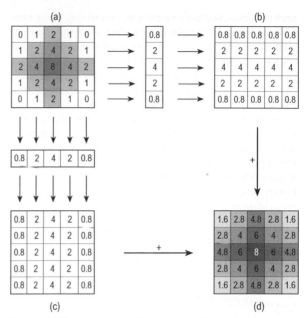

Figure 7.7 Reconstruction of a 5 × 5 matrix of values using back-projection (see text for explanation).

measurement, and these values are projected back as illustrated by the band of light grey in Figure 7.6b. A second projection at 90° provides a second band of grey as seen in Figure 7.6c, and progressive addition of projections produces the reconstruction shown in Figure 7.6d that clearly shows the hole positioned at the centre of the body but with a surrounding star-like pattern.

A second more mathematical illustration is given in Figure 7.7. In this case, the object is represented by a 5 × 5 matrix with cell values as shown (a). We consider just two projections that are represented by the sums of the values in each row and in each column. The summed values are 'projected' back as the average value of the five cells in each row and column (b) and (c), and the two back-projected images are then summed to give the final representation shown in the figure (d). In both examples, the final representation is not an accurate reproduction of the original. However, an approximate representation of the relative values in each cell is demonstrated, as shown by the shading in the figures.

Filtered back-projection

In the simplistic illustrations given above, the 'images' produced are effectively a heavily blurred version of the original object. To overcome this effect, a mathematical process called *filtering* is used. For each pencil beam measurement, the values that are projected back

into the overlying voxels use the data not just from the pencil beam itself but also from the neighbouring pencil beams. Data from the neighbouring beams can be either subtracted from or added to the projection to an extent that depends on the distance between the beams, the closest neighbouring beams having the greatest effect.

Filtered back-projection is the most common method used for image reconstruction. There are different filters and back-projection algorithms that may be applied that depend on the imaging task, for example to detect low-contrast detail or to enhance resolution in bone. It should be noted that although standard reconstruction algorithms are based on data collected from a full 360° rotation, it is possible to reconstruct from data collected over a reduced arc down to 180°. Such reconstructions may be used when imaging rapidly changing scenes, such as for CT fluoroscopy and for cardiac imaging.

Scanned projection radiographs

A standard feature on CT scanners is the facility to produce scan projection radiographs. These are known by a number of names, some proprietary, including scanogram, scout view and topogram. The scanned projection radiograph is a transmission image taken at a fixed projection angle. The collimator is generally set to the narrowest slice width, and the image is acquired as the patient table is moved through the gantry. The resultant image has a relatively poor spatial resolution when compared with a standard radiograph. However, one advantage of the technique is that there is minimal scatter. The appearance of the image is somewhat different to the conventional radiography, because there is no beam divergence along the z-axis. Scanned projection radiographs may in principle be taken at any projection angle, although in practice only the anteroposterior (or posteroanterior) and lateral views are normally required. The scans are used for planning the CT sequence, i.e. selecting scan start and end points and displaying scan slice positions.

Computed tomography fluoroscopy

Scanners commonly have the facility for so-called *CT fluoroscopy*; that is, a display of a CT image in real time. This is achieved through continuous rotation of the gantry without table movement. Using fast reconstruction techniques, generally from 180° datasets, frame rates of 5 frames s^{-1} or greater may be achieved. Most commonly, such techniques are used for biopsy needle placement. It should be noted, however, that although the effective dose may be less than for a standard diagnostic scan, there is the potential for relatively high patient skin doses because scanning is confined to a narrow region of the body. Operators have to adopt techniques that will minimize the risk of putting their fingers in the beam.

7.4 HELICAL AND MULTISLICE SCANNING

In the preceding section, the simplest form of CT scanner was described. It can be used to produce sequential transaxial slices with the patient being moved along the z-axis of the scanner between each succeeding slice. This is generally termed as *axial* scanning, although the term *step and shoot* may also be used. Scanning in this fashion is now a rarity other than for a few specific clinical protocols. Two significant developments will be considered here: helical scanning and multislice detectors.

7.4.1 Helical scanning

A major advance in scanner design was the introduction of *slip ring technology*. The X-ray tube has to be provided with a high voltage supply and the detectors have to pass their signals to the computer. If the equipment on the gantry was wired directly to external equipment, then the gantry would be able to rotate for not very much more than 360° without the cabling becoming entangled or overstretched. In older

equipment, following a single rotation of the gantry it would have to be returned to the start position, resulting in a delay of several seconds between each slice.

Slip ring technology was introduced in the early 1980s. In its simplest form, the slip ring comprises a metal ring mounted on the gantry. This is connected to the signal output from the detectors. Adjacent to the gantry there is a connector that is able to retain good contact with the ring as the gantry rotates. This connector takes the signal and passes it to the computer system for image reconstruction. To facilitate this, the detector signals have to be sent sequentially at very high frequency in order to accommodate the total number of individual detectors on the gantry and the sampling frequency. Additional rings are used to connect the X-ray generator to the external voltage supply. Connecting the system by slip ring rather than through hard wiring permits continuous, unidirectional rotation of the X-ray tube and detectors around the patient.

A basic advantage of continuous rotation is to permit faster rotation times; if the gantry can rotate through little more than 360°, then maximum rotation speed is severely limited, requiring 5 s or more per rotation. The more significant advantage is to permit continuous acquisition of data while the table moves the patient through the scan plane. Data for the complete volume to be imaged can be collected in a single exposure. This technique, introduced in the early 1990s, has been variously described as *volume*, *spiral* or *helical CT*; it is the last of these terms that will be used in this text. It has largely replaced conventional axial scanning.

A helical scan can be visualized, as in Figure 7.8a, as a ribbon wrapped around the body. If, for example, the scanner was set up with a slice width of 10 mm and it had a rotation time of 1 s and if the table movement were at a speed of 10 mm s^{-1} then, with the analogy of the ribbon wrapped round the patient, the edges of the 10-mm wide ribbon would be touching and there would be full coverage of the body. *Pitch* is defined as follows:

$$\text{pitch} = \frac{\text{tabletop movement per rotation}}{\text{slice thickness}}.$$

In the example given above, pitch = 1. For a pitch that is greater than 1, the ribbon edges would be separated; if less than 1, the ribbon edges overlap.

To reconstruct an image in helical scanning, the measured data have to be interpolated. For example, for the slice position marked in Figure 7.8b, the data to be used for the vertical downwards projection would be interpolated from data collected at positions

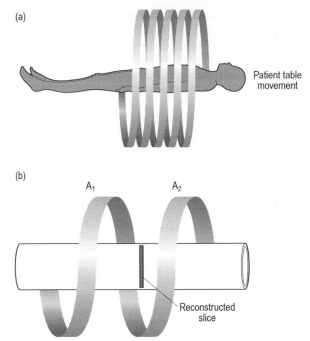

Figure 7.8 (a) The change in position of the collimated beam for a single-slice helical scanner, and (b) the method of interpolation from data collected at one angle on successive rotations of the gantry.

A_1 and A_2, the relative weight given to each being dependent on the relative distances from the plane of reconstruction. The position at which sections can be reconstructed can be anywhere within the scanned volume other than for a short distance at the start and at the end of the scan for which data are not available for interpolation. This means, for example, that if a 300 mm long volume is scanned with a 10 mm slice width and a pitch of 2, there will have been only 15 rotations (plus an extra one at each end for the purposes of interpolation). From the measured data, 30 contiguous sections, each 10 mm thick, can be reconstructed.

Although the position of the reconstructed sections can be selected retrospectively as required, the slice width cannot be less than the detector width. In the example given above, the data were collected for 10 mm thick voxels, and this is the size to which any reconstruction will match; it is not possible to extract finer detail. It is possible, however, to reconstruct on greater slice widths that are multiples of the detector width, effectively by adding adjacent slices. This technique is used with multislice scanners.

Helical scanning has a number of advantages in addition to those given above. The principal advantage is scan speed, which is beneficial for a number of reasons. For example, a scan of the chest at a pitch of 1.5 and with a slice thickness of 10 mm would take between 15 and 20 s at a rotation speed of 1 rotation s^{-1} (relatively slow for current technology). For many patients, this is possible in a single breath hold. This helps minimize the risk of *slice misregistration*. In sequential scanning, patients are asked to hold their breath for each separate slice. Because the depth of breathing is liable to vary over the time of the examination, anatomical detail, particularly close to the diaphragm, may shift in a direction parallel to the scanner axis between successive slices. This may cause a detail to be imaged on successive slices or to be missed entirely. With a single breath hold, such slice misregistration cannot occur. The other advantages of speed are patient throughput and the reduced use of contrast medium.

Increasing pitch above 1 is clearly advantageous both in reducing exposure time and in reducing patient dose (see section 7.7). However, as pitch is increased resolution is lost because of the need for greater interpolation, and it is a general rule that increasing pitch beyond 2 gives unacceptable image quality and for most clinical applications pitch is not increased beyond 1.5.

One of the consequences of helical scanning and the longer continuous exposure times associated with the technique (modern scanners generally have the capacity to expose continuously for 90 s or longer) is that a greater load is put on the X-ray tube. It is for this reason that tubes require to have the performance that was discussed in section 7.2.1.

7.4.2 Multislice scanners

In its original form, CT scanning was a two-dimensional imaging technique generating sectional views of the body on a transaxial plane. It could only be thought of as a three-dimensional technique in so far as multiple parallel sections could be imaged. True three-dimensional imaging requires isotropy; that is, the voxel size must be equal in all three dimensions. Under those circumstances, data generated in a three-dimensional matrix can be reconstructed on any plane and are not restricted to transaxial slices. In addition, with the development of ever more powerful image-processing software it is possible to display surface-rendered images, for example for reconstruction surgery, maximum intensity projections for angiography, and virtual endoscopy images, among many other potential applications.

The voxel size in the transaxial plane is determined by the matrix size and the field of view (FOV), but it is typically in the region of 1 mm (see section 7.5.1).

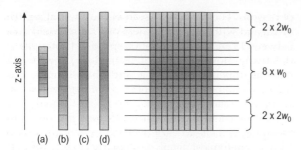

Figure 7.9 Detector configuration for an eight-slice scanner with 12 rows of detectors with four possible configurations, (a–d) – see text.

Single-slice helical scanners generally have the capability of collimating down to a slice width of 1 mm. Therefore a single-slice scanner theoretically has the capability of true three-dimensional imaging, but this is restricted by scanning time. Total scan time is limited to about 90 s because of X-ray tube limitations. Therefore with 1-s rotation speeds the volume to be imaged would be restricted to 90 mm if maximum resolution were to be achieved.

The key to true three-dimensional images lies with the multislice scanner. These scanners use solid state detectors with multiple rows of detectors. Figure 7.9 shows a typical detector configuration for an eight-slice scanner. The scanner has 12 curved detector rows with each row typically having about 800 detectors, as in the conventional scanner. Unlike the conventional scanner, however, each row is narrow, because the length of the detector along the z-axis determines the reconstructed slice width and not the collimated width of the fan beam. The detector rows are constructed to have the minimum possible gap between them consistent with a separator to prevent light crossover between detectors and to reduce the effects of scatter produced in the detectors. The configuration shown here is typical, with the central eight rows having half the length of the outer rows that are equally distributed on either side. The length of the individual detectors (parallel to the z-axis) in the central rows is typically between 0.5 and 1 mm. The detector rows may be used separately or in combination. Four possible combinations are shown in the figure. If the central detector length (w_0) were 1 mm, then the total detector length would be 16 mm. This configuration could give the following options: (a) 8×1 mm slices, (b) 8×2 mm slices, (c) 4×4 mm slices, or (d) 2×8 mm slices. Note that the dimensions given here are the size defined by the detector when projected back to the isocentre; the physical size is somewhat greater.

The eight-slice scanner described here is capable of producing scans at four slice widths: 1, 2, 4 or 8 mm. In each case, slice width is determined by the detector size and not by collimation. In theory, collimator length is set to 8 mm in option (a) above or to 16 mm for the other three options. In practice, the collimation will be somewhat greater in order to ensure that the outer two rows are uniformly covered by the X-ray beam.

An eight-slice scanner has been described here because of its relative simplicity. However, the rapid development in this technology has meant that scanners with increasing slice numbers have quickly become commonplace. Scanners with 16, 32, 40, 64 and even more rows of detectors are now available.

Multislice pitch

In single-slice helical CT, pitch is defined as the ratio of table movement during one full rotation to slice (or collimator) width. In multislice CT, it may be defined as:

$$\text{pitch} = \frac{\text{tabletop movement per rotation}}{\text{collimator length}}$$

That is essentially the same definition as single-slice helical pitch, except that slice width is replaced by the collimator length. Strictly, this should be written as nominal collimator length that is equal to the total detector length used for the scan. This is the preferred definition of pitch with values greater than 1, implying that there is a gap in data collection, whereas pitch less than 1 implies an overlap. However, some manufacturers have adopted an alternative definition in which the pitch is defined as the ratio of tabletop movement to slice width. The former definition may be referred to as *beam pitch* and the latter as *slice* or *row pitch*. In the example of the eight-slice scanner used to produce 8×1 mm slices, a beam pitch of 1 (i.e. 8 mm table movement per rotation) corresponds to a slice pitch of 8.

Multislice reconstruction

In principle, multislice and single-slice helical reconstruction techniques are the same. They involve interpolation of measured data between adjacent data-sets. However, in multislice scanning to reconstruct in a single plane within the scanned volume the data have to be interpolated for different pairs of detectors as the rotation progresses around the full 360° cycle. This is further complicated by the *cone beam effect* that is discussed in more detail in Box 7.2.

Box 7.2 Cone beam effect

Standard reconstruction algorithms assume that the X-ray beam is non-divergent in the z-direction. This is a reasonable assumption with a single-slice scanner, as shown in Figure 7.10a. The measurement made by the detector is due to voxels lying in a flat plane centred on the plane of rotation of the gantry. The figure shows two opposing projections. The beam length at the rotation axis that defines the slice width exactly matches the length of the voxel on axis. For a voxel displaced from the axis, the beam length is marginally smaller or larger than the slice width. This compromises the accuracy of calculation of CT number in that voxel, but even for a 10 mm slice, the maximum generally encountered on a single-slice scanner, this effect is marginal.

This may be compared with a multislice scanner. Figure 7.10b depicts the situation for an eight-slice scanner. The object on the rotation axis contributes to the ray sum of detector 2 and would be imaged on the slice plane defined by that detector, shown by the dashed line in the figure. However, the off-axis object that lies within the same slice plane contributes to the ray sums of detector 1 for the downwards projection, and detectors 2 and 3 for the upwards projection. In effect, the slice reconstructed from detector 2 relates to voxels within the shaded regions shown in the figure that would trace out a double cone in a full rotation.

The cone beam effect becomes more significant with increased numbers of slices and with increasing total detector length. Cone beam algorithms have had to be introduced to minimize the significance of this effect.

(a)

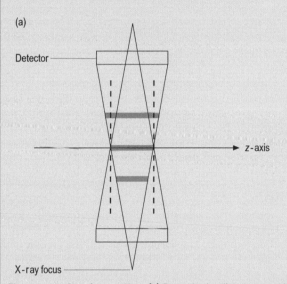

(b)

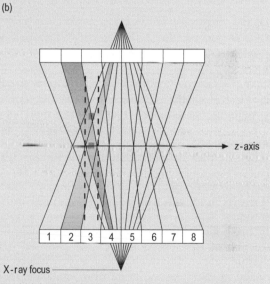

Figure 7.10 Cone beam effect. (a) For a single-slice scanner, the slice width is shown by the dashed lines and the minimal influence of beam divergence is shown by the voxel length defined by the upwards directed beam both on and displaced from the z-axis. (b) The effect of divergence in the reconstruction of out of plane slices for a multislice scanner; the dashed lines represent the plane reconstructed from detector 2.

Three-dimensional display techniques

A full discussion of image-processing and display techniques is beyond the scope of this text. However, some common techniques and the terminology to describe them are given in Box 7.3.

7.5 IMAGE QUALITY

7.5.1 Spatial resolution

The maximum high-contrast spatial resolution that may be achieved on a CT scan is about 20 lp cm^{-1},

---

Box 7.3 Three-dimensional image processing and display

There are a number of image-processing and display techniques that are commonly available for three-dimensional imaging with multislice computed tomography (CT) scanners.

- Multiplane reformatting permits display on any plane. This is commonly used to display images on the coronal and sagittal planes, but oblique plane display is also possible.

- Three-dimensional surface rendering is a technique in which the surface of a structure can be displayed. It is achieved by selecting a suitable range of CT numbers that are associated with that structure. Shading can be added to the reconstructed surface (shaded surface display) by considering the effect of light on the structure coming from a virtual light source.

- Maximum and minimum intensity projections (MIPs and MinIPs, respectively) are formed by projecting the volume of interest on to a viewing plane and

displaying the maximum (or minimum) CT number along each projected ray that forms the image. In effect, it has the appearance of a standard projection image with the background subtracted. MIP images may be used for CT angiography and MinIP for imaging the tracheobronchial region.

- Three-dimensional volume-rendering techniques such as MIPs are formed by projecting the volume of interest on to the viewing plane. However, instead of displaying the maximum voxel values along each ray path, selected ranges of CT numbers may be displayed with varying levels of opacity or with different colours to demonstrate, for example, not just the contrast-filled vessels but also adjacent structures.

- Virtual endoscopy is also a three-dimensional surface-rendering technique used to display the internal walls of body structures such as the colon. These may be referred to as fly-through projections.

---

although generally it is less than this. Note that resolution in CT is more commonly expressed in term of line pairs per centimetre rather than per millimetre, the unit that is generally used for radiography and fluoroscopy.

High-contrast spatial resolution within the scan plane is clearly limited by pixel size. Pixel size is dependent on matrix size and FOV. For example, a 512×512 matrix used with a 40 cm FOV has a pixel size of just under 0.8 mm, implying a resolution of about 6 lp cm^{-1}. However, because FOV is selectable, so in effect is pixel size. Therefore, although pixel size may determine the limit to resolution on a particular reconstructed image, it is not an intrinsic limitation; there are other factors that determine the maximum resolution that may be obtained for a particular scanner.

A second reconstruction parameter that can affect resolution is the algorithm used. Certain algorithms are designed specifically for bony structures and serve to enhance the edges of high-contrast structures. These algorithms provide improved spatial resolution at the cost of increased noise.

A factor intrinsic to the scanner is the width of the projection path of X-ray beam as it passes through the patient. This is affected by focal spot size, the geometry of the scanner (i.e. source to isocentre and source to detector distance), and the physical size of the sensitive area of the detector itself. A further factor is the

sampling frequency or number of projections sampled on each rotation. Within limits, spatial resolution increases with sampling frequency. The spatial resolution in the transaxial plane is not significantly different when comparing axial and helical scanning.

Spatial resolution in the z-direction, i.e. parallel to the rotation axis, depends on slice thickness. In single-slice helical scanning using the simple form of interpolation described in section 7.4, data collected outside the reconstructed section contribute to the transaxial image; the resolution in the z-direction is thus reduced. The greater the pitch, the greater is this effect. It is seen to a much lesser extent in multislice scanners because of the algorithms that are applied to overcome the cone beam effect.

7.5.2 Noise

Noise is a fundamental limit to the quality of the CT image, because it both reduces contrast resolution of small objects and worsens the spatial resolution of low-contrast objects. There are three sources of noise in CT images:

- quantum noise caused by random variations in the number of photons detected
- electronic noise produced in the measuring system

- structural noise that is affected by the reconstruction algorithm.

The least significant of these is electronic noise, and this will not be considered further.

Quantum noise may be reduced by increasing the number of photons contributing to each projection. There are three principal factors that affect quantum noise: mA, scan time and slice width. The first two of these are essentially linked; they both serve to increase mAs per rotation. Increasing slice width, while reducing noise, has an adverse effect on image quality because of the reduced spatial resolution and the increased partial volume effect. Signal to noise ratio (see Ch. 3.1.1), being directly related to the square root of the number of photons detected, is therefore increased by the square root of mAs and of slice width.

Quantum noise is influenced by kV. At increased kV, penetration is greater and therefore a greater number of photons are detected. Even if mA were reduced to restore dose to the same level as a scan at lower kV, the number of photons detected would be increased and noise consequently reduced. However, the influence of increased kV on noise may be offset by a reduction in contrast.

Field of view and matrix size also influence noise. For a reduced FOV or for a larger matrix, there is a smaller detector area defining each pixel. Thus there are effectively fewer photons per pixel and noise is therefore increased.

For single-slice scanners, pitch does not affect noise. At first sight, this may seem counterintuitive, because an increase in pitch reduces dose. The reason is that data are interpolated between successive rotations for a 360° scan and the same number of detected photons is effectively used in the reconstruction. The downside to increasing pitch is not an increase in noise; rather, it is an effective broadening of slice width that has an impact on spatial resolution and partial volume effect. The same is not true for multislice scanners. Reconstruction algorithms for multislice scanners also interpolate data between adjacent rotations. However, because of the cone beam effect, reconstruction is more complex than for the single-slice scanner. Interpolation involves not only the two detector rows spanning the reconstruction slice plane at the particular gantry angle; instead, data are used from all detector rows and, in the interpolation algorithm, values may be either added or subtracted at each projection angle. The net effect is to produce a scan slice that has minimal broadening in the z-direction, but this is at a cost of increasing noise with increasing pitch.

Noise becomes more apparent as window width is reduced. However, the noise is not increasing and the signal to noise ratio remains the same. Progressive reduction of window width will reveal low-contrast detail, but if the contrast between adjacent structures is comparable with the magnitude of the noise, no amount of windowing will improve the ability to resolve two structures.

7.6 IMAGE ARTEFACTS

- *Motion artefacts.* Cardiac motion produces streak artefacts (black and white bands). The reconstruction process is misled by a moving structure occupying different voxels during the scan. Mechanical misalignment and movement of the patient have similar effects.

- *High-attenuation objects.* Metal implants, dental amalgam, etc. give rise to streak artefacts that may obscure the area of interest. The streaks appear as dark and light lines emanating from the high-attenuation material. The effect is accentuated by motion. Small areas of bone or contrast medium can have a similar effect. Modern scanners commonly include metal correction algorithms that can be used to minimize the appearance of this artefact.

- *Photon starvation.* This is a variant of the streak artefact described above. A typical example might occur in the pelvis scan of a patient with bilateral hip implants. On the lateral projection, the X-ray attenuation through the two metal implants is very high and may be outside the dynamic range of the processing unit. As a result, the tissues between the hips are poorly represented in the displayed image and horizontal streaks appear across the image.

- *Beam hardening.* As the beam passes through the patient, the low-energy photons are filtered out and the beam becomes harder. This causes the attenuation coefficient and thus the CT number of a given tissue to decrease along the beam path. The reconstruction process assumes a homogeneous, i.e. monoenergetic, X-ray beam. The tissues towards the centre of the patient are invariably crossed by hardened beams, whereas those nearer the surface are for a significant part of the rotation time crossed by photon beams that have not been filtered to the same extent. The result is that CT numbers are lower in the centre of the patient than they should be. This effect may be described as cupping. In some situations, it may also result in dark streaks in the image. It can be corrected to some extent by a beam-hardening algorithm. The effect may also be reduced with the bow tie filter

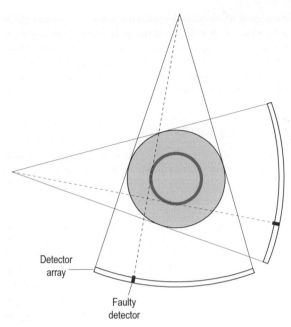

Figure 7.11 Formation of a ring artefact.

(section 7.2.2) that provides progressively increased filtration of the outer rays of the fan beam.

- *Ring artefact.* The ray passing from the tube focus to a particular detector in the row of detectors traces out a circle as the gantry rotates about the patient (Fig. 7.11). The CT numbers of the voxels that lie on that circle are calculated from the signal derived from that detector alone. Therefore, should that detector malfunction, the CT numbers in that ring will be incorrect and a light or dark ring will be seen in the image, depending on whether the detector is giving too low or too high a signal. It does not require a very big change in sensitivity of a single detector for a ring artefact to be visible. This effect can be seen on both single- and multislice scanners, although in the latter case larger changes in sensitivity are needed to make the artefact visible. An operational feature of CT scanners is that when they are switched on each day automatic calibration programmes are run to check and adjust the calibration of the detectors to ensure that they provide a balanced response.

- *Partial volume effect.* This was described in section 7.1.1.

- *Cone beam artefact.* The cone beam effect was described in section 7.4.2 and Box 7.2. If there is inadequate correction for this, an artefact is seen as a blurring at the boundaries between high-contrast details (e.g. at the boundary of bone and soft tissue).

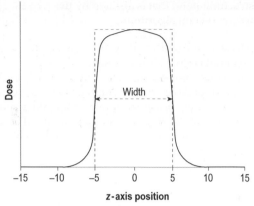

Figure 7.12 Dose profile of X-ray beam along the z-axis with an ideal square beam profile (dashed line).

7.7 DOSE

Computed tomography scanning is one of the highest dose techniques used in medical imaging. Within the UK, it has been shown to be responsible for 40% of the total population dose that is attributed to medical exposures, even though the number of CT examinations is only 4% of the total that use ionizing radiation. It is likely that the proportion of dose from CT will increase further with multislice scanners. Shorter scanning times permit greater patient throughput, thus increasing scanner availability; multislice scanners give somewhat higher doses than single-slice scanners; and three-dimensional imaging provides new clinical benefits and indications for using CT.

7.7.1 Dosimetry parameters

The *CT dose index* (*CTDI*) is a measure of dose from a single rotation of the gantry. Figure 7.12 shows a typical dose profile along the z-axis for an axial scan. It is drawn for a beam collimated to a width of 10 mm. It has a relatively flat peak, and the peak value is the maximum absorbed dose in the scan plane at the position of measurement. CTDI is defined as follows:

$$CTDI = \frac{\int D(z) \bullet dz}{T}$$

in which the dose at position z, $D(z)$, is integrated over the complete dose profile and divided by the nominal slice width, T.

The CTDI is measured using a pencil ionization chamber. This has a diameter that is typically about 8 mm and length of 100 mm, which is significantly greater than the maximum slice width that is to be measured. The measured dose multiplied by the length of the chamber represents the integration of

Table 7.2 DLP to effective dose conversion coefficients (E/DLP)

	E/DLP mSv (mGy cm)$^{-1}$
Head	0.0023
Chest	0.018
Liver	0.015
Abdomen and pelvis	0.017

DIP, dose–length product; E, effective dose.

Table 7.3 Typical doses for computed tomography scans

	CTDI$_W$ (mGy)	DLP (mGy cm)	E (mSv)
Head	60	700	1.5
Chest	14	400	7
Liver	16	350	5.5
Abdomen and pelvis	16	500	8.5

CTDI$_w$, CT dose index (weighted value); DLP, dose–length product; E, effective dose.

the dose profile, and division by the nominal width equals the CTDI.

The peak dose in the profile shown in Figure 7.12 is virtually independent of slice width; it depends only on scanner design, particularly filtration, and the kV and mAs settings. Therefore, provided that the collimation is accurate and the true profile width is equal to the nominal width, the integrated dose is directly proportional to width and CTDI is constant with width.

The CTDI is a useful parameter to assess the dose within the scan plane. If we consider the ideal square beam profile shown in Figure 7.12, it describes approximately the same area as the true profile, and therefore CTDI is a close approximation of the maximum dose at the position of measurement. There are internationally accepted standards for CTDI that involve measurement in cylindrical perspex phantoms. These have diameters of 16 and 32 cm to represent head and body scans, respectively. Measurements are made in the centre of the phantom and in several locations on the periphery in order to derive a weighted value ($CTDI_w$) for the complete cross-section that is an approximation to the average dose. For most standard scanning protocols, $CTDI_w$ is in the range 10–40 mGy (Table 7.3). Dividing $CTDI_w$ by pitch (beam pitch in the case of multislice scanners) gives $CTDI_{vol}$, which is an approximation to the average absorbed dose within the scanned volume. Maximum skin dose is approximately equal to $CTDI_w$ for scans of the head and about 20% higher for body scans. It can be seen that skin doses in CT are much higher than for radiographic examinations (Table 2.2) but not as high as doses from prolonged fluoroscopy.

The CTDI is useful for describing the dose efficiency of a scan protocol and for comparisons between scan models. However, it is less useful for a comparison of doses to individual patients, because attention also has to be given to the length of scan and to the number of times a particular region might be scanned (e.g. pre- and postadministration of contrast medium). *Dose–length product* (DLP) is defined as:

$$DLP = CTDI_{vol} \times L,$$

in which L is the total scan length. The length can be estimated from the total tabletop movement, but with helical scanning and particularly multislice helical scanning there is some over-scanning, with an additional part rotation at the beginning and end of the scan. This degree of over-scanning may be particularly significant for short scan lengths. Therefore more correctly length may be estimated from the number of rotations multiplied by collimated length and pitch.

Effective dose (E) can be derived from DLP using various published data sources. Conversion coefficients depend on the body region and on scanner design. Some approximate values are given in Table 7.2. It can be seen that the ratio E/DLP is much lower in the head than for regions in the trunk, and that it is also lower for the chest than for scans involving the pelvis. The differences are due to the distribution of the organs and tissues having the highest tissue weighting factors (w_T) that are used for the calculation of effective dose (Ch. 2.3.2). Tissues and organs in the head have relatively low weighting factors, whereas the highest w_T is for the gonads, resulting in the highest E/DLP factor being associated with scans of the pelvis.

Table 7.3 gives typical doses for some common CT examinations.

7.7.2 Factors influencing patient dose

It is not the intention here to consider how particular features of scanner design and construction (hardware and software) might influence patient dose. Such issues may influence the equipment selection process, but they do not affect the way in which equipment is used. The main concern of this text is the influence of operator-selectable parameters on dose. It needs to be recognized that selection of scanning parameters is interdependent; altering parameter A might well require adjustment of parameter B in order to maintain adequate imaging quality.

In setting up a new scan protocol, the parameters that the radiologist and radiographer may consider are likely to include:

- kV
- mA
- rotation time
- reconstructed slice width
- helical or axial acquisition
- pitch
- number of detector rows (multislice)
- reconstruction algorithm
- FOV.

In addition, the dose depends on scanned length (this is both protocol- and patient-dependent) and on patient build. The operator-selectable parameters above will be considered in turn.

Tube potential (kV) is commonly set to 120 kV, but for areas of high attenuation a higher setting may be used. Radiation output increases with kV (by about 40% for an increase of 20 kV), but attenuation in the patient is lowered. Therefore higher kV increases dose, but for the same level of noise in the image the mA may be reduced sufficiently to give an overall dose reduction to the patient.

The influence of mA and rotation time may be taken together as mAs per rotation. This is a key parameter to be selected when establishing a scanning protocol, because of the direct relationship between mAs and dose and the inverse dependence of noise on the square root of mAs. Scan protocols should be based on the maximum acceptable level of noise to give the optimum balance of image quality and dose.

Commonly, scanners include an option for mA modulation. In this technique, mA is adjusted with the aim of achieving a near constant detector signal so that changes in patient size through the scan region do not significantly influence the level of noise. The techniques used are manufacturer-dependent, but in principle the aim is to use higher mA on the thicker lateral projections compared with anteroposterior, and to adjust mA in accordance with changes in patient cross-section over the length of the scan and for patient to patient variations in build. Modulation is based on measured transmission through the patient, using either data from prescan scanned projection radiographs or from the previous rotation. Dose reduction in the range 10–40% may be achieved in comparison with constant mA techniques.

In a single-slice scanner, patient dose is generally independent of slice width. It was noted above that CTDI does not vary with slice width because the integration of the dose profile is normalized to slice width. Therefore DLP, the product of CTDI and scan length, should remain constant with changes in slice width. For example, a 200 mm long region may be scanned using 20 rotations and a 10 mm slice width or 100 rotations with a 2 mm slice width. The CTDI for the two geometries is the same as is the total scan length.

The first caveat to this general rule is that for some single-slice scanners the narrowest beam, nominally 1 mm, may be defined by post-patient collimation, and the beam size passing through the patient might be significantly greater. For such equipment, use of the narrowest slice width could produce a significantly increased dose. However, this is a very special case that only applies to a few single-slice scanners. It does not apply to multislice scanners.

The second caveat to the rule that slice thickness does not increase dose is to emphasize that this is only if the mAs is not changed. Reducing reconstructed slice thickness increases noise, as noted in section 7.5.2. Therefore as a general rule the use of narrower reconstructed slices is associated with an increase in dose, but this is not because of slice width per se; rather, it is due to the associated increase in mA.

The choice of helical rather than axial scanning does not influence dose other than the small amount of over-scanning at the start and end of the scan. The increase in dose is equivalent to an additional rotation of the gantry. Patient dose is inversely proportional to pitch, and therefore the use of a pitch of 1.5 rather than 1 leads to a 33% dose reduction.

In principle, the number of detector rows used together in a multislice scanner has no influence on dose, but some models of scanner have a better geometrical efficiency than others. Nor is there any direct influence of the reconstruction algorithm or the FOV. However, both of these last two do influence noise and image quality and will influence the choice of mA.

It is generally accepted that doses with multislice CT scanners are greater than with single-slice scanners. Some of these are intrinsic to the technology. One of these is the need for over-scanning at the start and end of each scan. This is true for helical scanning in general but is a larger effect for multislice because of the greater length of the detector. Of greater significance is over-collimation. For a single-slice scanner, the collimator length defines slice width. For an 8 mm slice the collimator is set precisely to 8 mm; if the beam width were any greater, a thicker slice would be produced. For the multislice scanner, the reconstructed slice width is defined by the length of the detectors in the detector rows. If, in the example given in section 7.4.2, the detector rows were combined to produce four 4 mm slices per rotation, the collimator width would have to be no less than 16 mm, otherwise the interpolation routines would be inaccurate. Therefore a tolerance is applied, and the overall beam length is likely to be about 2 mm greater than that required. This automatically increases dose to the patient by more than 10%.

Doses are also increased because of the method of use. Whereas previously it might have been standard practice to scan on 10 mm slice widths, it is now possible within shorter scanning times to produce 5 mm slices or less, thus providing potentially improved diagnostic information. However, reconstruction on thinner slices increases noise, and to compensate mAs, and thus dose, may be increased.

7.8 SUMMARY

- CT scanners generate images in transaxial slices.

- The CT number represents the average linear attenuation coefficient in the voxel.

- Contrast in the displayed image is enhanced by windowing.

- The scanner gantry carries the X-ray tube and generator and a curved bank of detectors.

- The image is reconstructed by filtered back-projection.

- Slip ring technology allows the gantry to rotate about the patient continuously.

- In helical scanning, the patient is moved through the gantry while the gantry rotates.

- Helical pitch is defined as the ratio of table movement per rotation and slice thickness.

- Multislice scanners have several rows of detectors (64 or more) that are able to collect data simultaneously.

- Multislice scanning can produce three-dimensional image data for reconstruction on any plane.

- Spatial resolution is limited to about 20 lp cm^{-1}.

- Quantum noise is the main limit to low-contrast resolution.

- Dose is generally higher for CT than other X-ray imaging techniques.

Chapter 8

Gamma imaging

8.1 RADIOACTIVITY

Stable nuclei

Nearly all the nuclides extant in the world are stable. Apart from the nucleus of ordinary hydrogen, which consists of a single proton, all the stable lighter nuclei contain nearly equal numbers of protons and neutrons. For example, the nucleus of a helium atom (otherwise known as an alpha particle) is a very stable combination of two neutrons and two protons. The heavier nuclei contain a greater proportion of neutrons.

Isotopes

Isotopes of an element are nuclides that have the *same* number of protons (atomic number), position in the periodic table, and chemical and metabolic properties but a *different* number of neutrons, mass number (protons plus neutrons), density and other physical properties.

The nuclei of all carbon atoms contain six protons. Ninety-nine percent of stable carbon nuclei are carbon-12, with six neutrons, while 1% are carbon-13, with seven neutrons. Carbon-11 (^{11}C), with only five neutrons, has a neutron deficit, while carbon-14 (^{14}C), with eight neutrons, has a neutron excess; both are artificially produced, unstable and radioactive. Note that all four nuclides are isotopes of carbon.

Radionuclides

Unstable nuclei, having a neutron excess or deficit, are radioactive and transform spontaneously (or decay) until they become stable nuclei, with the emission of any combination of alpha, beta and gamma radiation. Naturally occurring radionuclides such as uranium, radium, radon, ^{14}C and potassium-40 contribute to our background radiation exposure, whether external to the body or internal.

Production of radionuclides There are more than 2700 known radionuclides. A few of these are sufficiently long-lived to occur in nature. However, those used in medical imaging must be produced artificially, in the following ways.

- If an additional neutron is forced into a stable nucleus, so that it now has a *neutron excess*, the new nucleus is likely to be unstable. This process occurs in a *nuclear reactor*. For example, with molybdenum:

$$^{98}\text{Mo} + \text{n} \rightarrow {}^{99}\text{Mo}.$$

The atomic number of the nucleus remains unchanged, but its mass number has increased by one. Radionuclides produced in a nuclear reactor cannot be separated from the original stable nuclides, as they have the same atomic number and so the same chemical properties. They cannot be made carrier-free.

- If an additional proton is forced into a stable nucleus, knocking out a neutron so that it now has a *neutron deficit*, the new nucleus is likely to be unstable. For example, with oxygen:

$$^{18}\text{O} + \text{p} \rightarrow {}^{18}\text{F} + \text{n}.$$

The mass number of the nucleus has not changed, but its atomic number has increased by one to become fluorine. This process occurs in a *cyclotron*, which accelerates positively charged ions – protons, deuterons or alpha particles – on to the target material to produce radionuclides that are typically neutron-deficient.

Radionuclides produced in a cyclotron can be obtained carrier-free. They can be separated chemically from the original stable nuclides, as they have different atomic numbers and so different chemical properties. They are also short-lived (with half-lives ranging from less than a minute to a couple of hours; the term *half-life* is defined later), and so it is only possible to use them reasonably close to the cyclotron. Medical minicyclotrons have been designed specially for the production of short-lived radionuclides such as fluorine-18 (^{18}F) at or near the hospital site.

- Radioactive *fission products* may be extracted from the spent fuel rods of nuclear reactors.

$$^{238}\text{U} \rightarrow {}^{99}\text{Mo} + \text{other fission by-products.}$$

As the molybdenum is different chemically from the other products, it can be separated and prepared in a very pure form.

- In addition to the nuclear reactor and the cyclotron, some radionuclides are daughter products obtained from *generators* that contain a longer-lived radioactive parent. Useful daughter products are technetium-99m ($^{99}\text{Tc}^{m}$; see section 8.3) from a molybdenum-99 (^{99}Mo)/$^{99}\text{Tc}^{m}$ generator, and the positron emitter gallium-68 (^{68}Ga) from a germanium-68 (^{68}Ge/^{68}Ga) generator.

8.2 RADIOACTIVE TRANSFORMATION (DECAY)

Radionuclides with a neutron excess: β^{-} decay

Radionuclides with a neutron excess may lose energy and become stable by a neutron changing into a proton plus an electron. The electron is ejected from the nucleus with high energy and is referred to as a negative beta particle:

$$\text{n} \rightarrow \text{p} + \beta^{-}.$$

For example, iodine-131 (^{131}I), with atomic number 53, decays in this way to xenon-131, with atomic number 54. There has been no change of mass number, but the atomic number has increased by 1. Nearly always, the product or daughter nucleus is produced with excess energy. Usually, it loses this immediately, with the emission of one or more gamma photons, leaving the daughter nucleus with minimum energy, in the ground state.

Isomeric transition In the case of some radionuclides, the gamma ray is not emitted until an appreciable time after the emission of the beta particle. For example, when ^{99}Mo decays by the emission of a negative beta particle, the daughter nucleus technetium remains in the excited state for a variable length of time, which averages a matter of hours. It is said to be *metastable* and is written as $^{99}\text{Tc}^{m}$. Its decay to the ground state, technetium-99 (^{99}Tc), is most often with the emission of a gamma ray of energy 140 keV. ^{99}Tc has a very long half-life (see Table 8.1) but eventually decays to a stable nuclide, ruthenium-99.

$$^{99}_{42}\text{Mo} \xrightarrow[67\,\text{h}]{\beta,\gamma} {}^{99}_{43}\text{Tc}^{m} \xrightarrow[6\,\text{h}]{\gamma} {}^{99}_{43}\text{Tc}$$
$$\xrightarrow[2 \times 10^{5}\,\text{a}]{\beta,\gamma} \text{stable } {}^{99}_{44}\text{Ru}$$

Note the convention used:

$$\text{parent nuclide} \xrightarrow[\text{half-life}]{\text{emission}} \text{daughter nuclide}$$

Both $^{99}\text{Tc}^{m}$ and ^{99}Tc are said to be isomers, nuclei having different energy states and half-lives but otherwise indistinguishable as regards mass number, atomic number, numbers of protons and neutrons, and other properties.

Table 8.1 Half-lives of some radionuclides used in imaging

Half–life	Radionuclide
13 s	Krypton-81m
1 min	Rubidium-82
10 min	Nitrogen-13
20 min	Carbon-11
68 min	Gallium-68
110 min	Fluorine-18
6 h	Technetium-99m
13 h	Iodine-123
67 h	Molybdenum-99
67 h	Indium-111
73 h	Thallium-201
78 h	Gallium-67
5 days	Xenon-133
8 days	Iodine-131
200 000 years	Technetium-99

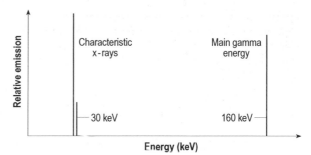

Figure 8.1 Photon line spectrum for iodine-123.

Whereas ^{99}Mo emits both beta and gamma rays, ^{99}Tc^m emits gamma rays only. The transformation,

$$^{99}\text{Tc}^m \rightarrow {}^{99}\text{Tc} + \gamma,$$

is an isomeric transition.

Another isomeric transition used in gamma imaging occurs when rubidium-81 decays to krypton-81:

$$^{81}_{37}\text{Rb} \xrightarrow[\;4.7\,\text{h}\;]{\beta^+,\gamma} {}^{81}_{36}\text{Kr}^m \xrightarrow[\;13\,\text{s}\;]{\gamma} {}^{81}_{36}\text{Kr}$$

$$\xrightarrow[\;2\times10^5\,\text{a}\;]{\gamma} \text{stable } {}^{81}_{35}\text{Br}$$

Radionuclides with a neutron deficit: β^+ decay or K-electron capture

β^+ decay   Radionuclides with a neutron deficit may lose energy and become stable by a proton within the nucleus changing into a neutron and a positive electron. The latter is ejected from the nucleus with high energy and is referred to as a positive beta particle (or *positron*). Mass and charge are conserved:

$$p \rightarrow n + \beta^+.$$

For example, ^{18}F, with atomic number 9, transforms into oxygen-18, with atomic number 8. There has been no change of mass number, but the atomic number has decreased by 1. The product or daughter nucleus, if left in an excited state, which is not the case here, loses its excess energy by the emission of one or more gamma photons until it reaches the ground state.

K-electron capture

Alternatively, the nucleus may increase its number of neutrons relative to the number of protons by capturing an extranuclear electron from the nearest (K) shell. Mass and charge are again conserved:

$$p + e^- \rightarrow n.$$

The daughter nuclide will emit K-characteristic X-rays when an electron from an outer shell fills the hole created in the K-shell. If the daughter nuclide is left in an excited state, it will also emit gamma rays. For example, iodine-123 (^{123}I) decays wholly by electron capture and emits 160 keV gamma and 28 keV X-rays but no positive beta particles.

Gamma rays

The gamma rays emitted during radioactive decay of a given radionuclide have at most a few specific energies (forming a line spectrum) that are characteristic of the nuclide that emits them. For example, ^{131}I emits mostly 360 keV gamma rays. Gamma rays have identical properties to X-rays, as described in Chapter 1.

Internal conversion   The gamma rays emitted by some nuclei do not leave the atom but are photoelectrically absorbed within its K-shell. As a result of this internal conversion, such radionuclides (e.g. iodine-125, ^{125}I) emit both photoelectrons and characteristic X-rays, usually of fairly low energy (less than 35 keV in this case). As an example, Figure 8.1 gives the simplified photon spectrum for another iodine isotope, ^{123}I, which is more useful for imaging than ^{125}I because of its higher-energy photon emission and shorter half-life (around 13 h).

Beta rays

Beta rays are emitted with a continuous spectrum of energies up to a maximum E_{max}, which is characteristic of the radionuclide. Their average energy is about $E_{max}/3$. When positive and negative beta particles travel through a material, being moving electrons they interact with the outer shells of the atoms they pass nearby and excite and ionize them. The track of the particle is dotted with ion pairs. When it has lost

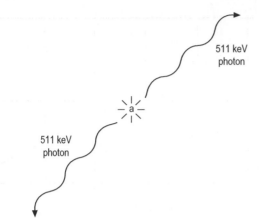

Figure 8.2 Positron annihilation: a is the point where positron meets electron and they annihilate.

the whole of its initial energy, it comes to the end of its range. The greater the initial energy of the beta particle, the greater its range. The range is inversely proportional to the density of the material. The most energetic beta rays have a range of a few millimetres in tissue.

Positron emitters
Positive electrons, being antimatter, have a very brief existence. When a positive beta particle comes to the end of its range, it combines with a nearby negative electron. The opposite charges neutralize each other, and the combined masses of the two electrons are wholly converted into energy. According to Einstein's formula ($E = mc^2$) for the equivalence between energy E and mass m, the mass of each electron is equivalent to 511 keV. When the positive and negative electrons annihilate each other, the energy is emitted as two photons of annihilation radiation (each of 511 keV) travelling in opposite directions (see Fig. 8.2). Positron emitters are used in positron emission tomography (PET) imaging (see section 8.5.2).

Radioactive decay
Radioactive disintegration is a stochastic process, governed by the statistical laws of chance. It is impossible to predict which of the unstable nuclei in a sample will disintegrate in the next second, but it is possible to be quite precise about the fraction that will do so on account of the large numbers of nuclei the sample contains.

Activity A radioactive nucleus does not make its presence known until it decays and emits a beta or gamma ray, or both. The quantity of radioactivity is

measured not by the 'population', the mass or number of radioactive atoms, but by the transformation rate, i.e. the number that disintegrate per second, also referred to as the decay rate.

The activity of a radioactive sample is the rate of disintegration, the number of nuclei disintegrating per second. The SI unit is the becquerel (Bq) = 1 disintegration s^{-1}. This is a very low activity – the natural radioactive content of the human body is about 2 kBq (2000 Bq). In imaging, most radionuclide administrations are measured in megabecquerels (1 MBq = 10^6 Bq), and the activity of radionuclide generators in gigabecquerels (1 GBq = 10^9 Bq). (A unit found in old textbooks is the curie, Ci: 1 mCi = 37 MBq.)

When the beta or gamma rays enter a detector, they may be registered individually as counts. The count rate (number of counts per second, cps) measured by a given instrument is less than the activity, because the greater proportion of the rays usually miss the detector and some pass through it undetected. However, there is a proportionality:

count rate ∝ activity ∝ number or mass of radioactive atoms in the sample.

The fundamental *law of radioactive decay* states that the activity of a radioactive sample decreases by equal fractions (percentages) in equal intervals of time. This is referred to as the exponential law.

Physical half–life The half-life ($t_{1/2}$) of a radionuclide is the time taken for its activity to decay to half of its original value. For example, two successive half-lives reduce the activity of a radionuclide by a factor of $2 \times 2 = 4$. Ten half-lives reduce the activity by a factor of $2^{10} \approx 1000$.

This half-life is more properly called the physical half-life. It is a fixed characteristic of the radionuclide; cannot be predicted for a given radionuclide in any way; and is unaffected by any agency such as heat, pressure, electricity or chemical reactions. It can range from fractions of a second (useless in imaging) to millennia in the case of ^{99}Tc (also useless in imaging). Examples are given in Table 8.1.

Exponential decay However long the time, the activity of a radioactive sample never falls to zero. A graph of radioactivity versus time shows this clearly. If the graph is plotted using linear scales for both axes, it is referred to as an exponential curve. If, however, the activity is plotted on a logarithmic scale, a straight line graph results (Fig. 8.3), making it easier to read off the half-life.

Such graphs are useful in calculating the activity that must be prepared at a particular time for use at a subsequent time, and how long it is necessary to store

Figure 8.3 Exponential decay. Activity on a logarithmic scale against time on a linear scale.

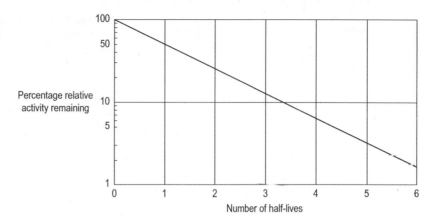

radioactive material before it becomes sufficiently harmless to be disposed of safely.

Effective half–life   When a radionuclide is used in imaging, it usually forms part of a salt or organic compound, the metabolic properties of which ensure that it concentrates in the tissues or organ of interest. A pharmaceutical that has been labelled with a radionuclide is referred to as a radiopharmaceutical.

If the pharmaceutical alone is administered, it is gradually eliminated from the tissues, organ and whole body by the usual metabolic processes of turnover and excretion. Such a process can be regarded as having a biological half life, t_{biol}.

If the radionuclide is stored in a bottle, its activity decays with its physical half-life, t_{phys}.

If the radiopharmaceutical is administered to a person, the radioactivity in specific tissues, an organ or the whole body decreases because of the simultaneous effects of radioactive decay and metabolic turnover and excretion. The radiopharmaceutical can be regarded as having an effective half-life, t_{eff}.

The effective half-life is shorter than either the biological or physical half-lives. In fact:

$$1/t_{eff} = 1/t_{biol} + 1/t_{phys}.$$

It depends on the radiopharmaceutical used and the organ etc. involved and can vary from person to person, depending on their disease state.

8.3   RADIOPHARMACEUTICALS

Desirable properties
Desirable properties of a *radionuclide* for imaging are as follow.

- A physical half-life of a few hours, similar to the time from preparation to injection. If the half-life is too short, much more activity must be prepared than is actually injected.

- Decay to a stable daughter or at least one with a very long half-life (e.g. ^{99}Tc has half-life of about 200 000 years).

- Emission of gamma rays (which produce the image) but no alpha or beta particles nor very low-energy photons (which have a short range in tissue [see Ch. 2.2] and deposit unnecessary dose in the patient). Decay by isomeric transition or electron capture is therefore preferred.

- Emission of gamma rays of energy 50–300 keV and ideally about 150 keV – high enough to exit the patient but low enough to be easily collimated and easily detected.

- Ideally, emission of monoenergetic gamma rays so that scatter can be eliminated by energy discrimination with a pulse height analyser (PHA).

- Easily and firmly attached to the pharmaceutical at room temperature but has no effect on its metabolism.

- Readily available at the hospital site.

- A high specific activity, i.e. high activity per unit volume.

In addition, the *radiopharmaceutical* should:

- localize largely and quickly in the target, the tissues of diagnostic interest
- be eliminated from the body with an effective half-life similar to the duration of the examination, to reduce the dose to the patient
- have a low toxicity
- form a stable product both *in vitro* and *in vivo*
- be readily available and inexpensive per patient dose.

The decay during transport and storage of a short-lived radionuclide is reduced if it can be supplied with its longer-lived parent in a generator.

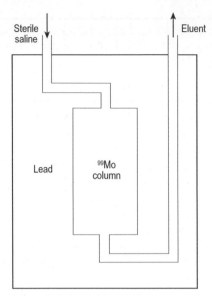

Figure 8.4 A technetium-99m generator.

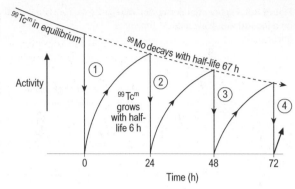

Figure 8.5 Decay of activity of molybdenum-99 and growth and regrowth of activity of technetium-99m in a generator that is eluted daily.

Technetium generator

Technetium-99m is used in 90% of radionuclide imaging, as it fulfils most of the above criteria. With its gamma energy of 140 keV, it is easily collimated and easily absorbed in a fairly thin crystal, thus giving good spatial resolution. With its short half-life (6h) and pure gamma emission, a reasonably large activity can be administered, reducing noise in the image. It is supplied from a generator shielded with lead. As the simplified cross-section in Figure 8.4 shows, this contains an exchange column of alumina beads on which have been absorbed a compound of the parent ^{99}Mo (which can be produced in a reactor and has a 67h half-life).

When the generator is delivered, the activity of the daughter ^{99}Tc^m has built up to its maximum, equal to that of the parent ^{99}Mo. The daughter is decaying as quickly as it is being formed by the decay of its parent. It is said to be in transient equilibrium with the parent. The daughter and parent decay together with the half-life of the parent, 67h (left-hand side of Fig. 8.5).

The technetium is washed off the column (*eluted*) as sodium pertechnetate with sterile saline solution. This flows under pressure from a reservoir through the column into a rubber-capped sterile container. The precise design of the generator and pressure system depends on the manufacturer. Elution takes a few minutes and leaves behind the molybdenum, which is firmly attached to the column.

Thereafter, the eluant decays with its own half-life of 6h. At the same time, after the elution at (1) in

Figure 8.5, the ^{99}Tc^m in the column increases with the same half-life of 6h. After 24h, the activity has grown again to a new maximum (equilibrium) value. (After 6h, it has reached 50% of the maximum; after 12h, 75%; and so on.)

Figure 8.5 plots the activity of ^{99}Mo (dashed line) and ^{99}Tc^m (solid line) against time, following the first elution (1) at time 0. Elution can be made daily, although it will be seen that the strength of successive eluants (2, 3, ...) diminishes in line with the decay of ^{99}Mo. After a week, the generator is usually replaced and the old one is returned for recycling. If necessary, the column can be eluted twice daily.

Uses of technetium-99m

Sodium pertechnetate-99m is used for imaging the tissues, which take it up on account of its similarity to iodide and chloride ions: the thyroid (by which it is trapped but not fully metabolized), the gastric mucosa (localization of Meckel's diverticulum) and the salivary glands. Blocked from the thyroid by administration of potassium perchlorate, it can be used for cerebral blood flow and testicular imaging and, mixed with bran porridge, for gastric-emptying studies.

Technetium can easily be labelled to a wide variety of useful compounds, for example:

- methylene diphosphonate (MDP), for bone imaging
- hexamethyl propylene amine oxime (HMPAO), for cerebral imaging
- dimercaptosuccinic acid (DMSA) and mercaptoacetyltriglycine (MAG3) for renal studies
- iminodiacetic acid (HIDA) for biliary studies
- human serum albumin (HSA) colloidal particles, 0.5 μm in size, which are phagocytosed in

reticuloendothelial cells – imaging of liver, spleen and red bone marrow

● HSA macroaggregates – 15 to 100 μm microspheres that temporarily block a small fraction of the capillaries in lung perfusion imaging

● diethylene triamine pentacetic acid (DTPA) aerosol (5 μm particles) in lung ventilation studies

● autologous red cells, for cardiac function

● heat-damaged autologous red cells, for imaging the spleen

● sestamibi or tetrofosmin, for cardiac perfusion imaging.

Other radionuclides and their uses

Iodine is avidly trapped and metabolized by the thyroid, which was the first organ ever imaged, and ^{131}I was the first radionuclide used for imaging. It was cheap, highly reactive and an excellent label. It is produced in a reactor and has a long shelf life (half-life 8 days) but emits beta rays as well as rather energetic (mainly 364 keV) gamma rays. It has therefore largely been replaced for imaging by ^{123}I, which is more expensive, is cyclotron produced, has a half-life of 13 h, and decays by electron capture, emitting 159 keV gamma rays. It is also more expensive than, but otherwise superior to, ^{125}I, with its long half-life (60 days) and low photon energy (around 30 keV). It may be labelled to hippuran for renal studies, being cleared by both glomerular filtration and tubular secretion. Note, however, that both ^{131}I and ^{125}I are used for therapy, for thyroid ablation and as brachytherapy seeds, respectively.

Xenon-133 (^{133}Xe) is produced in a reactor, has a half-life of 5.2 days and emits beta rays and rather low-energy (81 keV) gamma rays. It is an inert gas, although somewhat soluble in blood and fat, and is used, with rebreathing, in lung ventilation imaging.

Krypton-81m ($^{81}Kr^m$), another inert gas, is generator-produced, has a half-life of 13 s and emits 190 keV gamma rays. The generator is eluted with compressed air, the patient inhaling the air–$^{81}Kr^m$ mixture in pulmonary ventilation studies. The short half-life (4.7 h) of the parent, ^{81}Rb, presents transport difficulties, and means that it must be used the day it is delivered.

Gallium-67 (^{67}Ga) is cyclotron-produced, has a half-life of 78 h, and decays by electron capture, emitting gamma rays of three main energies (93, 185 and 300 keV). Gallium citrate is used to detect tumours and abscesses, as it binds to plasma proteins.

Indium-111 (^{111}In) is cyclotron-produced, has a half-life of 67 h, and decays by electron capture, emitting 173 and 247 keV gamma rays. It is used to label white blood cells and platelets for locating abscesses and thromboses, respectively.

Indium-113m is sometimes used instead of ^{111}In, is generator-produced, has a half-life of 100 min, and emits only gamma rays, but they have a high energy (390 keV).

Thallium-201 (^{201}Tl) is cyclotron-produced, has a half-life of 73 h, and decays by electron capture, emitting 80 keV X-rays. An analogue of potassium, it is used as thallous chloride in myocardial perfusion imaging, where its half-life is well suited to repeated imaging over a few hours.

Positron emitters are needed for PET (see section 8.5.2). The most common PET radionuclide is ^{18}F, with a half-life of 110 min, often used in the form of ^{18}F 2-fluoro-2-deoxyglucose (2-FDG) for brain and heart metabolism as well as epilepsy and tumour detection. Other radionuclides used for PET are ^{11}C, nitrogen-13, oxygen-15 and rubidium-82 (^{82}Rb), but these have very short half-lives: 20 min, 10 min, 2 min and 75 s, respectively. The last of these, ^{82}Rb, produced from a strontium-82 generator that lasts about 1 month, can be used for myocardial perfusion imaging. Perhaps a more useful radionuclide is technetium-94m, cyclotron-produced with a half-life of 50 min, as it can be used to label many pharmaceuticals already available for $^{99}Tc^m$ imaging.

Preparation of radiopharmaceuticals

This usually involves the simple mixing or shaking at room temperature of the radionuclide (e.g. $^{99}Tc^m$ as sodium pertechnetate) with the compound to be labelled (e.g. MDP) and other necessary chemicals. Shielded syringes are used to transfer the components between sterile vials. The manipulations are carried out under sterile conditions in a workstation, for example a glove box or a sterile laminar down-flow cabinet that admits the entry of hands etc. through a curtain of air flowing down across the open face of the cabinet. The cabinet is located in a room that is under a positive pressure of filtered sterile air.

All surfaces are impervious: continuous floors, gloss-painted walls, and formica-topped or stainless steel benches. Entry is via an air lock and changing room. Normal sterile procedures are followed. The radiopharmacy must meet the conditions of both the Medicines Act and the Ionising Radiations Regulations in the UK, or the relevant regulations in other countries.

With preparation time being necessarily short for PET radiopharmaceuticals, automated synthesis devices using microprocessor control are commonly used. These also greatly reduce the radiation exposure of the staff.

Quality control includes testing for:

● radionuclide purity – for example testing for contamination with ^{99}Mo, which would give an unnecessary dose to the patient, by measuring any gamma radiation from ^{99}Mo after blocking off the gamma rays from ^{99}Tc^m with 6 mm lead

- *radiochemical purity* – for example testing for free pertechnetate in a labelled ^{99}Tc^m compound using chromatography

- *chemical purity* – for example the spot colour test for alumina, which may have come from the ^{99}Mo column and would interfere with labelling

- *sterility testing and pyrogen testing* – the results of which are available only retrospectively, for example after the main part of the eluant has been used

- *response of the radionuclide calibrator* (see section 8.7) – for example to a standard source with a long half-life.

8.4 PLANAR IMAGING

The patient is given an appropriate radiopharmaceutical, usually by intravenous injection. The function of the pharmaceutical is, ideally, to concentrate in the organ or tissues of interest. The role of the radionuclide is to signal the location of the radiopharmaceutical by the emission of gamma rays. The radionuclide most commonly used, ^{99}Tc^m, emits 140 keV gamma rays. These are detected by a gamma camera, and an image of the radioactive distribution is produced on a monitor screen. As gamma rays cannot be focused, instead of a lens a multihole collimator is used to delineate the image from the patient.

A gamma camera has heavy lead shielding to attenuate unwanted background gamma radiation coming from the patient generally, any other sources in the room, and building materials. The following sections describe the components of a typical gamma camera with a circular head for imaging ^{99}Tc^m.

The multihole collimator

The patient is positioned, as shown in Figure 8.6, close to the collimator. This consists of a lead disc, typically 25 mm thick and up to 400 mm in diameter. It is drilled with some 20 000 closely packed circular or hexagonal holes, each about 2.5 mm in diameter. They are separated by septa 0.3 mm thick that absorb all but a few per cent of the rays attempting to pass through them obliquely. (The half-value layer of lead for ^{99}Tc^m gamma rays is 0.3 mm.)

Each hole only accepts gamma rays from a narrow channel, thus locating any radioactive source along its line of sight. For example, in Figure 8.6, ray a is accepted by the collimator and ray b rejected. However, other rays, such as c, can be scattered in the body and then pass through the collimator. These rays will have less energy and so can be rejected later by energy discrimination (see under *Pulse height analyser*, below). Other types of collimator are described in a later paragraph.

The crystal

Instead of using a large number of tiny detectors, behind the collimator there lies a single large phosphor crystal some 500 mm in diameter and 9–12 mm thick, usually made of sodium iodide (activated with a trace of thallium), NaI(Tl). Having a high atomic number ($Z = 53$) and density, it absorbs about 90% of ^{99}Tc^m gamma rays, principally by the photoelectric process, but only some 30% of those from ^{131}I. It is fragile and easily damaged by temperature changes. To protect it from light and moisture in the atmosphere (it is hygroscopic), it is encapsulated in an aluminium cylinder with one transparent face.

Each gamma photon (such as photon a in Fig. 8.6), when absorbed by the crystal, produces a flash of light, shown by the dashed lines in the diagram. The flash contains some 5000 light photons, which travel in

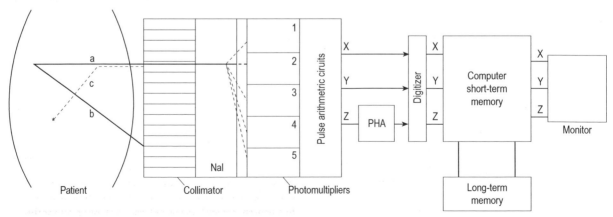

Figure 8.6 A gamma camera with a parallel hole collimator. PHA, pulse height analyser.

all directions and last less than a microsecond. About 4000 of them emerge via the transparent face, having been reflected off the other faces, which are coated with a reflecting titanium compound. The distribution of light leaving the face of the crystal depends on which collimator hole the gamma ray passed through and is measured by up to 91 matched photomultipliers, closely packed in a hexagonal array. Five of these are shown, diagrammatically, in Figure 8.6. A light guide, a flat transparent plate, can maximize transfer of light from the crystal to the photomultipliers.

Photomultipliers

Each photomultiplier (Fig. 8.7) consists of an evacuated glass envelope containing (on the left) a photocathode coated with a material that absorbs light and emits photoelectrons – one electron per 5 or 10 light photons. These are accelerated toward a positive anode (on the right). On route, they impinge on a series of dynodes that are connected to progressively increasing positive potentials. Four such dynodes are shown in the diagram.

When each electron strikes a dynode, it knocks out some three or four electrons, which are then accelerated, as shown, to strike the next dynode. In this way, after 10 stages, the electrons have been multiplied by a factor $4^{10} \approx 10^6$. Thus each initial flash of light produces a pulse of charge or voltage large enough to be measured electronically. The amplification factor is very sensitive to changes in the overall voltage (about 1 kV), which has to be highly stabilized.

Pulse arithmetic (position logic)

Returning to Figure 8.6, the light pulse illuminates differentially the array of photomultiplier tubes. It produces the largest electrical pulse in the photomultiplier (no. 2) nearest to the collimator hole through which the gamma ray a passed, and smaller pulses in adjacent photomultipliers. A microprocessor chip, the pulse arithmetic circuit, combines the pulses from all the photomultipliers according to certain equations.

This yields three voltage pulses (X, Y and Z), which are proportional to:

- The horizontal and vertical coordinates (X, Y) of the light flash in the crystal, the hole through which the gamma ray has passed, and so the (X, Y) position in the body of the radioactive atom that has emitted it.

- The photon energy of the gamma ray (Z). For this purpose, the pulses from all the photomultipliers are simply summed as if there were one large photomultiplier, measuring all the light produced by the gamma ray in the phosphor crystal. The size or 'height' of the Z-pulse (so many volts) is proportional to the gamma ray energy (in keV) absorbed by the crystal. For convenience, the pulse height is generally stated in the corresponding keV.

Pulse height spectrum

The account so far ignores two facts:

- gamma rays are scattered in the patient, so that gamma rays that have originated outside the line of sight of the collimator can enter a collimator hole and, as they have been scattered, do so with reduced energy (ray c in Fig. 8.6)

- gamma rays may lose energy through Compton interactions in the crystal before escaping from the crystal, and so produce pulses of reduced height.

When a large number of gamma rays are emitted in succession from a patient, the Z pulses therefore vary in height. Taking $^{99}Tc^m$ as an example, Figure 8.8 illustrates a sequence of such pulses; it plots the pulse height (proportional to the photon energy) against time. Only the pulses that fall inside the PHA window, set around the photopeak for $^{99}Tc^m$, are selected to form the gamma image. Figure 8.9 plots the relative number of pulses (counts) having various heights or

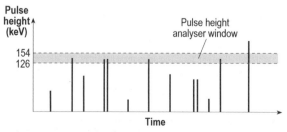

Figure 8.8 Graph against time of 'height' or voltage of pulses coming in succession from a photomultiplier coupled to a phosphor crystal. The pulse height analyser is set for the detection of photons from technetium-99m.

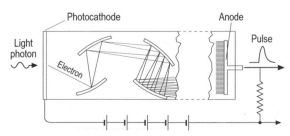

Figure 8.7 Photomultiplier tube.

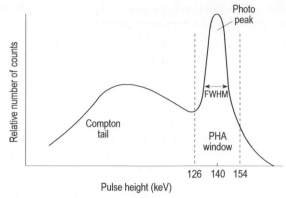

Figure 8.9 A pulse height spectrum showing the relative frequency of pulses of various heights.
FWHM, full width at half maximum; PHA, pulse height analyser.

energies in a given period of time. This pulse height spectrum is made up of the following.

- A *photopeak*, on the right, comprising pulses produced by the complete photoelectric absorption in the crystal of those gamma ray photons that have come from the patient without suffering Compton scattering within the patient. They vary somewhat in height, lying within a 'window' shown by the horizontal dashed lines in Figure 8.8 and vertical dashed lines in Figure 8.9.

    This spread of energies in the photopeak is caused by statistical fluctuations in both the number of light photons produced in the crystal by each gamma ray photon, and the number of electrons produced in the photomultiplier by each light photon. This also contributes to the short tail on the right.

- A *tail*, on the left, containing pulses of lower energy, mostly produced by those gamma rays that have suffered Compton interactions in either the patient or the crystal. (There is also, not shown in Fig. 8.9, a subsidiary iodine escape peak at 30 keV below the photopeak, due to some of the K-characteristic rays from iodine escaping from the crystal.) Only pulses in the photopeak are of use in locating the position of the radioactivity in the patient, and a PHA is used to reject those in the Compton tail.

Pulse height analyser

As shown in Figure 8.6, the Z-pulses enter a PHA, which is set by the operator to reject pulses that are either lower than a preset value or higher than another preset value. It lets through only those pulses that

lie within a window of, say, ±10% of the photopeak energy. The pulses so selected are referred to as counts. As Figure 8.8 illustrates, any high-energy pulses (e.g. cosmic rays or as a result of pulse 'pile-up', i.e. two or more gamma rays being detected simultaneously) are also rejected.

In the case of $^{99}Tc^m$, the window might be set at 126–154 keV, centred on 140 keV (Fig. 8.8). Even so, because a 140 keV photon will lose only 10 keV of energy even when scattered through 45°, some scattered photons may 'pass through' the window, produce counts and so degrade the image. In the case of ^{67}Ga or ^{111}In, two or three windows must be used simultaneously, each selecting one of the emitted gamma ray energies.

The X-, Y- and Z-pulses are next sent, as shown in Figure 8.6, via analogue to digital converters into a computer. This enables dynamic and gated studies to be undertaken as well as a range of image processing.

The computer

After digitizing the pulses with an analogue to digital converter, the X-, Y- and Z-pulses pass to a computer that records each Z-pulse as a count in a memory location corresponding to the X- and Y-coordinates. As the pulses arrive at random, the counts build up in each location and are stored as a digital image in a matrix (e.g. of 128 × 128 pixels). Once complete, the image is displayed on a monitor screen (e.g. as a 128 × 128 matrix of 3 mm pixels). The brightness of each pixel depends on the number of counts stored in the corresponding memory location, i.e. in proportion to the number of gamma rays that have emanated from the corresponding area of the patient and to the activity therein located.

Note that, if counts were acquired for too long, the memory locations would become full (an 8-bit memory can hold 2^8 counts) and the monitor screen would become more or less uniformly bright. If they were acquired for too short a time, the image would be grainy. Typically, a total of 500 000 or 1 million counts are acquired for each image frame.

Before (or after) initial display, the stored image can be manipulated and improved in the usual ways for any digital image. Background can be suppressed, blurring reduced, contrast enhanced by windowing, noise reduced by averaging, and the matrix increased and made less evident by pixel interpolation. Quantitative data can be extracted (e.g. a plot of activity along a selected line). Separate images of two radionuclides, administered at the same time, can be obtained with different settings of the PHA. Indeed, one image can be subtracted, pixel by pixel, from the other, similarly to digital subtraction angiography.

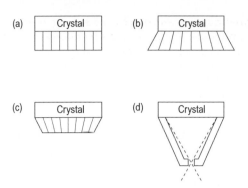

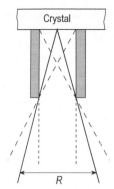

Figure 8.10 Types of collimator: (a) parallel hole, (b) divergent hole, (c) convergent hole, and (d) pinhole.

Figure 8.11 Spatial resolution of a single-hole collimator.

Types of gamma camera

The 400 mm general purpose camera described above has been optimized for $^{99}Tc^m$. Mobile gamma cameras have been designed for cardiac imaging. These generally have a 250 mm field and a crystal 5 mm thick, which give good spatial resolution with the 80 keV gamma rays from ^{201}Tl. Being easy to position, it is used in cardiac stress laboratories and intensive care units.

A large field of view (FOV: 500 mm) camera can take in the whole width of the patient and is used in bone and gallium imaging. A scanning gamma camera, in which the camera head transverses along the long axis of the supine patient, effectively increases the image matrix.

Collimators

Most commonly used with a 400 mm camera is the parallel hole collimator (Figs 8.6 and 8.10a). The FOV and the in-air sensitivity are the same at all distances from the collimator face.

With a smaller-diameter camera, a larger FOV can be obtained by a divergent hole collimator (Fig. 8.10b), which minifies the image, allowing a large organ such as the lung to be imaged with a small crystal such as in a mobile gamma camera. A convergent hole collimator (Fig. 8.10c), in which the holes converge to a point in the patient, magnifies the image but reduces the FOV and may be useful when imaging children or small organs. Spatial resolution deteriorates slightly towards the edge of the field.

Both of these special collimators, b and c in Figure 8.10, suffer from geometrical distortion: the back of an organ is minified or magnified differently from the front, and the FOV and in-air sensitivity both vary with distance.

A pinhole collimator (Fig. 8.10d), a cone of lead with a single hole a few millimetres in diameter at its apex, can be used to produce a magnified but inverted image of a superficial small organ such as the thyroid.

The sensitivity of a collimator measures the proportion of gamma rays falling on it from all directions that pass through the holes. It is typically only a fraction of 1%. The more holes there are, or the wider they are or the shorter they are, the greater the sensitivity, the less radionuclide needs to be administered, and so the less the patient dose.

Spatial resolution Figure 8.11 illustrates one of the holes in a parallel hole collimator, lying between the crystal and the surface of the patient. Gamma rays originating anywhere between the inner dotted lines 'illuminate' the whole of the 'visible' crystal surface and produce a maximum signal. Gamma rays originating anywhere outside the outer dashed lines are cut off by the lead septa and produce no signal. Gamma rays originating from any points along the solid lines illuminate exactly half of the crystal face. R is a measure of the spatial resolution of the collimator. R is larger, i.e. the resolution is worse, when the distance of the source from the face of the collimator is increased. Resolution is best close to the collimator, and the patient should be positioned accordingly.

The wider the holes or the shorter they are, the more gamma rays are seen and so the greater the sensitivity but the worse the spatial resolution. It follows that the better the resolution, the less the sensitivity. It is not possible to *maximize* both sensitivity and spatial resolution (unless something else is sacrificed, e.g. FOV), and an optimum compromise must be made. This is a major limitation to the performance of a gamma camera.

Types of collimator *Low-energy collimators* have thin septa (0.3 mm) and can be used with gamma rays of up to 150 keV (e.g. with $^{99}Tc^m$). A *general purpose* collimator might have 20 000 holes each 2.5 mm diameter, a resolution (10 cm from the face) of 9 mm, and sensitivity 150 cps MBq^{-1}. A *high-resolution* collimator would have more and smaller holes and lower sensitivity. It can be used where high resolution is required and the amount of radioactivity and the imaging times needed are acceptable. A *high-sensitivity* collimator would have fewer and larger holes and poorer resolution. It can be used in dynamic imaging where short exposure times are necessary and the poorer resolution must be accepted. *Medium-energy collimators*, for use up to 400 keV (e.g. with ^{111}In, ^{67}Ga and ^{131}I), have thicker septa (1.4 mm) and consequently fewer holes and lower sensitivity (see also section 8.6).

Dynamic imaging

The function of kidneys, lungs, the heart, etc. can be studied by acquiring a series of separate image frames in suitably rapid succession. The images can be retrieved from the computer stored in sequence and either recorded side by side on a single film in a multiformat camera, or repeatedly displayed *seriatim* on the screen as a cine loop.

Regions of interest (ROI) (e.g. kidneys) can be defined by cursors, and the total counts therein measured on each frame and displayed as a function of time (e.g. a renogram). An area of interest between the kidneys can be defined and used for background subtraction to improve the signal to noise. An example of the uptake and excretion of iodine-labelled hippuran is shown in Figure 8.12.

In typical multiple-gated (MUGA) cardiac studies, separate images, each lasting 40 ms, are acquired at 20–30 different points in each cardiac cycle. At each such point, several hundred successive images are added, pixel by pixel, to improve statistics and so reduce noise.

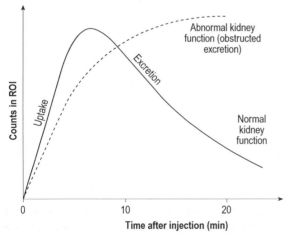

Figure 8.12 Renogram using iodine–123-labelled hippuran. ROI, region of interest.

Each sequence is initiated by the R-wave from an electrocardiogram. The images can be recorded separately in a multiformat mode or displayed as a video of the pulsating heart. Quantitative data about heart function, such as left ventricular ejection fraction (LVEF) and peak left ventricular filling rate, can also be extracted.

8.5 TOMOGRAPHY WITH RADIONUCLIDES

Conventional planar gamma imaging, so far described, produces a two-dimensional projection of a three-dimensional distribution of a radiopharmaceutical; the images of organs are superimposed, depth information is lost and contrast is reduced. These deficiencies are addressed in emission tomography, which uses the same principles as X-ray or transmission computed tomography (CT) to reconstruct the images of a series of parallel body sections. There are two methods: *single-photon emission computed tomography* (*SPECT* or *SPET*) and PET.

8.5.1 Single–photon emission computed tomography

In its simplest form, a gamma camera with a parallel hole collimator rotates slowly in a circular orbit around the patient lying on a narrow cantilever couch. Every 6°, the camera halts for 20–30 s and acquires a view of the patient; 60 views are taken from different directions, each, however, comprising fewer counts than in conventional static imaging. Some 3 million counts are acquired in an overall scanning time of around 30 min. Image acquisition time is halved or the sensitivity improved by using a dual- or triple-headed camera.

Figure 8.13 shows just two positions of the single camera, which is represented schematically by its equivalent pixel matrix. Each column set of pixels, two or three pixels wide, like the one identified in the diagram, corresponds to a transverse slice through the patient. Each pixel corresponds to a line of sight, along which the counts from the radionuclide are summed – the emission analogue of a pencil beam in X-ray CT.

The considerable amount of gamma ray *attenuation* that takes place in the patient would result in fewer counts from the centre than from the edges. Allowance for this is made, by means of an algorithm for gamma attenuation through the tissues, in reconstructing the image. An approximate method of attenuation correction is to add the counts, pixel by pixel, in each pair of opposing views (Fig. 8.13). The combined counts are then more nearly the same, whether the same amount of activity is near the centre (a in Fig. 8.13) or near the edge of the patient's transverse section (b).

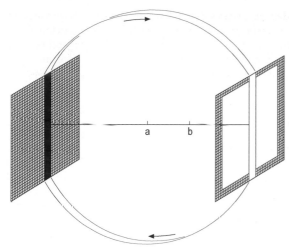

Figure 8.13 A single-photon emission computed tomography imaging system.

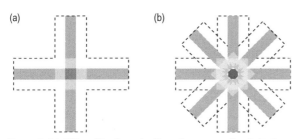

Figure 8.14 Filtered back-projection of a source of activity in the patient (a) after two angle projections and (b) after four angle projections.

The 60 sets of data (or two-dimensional projections) are synthesized into a set of transverse images by methods similar to those used in X-ray CT – *filtered back-projection* (see Ch. 7.3). This mathematical 'filtering' process can perhaps be understood more easily here than in the X-ray case. Figure 8.14 shows a single source of activity with differing amounts of *negative* counts projected in 'stripes' along either side of the stripes of true positive counts. A sufficient number of projections taken all around the patient add up to form the image free of star artefacts, with the background also reduced by the negative counts to give much improved contrast. However, an area of very high activity (e.g. the bladder or the injection site) can cause streaking of the image and even hide adjacent areas of activity. This is a limitation of filtered back-projection. An alternative algorithm, *iterative reconstruction*, whereby the image activity content is adjusted in steps until the calculated activity in the image is as close as possible to the measured activity

(counts), is less sensitive to such artefacts and can also correct accurately for attenuation. Other advantages of iterative reconstruction include insensitivity to noise and the ability to reconstruct an image even when data acquisition is incomplete. This can occur if the camera cannot be rotated all around the patient so the projections are missing at some angles.

A stack of 20–30 parallel transverse sections can be imaged simultaneously in SPECT. If required, sagittal, coronal and oblique sections can be derived from the transverse sections. It is also possible to display a continuously rotating three-dimensional representation, as in multislice X-ray CT.

The SPECT images can be severely photon-limited. *Noise* is high because of the limited number of counts in each voxel. Very few of the photons emitted in the patient are collected by the collimator holes corresponding to each slice. Photons are collected for only 20–30 s for each image, and the long overall imaging time is limited by patient movement, although movement compensation techniques can be used during image reconstruction. Making the slices thicker could reduce noise, but that would increase partial volume artefacts. The need to reduce noise often limits the pixel matrix to 64×64 and the number of views to 60, i.e. 30 pairs. Noise can also be reduced by mathematical filtering, but again at the cost of reduced spatial resolution, or by using iterative reconstruction.

Each slice is therefore reconstructed typically from only 64 measurements in each of 30 or more angular positions. On account of this and the need to use high-sensitivity collimators, the *spatial resolution* in the reconstructed image may be no better than 18 mm, i.e. about $3 \times$ pixel size. This is worse than a conventional gamma image and much worse than X-ray CT.

The image reconstruction process often magnifies the effect of noise and also of any non-uniformity in the field. Automatic balancing of the photomultipliers is desirable. The photomultipliers would be affected by changes in their orientation, as the camera rotates, if they were not shielded from the earth's magnetic field. For similar reasons, the gantry must be extremely well made. Maintenance and quality assurance are both particularly important.

The camera must move on a sufficiently large circular orbit to miss the patient's shoulders. An elliptical orbit is sometimes used to minimize the gap between the collimator and the patient and so improve resolution. Rotation of 180° is a useful option (e.g. in cardiac tomography). Some dedicated equipment uses three or four gamma cameras equally spaced around the rotating gantry, thus improving sensitivity. The increased sensitivity can be used for faster patient throughput or to improve the resolution.

As indicated above, SPECT studies can be presented either as a series of slices or as a *three-dimensional display*. The latter is particularly effective when the image is rotated continuously on the computer screen, as persistence of vision helps to reduce the effects of image noise. Thallium studies of myocardial infarctions and ischaemia are major uses of SPECT, along with quantitative cerebral blood flow. Other applications, such as the detection of tumours and bone irregularities, are increasing in clinical usefulness, particularly when SPECT is combined with CT to correct for tissue attenuation.

Gated acquisitions are also possible with SPECT as in planar imaging (e.g. MUGA studies). Cardiac gated myocardial SPECT can be used to obtain quantitative information about myocardial perfusion, thickness of the myocardium, left ventricular ejection fraction, stroke volume and cardiac output. Indeed, SPECT is probably the clinical standard for assessment of myocardial ischaemia, although PET now offers more accuracy and better spatial resolution.

8.5.2 Positron emission tomography

The most common positron emitter used in PET is ^{18}F. When ^{18}F emits a positive beta particle (positron), this travels for about 2 mm through the patient before being annihilated by a negative electron. Their combined mass (positron plus electron) is converted into two energetic photons, each of exactly 511 keV, emitted simultaneously and in practically opposite directions (but not exactly so, if the positron is moving when annihilated). PET imaging (Fig. 8.15) is based on detecting these two annihilation photons in coincidence and identifying their origin in the patient to locate the radioactive source.

A *positron* or *PET camera* comprises a ring, hexagon or other polygon surrounding the patient and composed of a very large number of solid scintillation detectors (10 000–20 000), often of bismuth germanate

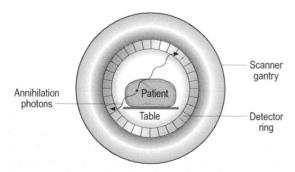

Figure 8.15 Cross-section through a patient inside a positron emission tomography scanner.

(BGO). Other efficient scintillators, such as lutetium oxyorthosilicate (LSO) or gadolinium oxyorthosilicate (GSO), are also in use. The ideal choice would be readily available, cheap to produce, and easy to manufacture into crystal blocks, with:

- high detection efficiency – to absorb and convert 511 keV photons into light
- very short scintillation decay time
- good energy resolution.

As usual, a compromise is necessary; see Table 8.2, which also shows a comparison with sodium iodide, which is normally used in gamma cameras.

Positron emission tomography detectors are commonly made in block format, coupled to photomultiplier tubes (see Fig. 8.16). Note that the detector material, configuration, number of detector blocks and number of photomultiplier tubes depend on the manufacturer, but the principles of operation are the same.

If, as in Figure 8.17, the annihilation photons from the event at (a) enter detectors A and B, they produce simultaneous (coincident) pulses, which are then accepted and combined by the electronics. Any pulses that do not coincide in time are ignored by the electronics, as are any single photons of background radiation. These two detectors therefore measure only the sum of the activity present along a line AB, called the line of response (LOR) – and similarly for each of the many pairs of detectors – which is just the information required for tomographic reconstruction, as in CT or SPECT. However, as the detection mechanism is different, so is the data acquisition (see below).

Each detector can operate in coincidence with perhaps half of the detectors that face it in the ring, so that the patient is criss-crossed by hundreds of LORs, just some of which are shown in the single ring of Figure 8.17. There are three types of coincidences that can occur: true, as in Figures 8.17 and 8.18 a; random, from independent events, as in Figure 8.18 b, that may not occur in the same plane (ring); and scatter, as in Figure 8.18 c, that may also be cross-plane. To reduce the random and scatter events from adjacent rings, narrow lead or tungsten septa (about 1 mm thick by up to 10 mm deep, Fig. 8.19) can be used between each ring of detectors to act like a parallel antiscatter grid in radiography. In modern PET scanners with block detectors set in a series of rings, data acquisition is fast and contiguous. The axial FOV is given by the width of the complete set of rings. As in CT, the patient is moved along the axis of the scanner to obtain the next set of sequential transverse slices.

In data acquisition, the summed count of each LOR is plotted as a function of its angle to and shortest

Table 8.2 Properties of some scintillation detectors compared with sodium iodide

Property or material	Bismuth germanate	Lutetium oxyorthosilicate	Gadolinium oxyorthosilicate	NaI(Tl)
Effective atomic number	75	66	59	51
Relative light output	15	75	25	100
Decay time	300 ns	40 ns	60 ns	230 ns
Typical energy resolution at 511 keV[a]	25%	25%	15%	10%

NaI(Tl), sodium iodide activated with a trace of thallium.
[a]For commercial scanners.

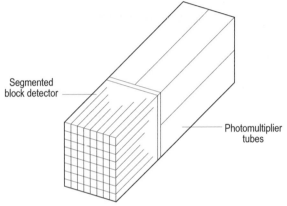

Figure 8.16 Block detector configuration commonly used in positron emission tomography scanners, with opaque reflective layers in the slots between the segments.

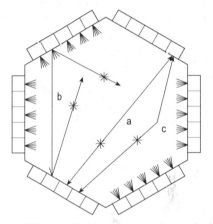

Figure 8.18 Different coincidence events: a, true coincidence; b, random coincidence; and c, scatter coincidence.

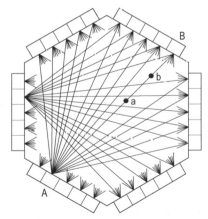

Figure 8.17 A positron emission tomography imaging system showing some lines of response. The event at a is detected at A and B in coincidence.

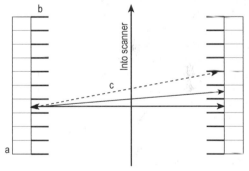

Figure 8.19 Adjacent rings of detectors, a, with interplane septa, b, to reduce detection of cross-plane coincidences, c.

distance from the centre of the scanner (see Fig. 8.20). Each detector pair receiving a coincidence from the same location in the patient will contribute to a point on the same half *sine wave*, as in Figure 8.20b. Thus the composite intensity plot (Fig. 8.20c) is called a

sinogram and comprises a number of blurred sine waves with different amplitudes and phases. Each time a coincidence occurs for a given LOR (or detector pair), this is added to that pixel in the sinogram. The fan angle of LORs from any given detector is plotted as a diagonal across the sinogram. Each horizontal row of the sinogram corresponds to all the LORs,

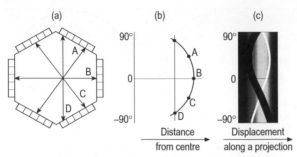

Figure 8.20 Sinogram production. (a) Four lines of response (A–D) from one source of activity, (b) plotted on a sine wave, and (c) combined in the sinogram with multiple sine waves from all other data points for all the sources of activity in the image slice to be reconstructed.

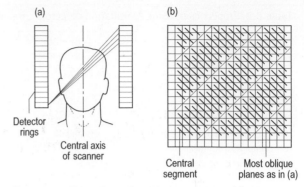

Figure 8.21 Three-dimensional data acquisition: (a) oblique planes and (b) a Michelogram organized into five segments.

parallel to each other at the *same angle* of orientation, and can be converted into the projection of the slice associated with that angle (see Fig. 8.20b). Each transverse slice through the patient has its own sinogram, which comprises all the data for that slice across all projection angles (see Fig. 8.20c). (Note that this contrasts with SPECT, for which the data in each acquired two-dimensional projection image are from all slices at that angle.) The set of acquired PET sinograms is computer-analysed to give a series of *projection views* like those acquired for SPECT.

The reconstruction algorithm includes a correction for *tissue attenuation.* Indeed, because the combined distance travelled in tissue by the two photons is the same whether the annihilation took place at, for example, a or b in Figure 8.17, attenuation depends only on the patient's dimensions and tissue structures. A transmission scan of the patient enables this correction to be made. This is usually made immediately before or after the emission scan using a long-lived radioactive source (^{68}Ge or caesium-137, ^{137}Cs) located in the scanner gantry (or the CT scan for PET–CT, see later). The source is rotated around the patient and the paired detectors' response is compared with an earlier scan made without the patient. As the attenuation correction is comparatively large at 511 keV, it significantly improves the contrast and detail in the PET images.

When the detectors are in a circle, the LORs of the detector pairs are bunched together at the sides of the gantry and more uniformly spaced at the centre. An *arc correction* compensates for this effect, which is more important for large organs where the LORs are likely to be away from the centre.

Data acquisition depends on the scanner and can be in two-dimensional mode, as described above, using septa and producing sinograms. However, greater sensitivity, up to 6 times that of two-dimensional,

can be gained by not using septa and collecting data from all the rings at once in so-called three-dimensional mode, although this obviously increases the scatter fraction, actually from 10 to about 40%. This is called three-dimensional because detection is not just from the two-dimensional array from the ring around the patient but also includes the other rings located axially into the gantry (see Fig. 8.21). Data are acquired into a three-dimensional sinogram, sometimes called a *Michelogram*, whereby several (typically five) axially angled views of the patient are collected at each projection angle. Whereas two-dimensional data can be reconstructed into independent parallel slices, three-dimensional data must be rebinned to resemble two-dimensional data before this can be done. Alternatively, a special three-dimensional reconstruction algorithm is used. Some scanners that can retract the septa can be operated in either mode. (Note that two-dimensional and three-dimensional refer to the data acquisition mode and not to image reconstruction; either mode can be used to produce three-dimensional images from the sets of transverse slices, as for CT and magnetic resonance imaging, MRI.)

The main positron emitter used in PET imaging is ^{18}F (half-life 110 min), primarily used to label deoxyglucose (FDG). Other useful radionuclides are ^{68}Ga (68 min) and ^{82}Rb (1 min), particularly as these two are produced by radionuclide generators (see section 8.1). The effective dose to the patient (see section 8.7) is much the same as in routine gamma imaging, as the short half-life of the positron emitters compensates for the beta energy deposition.

Dual-headed conventional gamma cameras used for planar imaging or SPECT can have integrated coincidence circuitry to enable them to function also as PET scanners. Data are acquired by rotating the cameras around the patient, *without* the collimators in

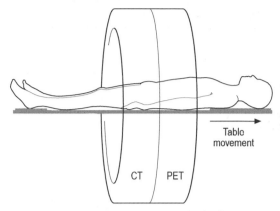

Figure 8.22 A positron emission tomography (PET)–computed tomography (CT) combined imaging system.

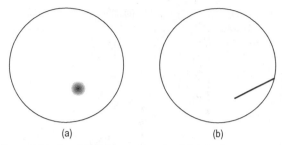

Figure 8.23 Flood field images showing (a) defective photomultiplier tube and (b) damaged crystal.

place. The sensitivity of the sodium iodide crystals for the 511 keV photons is much lower than for BGO (see Table 8.2), so a thicker crystal will give better results, and the higher background noise level reduces overall contrast in the image. The spatial resolution is also poor compared with a purpose-built PET scanner. Note that PET imaging has stimulated the production of pharmaceuticals labelled with ^{123}I and ^{99}Tc^m, which can cross the blood–brain barrier, for use in SPECT – which can be a simpler and cheaper alternative to PET for cerebral blood flow imaging.

Positron emission tomography images (as with all gamma images) give functional and physiological information. To be able to locate and visualize this information within the patient's anatomy, PET (and SPECT) images are usefully fused with CT images or MRI images. Combining two sets of such digital images is often complicated by the need for adjustment of matrix size, matching rotational position, the transverse plane and coregistration to enable one to one spatial matching of the images. Commercial image fusion software is available to do this. However, spatial matching when images are obtained at different times on different equipment also has uncertainties because of patient positioning, movement, etc., and even the best algorithms used can produce fused images that are misaligned by several millimetres.

To overcome these problems, integrated PET–CT systems are used (Fig. 8.22). Both detection systems are mounted on the same support, adjacent to each other, so that the single patient table moves along the central axis. Once the CT scan is complete, the patient table moves into position for the PET data collection; almost perfect matching of the images is obtained, except for involuntary patient movement. The CT scan can also be used for the PET attenuation corrections,

and so a whole body study with the two sets of images can be obtained in less than 30 min. The combined images are particularly useful in oncology, both for diagnosis and for accurate tumour location and follow-up. Carefully gating image acquisition to the cardiac cycle can also produce useful fused images in cardiology.

8.6 CHARACTERISTICS AND QUALITY ASSURANCE OF GAMMA IMAGES

Uniformity of detector response
A conventional gamma camera should give a uniform response to a uniform field. A flood field or sheet phantom is used to check this. It consists of a flat sealed plate, larger than the FOV and usually filled with cobalt-57 (^{57}Co), which has a similar gamma emission to but is longer-lived than ^{99}Tc^m. This should give a uniform image with the collimator in place: a defective photomultiplier will be seen as an area of reduced counts in the image (Fig. 8.23a). A cracked crystal will show as a linear defect (Fig. 8.23b). Non-uniformity caused by the usual slight differences in the performance of individual photomultipliers is analysed by counts in each pixel, and image data acquisition can be compensated automatically from this analysis. However, regular checks are needed to monitor any deterioration in the photomultipliers.

Background radiation checks are useful to identify contamination of the gamma camera or its collimator, or even the presence of a local unshielded source. A high reading obtained whatever the camera orientation indicates contamination on the crystal or the camera head; subsequent high readings, obtained once the collimator is in place, indicate collimator contamination.

The detector uniformity of a PET scanner is checked using either a long-lived source (^{68}Ge or ^{137}Cs) mounted on the gantry and rotating it around the field to expose all the detectors uniformly, or a standard phantom with a centrally located positron

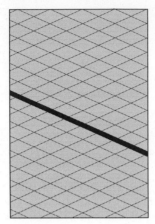

Figure 8.24 Defective detector block showing as a diagonal streak in the positron emission tomography sinogram.

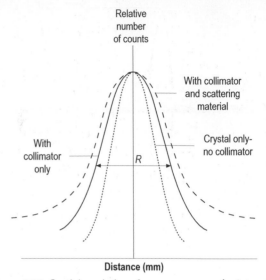

Figure 8.25 Spatial resolution of a gamma camera (*point spread function*) under different conditions. (Each curve is plotted relative to its own maximum value.)

source. The sinogram should be uniform, any malfunctioning detector block appearing as a diagonal streak covering all the angles with each detector block in coincidence with it (Fig. 8.24).

Spatial resolution

This is the ability of the system to produce distinct images of two small radioactive sources, and is often defined as the *minimum distance* at which the two sources can still be resolved. *Intrinsic resolution* refers to the camera (crystal, photomultipliers and position logic circuits) in the absence of the collimator and patient. When a single gamma photon is absorbed at a point in the crystal, the 4000 or so photons of emerging light eject only a total of 400 or so electrons from the photocathodes of all the photomultipliers. In Figure 8.6, photomultipliers numbered 1 and 3 should receive equal numbers of photons and produce identical pulses. However, on account of the small numbers of light photons and electrons involved, there are significant statistical variations in the relative numbers and so a difference in the heights of the pulses they produce. This leads to errors in the X- and Y-coordinates assigned to the event, and so causes blurring of the image. Intrinsic resolution could be improved by using a thinner crystal, so that the light has less distance to travel before reaching the photomultiplier tube. However, this results in a consequent reduction in sensitivity, especially if the camera is used for imaging medium and high-energy photons as well as the lower-energy photons from $^{99}Tc^m$.

Collimator resolution   The intrinsic blurring of the camera is increased (as for radiographic blur) by the scattering of gamma rays in the patient (see Fig. 8.25 for the resolution measured with a point source).

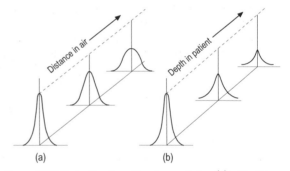

Figure 8.26 Reduction in collimator resolution (a) with distance in air and (b) with organ depth.

The collimator helps to reduce this blurring but compounds the intrinsic resolution with its own, which is determined by its thickness and the spaces between the collimator septa. Smaller spaces give better collimator resolution but lower sensitivity, and *vice versa*. Collimator resolution worsens with the distance in air of a source from the collimator, as shown in Figure 8.26a, where the *area* under each *point spread function* (the number of counts) remains constant. Figure 8.27 illustrates the change in resolution at different distances for different collimator types.

System resolution   When the radioactive source is inside the patient, the attenuation in the patient's tissues will reduce the number of counts reaching the collimator and the scatter will 'blur' the image. The more tissue, the bigger the spread of the point spread function and the smaller the area. Figure 8.26b

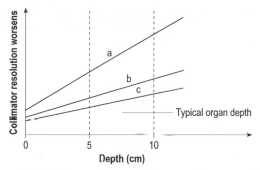

Figure 8.27 Relative resolution of different collimators: a, high sensitivity; b, standard; and c, high resolution.

shows the effects of attenuation (including scatter). Consequently, system resolution is worse for organs at depth, particularly for large patients.

Testing the resolution Resolution can be tested by imaging a small point source as above, but it is easier in practice to make and image a line source. The computer plots the counts along a line of pixels at right angles to a thin tube filled with ^{99}Tc^m. This graph (similar to Fig. 8.25) is then called the *line spread function*.

The line source can be placed:

- Against the face of the collimator in air (solid curve). The spread of the curve (measured halfway up and called the full width at half maximum, FWHM) corresponds to R in Figure 8.25 and is typically less than 5 mm. The FWHM is a measure of the system resolution at the face of the collimator.

- At 50 mm from the uncollimated camera head with the source itself collimated (dotted curve). The FWHM of this curve measures the intrinsic resolution, typically between 1 and 2 mm.

- At 10 cm deep in a scattering medium while using the collimator, for system resolution (dashed curve). (The depth is chosen to match that of the organs being imaged typically.) The FWHM of this curve measures the system resolution at that depth, typically 10 mm. Resolution is therefore not improved by using a smaller pixel size than 3 mm (e.g. in a 128 × 128 matrix).

Alternatively, spatial resolution can be tested with a bar test pattern – made of strips of lead placed on a sheet source. This can be used for system or intrinsic measurements. For system, the bar phantom is placed between the flood source and the multihole collimator. For intrinsic, the bar phantom is placed on the collimator, and a point source at a distance is used to produce the uniform photon flux at the surface of the camera. In practice, the overall system resolution is

no better than 5 mm, but the value of gamma imaging lies in evaluating function rather than anatomy that needs high resolution.

Spatial resolution in PET is worsened by Compton scatter of the annihilation photons in the body (see Fig. 8.18), although the full width at tenth maximum is affected much more than the FWHM by both scattered and random events. Overall resolution depends on the width or acceptance angle of the detectors and can be 8 mm at the edge of the FOV and half this in the centre, whereas in SPECT it worsens with increasing depth. It is usually measured using point or line sources, often of ^{68}Ge or sodium-22, spaced apart inside the FOV and for at least two axial positions in the scanner. The FWHM of these *point spread functions* are used to produce the transverse radial, transverse tangential and axial resolutions. When a line source is used, the transverse measurements are obtained with the source parallel to the central axis, and the axial measurements are obtained with the source parallel to a transaxial plane.

Sensitivity and energy resolution

The *sensitivity* (in cps MBq^{-1}) or *efficiency* (quoted as a percentage) of a gamma camera is dependent on both the detector and the collimator. The intrinsic detection efficiency is almost 100% up to 100 keV. Above this, it depends on the crystal thickness. The collimator sensitivity is a function of how many gamma rays will pass through, and so depends on the septa thickness. Thicker septa are needed at higher gamma energies for adequate resolution. The sensitivity of the collimator is approximately proportional to the square of its spatial resolution.

The system sensitivity is measured with a smaller version of the flood field or sheet phantom and expressed as total counts per second per megabequerel of activity (cps MBq^{-1}). As the crystal efficiency is quite high, it is the collimator that determines overall efficiency. Up to a point, using a thicker crystal increases sensitivity at the expense of poorer resolution; more importantly, so does using a collimator with larger holes. The choice of collimator is always a compromise between sensitivity and spatial resolution. Figure 8.27 illustrates the importance of the names given to collimators.

The energy resolution is the ability to distinguish between separate gamma rays of different energies. Its importance lies in the fact that the better the energy resolution, the better the rejection of scatter and the better the spatial resolution. As remarked earlier, when a crystal absorbs a single gamma photon the resulting 4000 light photons emerging from the crystal eject only a total of 400 or so electrons from the photocathodes of

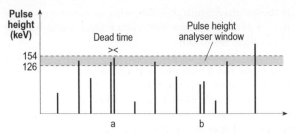

Figure 8.28 Illustration of pulses to show dead–time effects.

all the photomultipliers. Statistical fluctuation in such a small number produces the range of pulse heights seen in the photopeak (see Fig. 8.9) as plotted by the PHA or multichannel analyser. The FWHM of the photopeak is defined as the energy resolution and is typically 12% of the peak energy at 140 keV.

Setting a narrower PHA window improves the scatter rejection but reduces the sensitivity and increases imaging time. The energy resolution is better for high-energy gamma photons (being detected in a thick crystal) because they each produce more light photons. In a conventional gamma camera, it is therefore better with $^{99}Tc^m$ than with ^{201}Tl. However, for PET scanning using BGO crystals, the energy window is about 300 keV wide, centred around the annihilation photon energy 511 keV. This larger energy window is necessary mainly because the light yield for BGO is much less than for NaI(Tl). The energy resolution is also affected by the effective atomic number (and hence stopping power) and the crystal thickness.

For PET scanners, the system sensitivity is measured using a long tube filled with a low activity of a positron emitter suspended at the centre of the transverse FOV and parallel to the scanner axis. Data within an energy window set about 100 keV above and below the 511 keV level are collected in sinograms, with different thickness of metal sleeve around the source tube. These are analysed and summed for all slices to give the total count rate for each sleeve, and the result is extrapolated to zero sleeve thickness. The sensitivity obtained on axis is about 5 cps Bq^{-1} per mL for two-dimensional systems and about four times better than this for three-dimensional systems.

Temporal resolution: dead time and lost counts
The flash of light produced by a gamma photon in the crystal detector has a scintillation decay time of a fraction of a microsecond. The total time for the electronics to register the output of the photomultiplier tube for each such event, from light production through pulse production to count registration, is called the *dead time*. During that period, the counting circuit does not

recognize other independent pulses and is said to be 'dead'. Due to the stochastic nature of radioactive decay, counts arrive at irregular intervals, as reshown in Figure 8.28 for $^{99}Tc^m$. If a second gamma photon enters the detector during the dead time, the two flashes of light overlap and they are treated as one. If the system is set up as non-paralysable, the second pulse is ignored, but if it is paralysable the two pulses will be added. In the latter case, if the combined pulse in Figure 8.28 A is too large, the PHA will reject it. If two Compton-scattered photons are summed and their combined energy falls within the PHA window, they will be recorded as a single event but their location will be falsely recorded. For example, if two Compton-scattered photons (of say 60 and 80 keV) enter the gamma camera crystal within 1 μs of each other, as in Figure 8.28 B, they will be recorded as a single photon of 140 keV. This will pass through the PHA and produce a spurious event in a false location. At the high count rates in cardiac imaging, this may cause deterioration of the spatial resolution.

Also, at high count rates a significant proportion of the gamma photons may be missed altogether, the pulses pile up, the counts are *lost* and so the count rate is underestimated. Typically, there might be a 20% dead-time loss at 40 000 cps and more at higher count rates. A correction can be made to compensate for dead-time losses, using measurements of count rate for the detector system as a function of activity. In addition, there are electronic means of reducing dead-time losses by using buffers to store the overlapping events, pulse pile-up rejection circuits and high-speed electronics. In PET, using a detector with a fast scintillation decay time is obviously advantageous (see Table 8.2).

Noise: quantum mottle and contrast
When a flood field or sheet phantom is imaged for too short a time, the image shows a characteristic mottled appearance. This is because of the statistical nature of radiation emissions making the counts fluctuate from pixel to pixel. A computed analysis of counts per pixel to give the mean and standard deviation identifies the signal to noise ratio (SNR). This is defined as the mean divided by the standard deviation. The greater the number of counts, the smaller the standard deviation and the greater the SNR. However, noise in gamma imaging is generally high because of the inherently small signal from a necessarily limited amount of radioactivity.

In PET imaging, the noise-equivalent count rate is a measure of the true coincidences against the total coincidences and is proportional to the SNR in the final image. The true coincidences are obtained by subtracting the random and scatter coincidences from the total coincidences measured using a standard phantom centred in the FOV. Maximizing the noise-equivalent count rate will minimize image noise.

The *contrast* in an image depends on the relative difference in radionuclide concentration in normal and pathological tissue. Most important is the number of counts acquired per unit area in the area of interest. To detect hot spots and cold spots of about 10% against the background activity in the body needs a noise level of less than 3%. The noise level can be reduced (and hence SNR increased) only at the expense of either increased patient dose or worsened spatial resolution. Patient motion will reduce image contrast, so keeping the patient comfortable is important also for image quality.

Using more radioactivity could reduce noise. However, there are a number of constraints.

- The amount of radioactivity that may be administered to a patient is limited by the acceptable radiation dose to the patient.

- Activity is distributed through the body; typically, only some 20% is concentrated in the organ of interest.

- Gamma rays are emitted isotropically, and only a small fraction pass through the gamma camera collimator holes, which cannot be made too large if high resolution is required.

- Gamma rays could be collected for any length of time without further dose to the patient, but the imaging time is limited by:
  — the ability of the patient to stay still
  — the biological removal of the activity from the organ of interest
  — the workload required of the camera
  — the need for multi-imaging for dynamic studies (e.g. for cardiac imaging).

Noise is the principal factor in determining the quality of gamma images. The total counts acquired per image slice are subdivided among the image pixels. If there are only about 100 counts per pixel, the pixel to pixel noise is 10%. Gamma imaging is therefore said to be *noise-limited* or *dose-limited*. The count rate is maximized and the patient dose minimized by a judicious choice of radiopharmaceutical.

8.7 DOSE TO THE PATIENT

Administering a radioactive material to the patient necessarily gives the patient a radiation dose. The organ of interest that takes up the radionuclide (referred to as the source organ) will receive a dose, but it also acts as a source of irradiation for other so-called

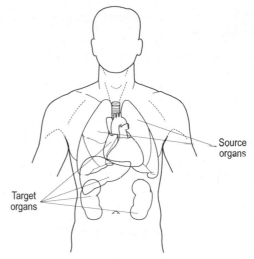

Figure 8.29 How activity in source organs can contribute to patient dose in both source (lungs) and target organs (heart, liver and kidney) in a ventilation study.

target organs and tissues in the body. An example of the source and target organs in lung ventilation studies is shown in Figure 8.29.

Dose to an organ
The absorbed dose delivered to an organ by the activity within it increases in proportion to:

- the activity administered to the patient
- the fraction taken up by the organ
- the effective half-life of the activity in the organ
- the energy (keV) of beta and gamma radiation emitted in each disintegration.

It also depends on how much of that energy escapes from the organ, and so does not contribute to the absorbed dose within the organ but will irradiate other tissues. Almost all the energy of a beta ray is deposited inside the organ, and very little escapes. Some of the energy of a gamma ray is deposited in the organ and some leaves it, to an extent depending on the size of the organ and how energetic the gamma ray is.

The calculation of internal absorbed dose is complicated and often uses Monte Carlo methods (a mathematical technique that considers the fate of individual photons whose behaviour is determined in terms of probabilities) and mathematical simulations of patient anatomy based on CT images. It must also take account of the additional dose delivered to the organ by gamma rays coming from activity in surrounding tissues and organs. The American Society of Nuclear Medicine has developed a method to calculate organ dose, which is referred to as the Medical

Table 8.3 Organ dose and organ-weighted effective dose for bone marrow imaging using a technetium-99m colloidal injection

Main source and target organ(s)	Organ absorbed dose (μGy MBq^{-1})	w_T	Effective dose contributions, organ-weighted using w_T (μSv MBq^{-1})
Spleen	110	0.025[a]	2.8
Liver	66	0.05	3.3
Red marrow	13	0.12	1.6
Stomach	7.1	0.12	0.9
Colon	3.8	0.12	0.5
Lungs	5.7	0.12	0.7
Bone surfaces	9.8	0.01	0.1
Breasts	1.9	0.05	0.1
Other	Various	0.025	0.1
Total effective dose (whole body)	–	–	10.1

[a]Spleen is a remainder organ. For internal radiation dosimetry, the remainder organ receiving the highest dose is assigned half the remainder tissue-weighting factor.

Internal Radiation Dose (MIRD) scheme. This assumes that there are source organs, which accumulate the activity, and target organs, which are irradiated by the source organs. Table 8.3 shows, in the organ dose column, that the three source organs in bone marrow imaging – liver, spleen and red bone marrow – receive the highest doses after a ^{99}Tc^m colloidal injection, but there are at least five other target organs that receive significant doses. The calculation is obviously approximate, as uptake depends on body size and weight, disease, age, sex, diet and drugs. However, the estimations are usually within a factor of 3 of an individually calculated patient dose based on activity uptake as measured from their gamma images.

Effective dose to the body

Unlike imaging with X-rays, the dose delivered by a radionuclide examination is unaffected by the number of images taken, neither is it confined to the region of diagnostic interest. After an intravenous injection, most tissues may receive some dose, but the organs of interest and the organs of excretion generally receive the highest doses.

The distribution of a dose is non-uniform and specific to the examination, but an average dose to the body as a whole can be calculated to give a measure of risk. This is termed the *effective dose* (E), which has the unit sievert (Sv; see Ch. 2.3.2). It is calculated using the differing sensitivities of the various organs and tissues to irradiation, by weighting each organ-absorbed dose with a tissue-weighting factor, w_T, to produce an equivalent dose. These are then summed to give the effective dose per MBq activity administered. Thus, in Table 8.3, if 400 MBq is the administered activity, the effective dose is 4 mSv.

Typical activities and doses

Most nuclear medicine investigations deliver an E of less than 5 mSv, which is of the order of the variation, from place to place and individual to individual, in the annual dose of natural radiation. Some, such as bone or static brain imaging, deliver doses in the region of 5 mSv. A few examinations, such as tumour or abscess imaging with ^{67}Ga, deliver higher doses and should be undertaken only when other imaging modalities are inappropriate. Table 8.4 gives some typical effective doses for given levels of activity administered.

The activity of each administration of radiopharmaceutical is kept within the limits set in each country, for example in the UK by the Administration of Radioactive Substances Advisory Committee (ARSAC) of the Department of Health (see Ch. 2.7.2). The activity should be checked and recorded before administration. The vial is placed in the 'well' of a large re-entrant ionization chamber, the *radionuclide* or *dose calibrator*. The ionization current produced by the gamma rays is proportional to the activity of the sample (provided that there are no dead-time effects), but it also depends on the sensitivity of the well chamber to the gamma energy of the radionuclide being assayed and to the geometry of the source within the calibrator. Thus the radionuclide and the vial or syringe type is selected on the control panel, and the activity in megabecquerels is displayed on a digital read-out. The accuracy of the radionuclide calibrator must be checked regularly using a reasonably long-lived source, such as ^{57}Co. The calibrator can also be used to check radionuclide purity (see section 8.3).

In order to minimize patient dose, patients should drink a good deal of water and empty the bladder

Table 8.4 Some typical radionuclide administrations for adults and consequent effective doses

Site	Agent	Activity (MBq)	Effective dose (mSv)
Bone	Technetium-99m diphosphonates	600	5
Lung ventilation	Technetium-99m DTPA aerosol	80	0.5
	Krypton-81m gas	6000	0.1
Lung perfusion	Technetium-99m HSA macroaggregates	100	1
Kidney	Technetium-99m DTPA gluconate	300	2
	Technetium-99m MAG3	100	0.7
Infection	Gallium-67 citrate	150	15
	Indium-111 leucocytes	20	7
Tumour	Iodine-123 MIBG	400	5
Thyroid	Iodine-123 iodide	20	4
Heart	Technetium-99m MIBI	400	3
	Thallium-201 chloride	80	18
Brain	Fluorine-18 FDG	400	8

DTPA, diethylene triamine pentacetic acid; FDG, fluoro-2-deoxyglucose; HSA, human serum albumin; MAG3, mercaptoacetyltriglycine; MIBG, meta-iodobenzylguanidine; MIBI, methoxy isobutyl isonitrile.

frequently to reduce the dose to the gonads and pelvic bone marrow. As fetal doses should also be constrained, ARSAC gives guidance recommending that female patients should avoid conception for an appropriate period following administration of long-lived (half-life more than 7 days) diagnostic radionuclides, while male patients do not need to be given any particular advice concerning diagnostic examinations. If a patient is or may be pregnant, certain examinations may result in a fetal dose greater than 10 mSv and should be avoided. Equally, if a patient is breast feeding, her infant will be exposed to a radiation dose from the activity secreted in her milk. An interruption in feeding may be recommended, and advice should be sought.

8.8 PRECAUTIONS NECESSARY IN HANDLING RADIONUCLIDES

When handling radionuclides, in addition to the hazard from external radiation there is also a potential hazard from internal radiation due to accidental ingestion or inhalation of the radionuclide or its entry through wounds. It is therefore important to avoid contamination of the environment, the workplace and persons, and to control any spread of radioactive materials. Generally, the risk from contamination is greater than that from external radiation.

Segregation

A nuclear medicine facility must have identified and preferably separate areas for:

- the preparation and storage of radioactive materials

- the injection of patients
- patients to wait (to allow uptake of the radiopharmaceutical into the organ of interest)
- imaging
- temporary storage of radioactive waste.

Patients containing radioactivity are a source of external radiation. They should be spaced apart in the waiting area. Departmental layout should make use of the inverse square law to reduce the effect of background radiation from other patients and sources, particularly in the imaging areas.

Personal protection

Use should be made of distance, shielding and time. Staff should enter areas where there is radioactivity only when it is strictly necessary; all procedures must be carried out expeditiously and efficiently. Departmental local rules must be followed. Some general guidance follows.

Radionuclides are contained in shielded generators or in bottles inside lead pots. Where feasible, bottles and syringes are handled with long-handled forceps (tongs). Manipulations, such as the labelling of pharmaceuticals and the loading of syringes, are carried out with the arms behind a lead barrier that protects the body and face, and over a tray, lined with absorbent paper, to catch any drips.

Syringes are protected by heavy metal, tungsten or lead glass sleeves (which can reduce radiation doses to the fingers by 75%) and are carried to the patient in special containers or on a disposable tray. Before injection, syringes are vented into swabs or closed containers and not into the atmosphere.

To avoid accidental ingestion, waterproof (double latex) surgical gloves are worn when handling radionuclides. Cuts and abrasions must be covered first. There must be no eating, drinking or facial contact. Hands and work surfaces are routinely monitored for radioactive contamination, and the air in radiopharmacies should also be sampled and monitored. Staff will be monitored for external radiation doses to the body and possibly also the hands. Staff may also be monitored for internal contamination. Swabs are taken from the radiopharmacy workstation to monitor for radioactive and bacterial contamination. Note that lead-rubber aprons are ineffective against the high-energy gamma rays of $^{99}Tc^m$.

Hands should be washed regularly at special hands-free designated (for disposal of radioactivity) washbasins. Whenever there is a spillage, however slight, decontamination procedures must be followed. This normally involves the use of water, mild detergents and swabs, which are then sealed in plastic bags and disposed of as radioactive waste in marked bins. Any use of a nailbrush should be gentle; if contamination is obstinate, special detergent solutions may be necessary.

Patient protection

Every radionuclide should be checked for activity before administration, using a radionuclide (well) calibrator. The patient's identity must be checked against the investigation to be made and the activity to be administered, and this must be recorded. Particular care should be taken to avoid contamination during oral administrations. Special circumstances apply for pregnant patients and those with babies whom they are breast feeding (see section 8.7).

Dealing with a radioactive spill

In the case of a radioactive spill, vomiting, incontinence, etc., clear the area of non-essential persons. Wearing gloves, aprons and overshoes, mop the floor with absorbent pads and seal the swabs in designated plastic bags. If necessary, continue with wet swabs. Continue until monitoring shows the activity to be at a satisfactorily low level. If necessary, cordon off the area or cover it with impervious sheeting until sufficient decay has occurred. Contaminated materials are treated as waste.

Disposal of radioactive waste

Disposal of radioactive waste follows the two principles of:

- containment and decay
- dilution by dispersal to the environment.

Special rules and authorizations cover the accumulation, storage and disposal of radioactive waste. In the UK, these are laid down in the Radioactive Substances Act (Ch. 2.7.1). Every hospital is subject to strict limitations on the amount that can be disposed of by each of the following routes.

Gaseous waste can be vented to the atmosphere; in lung ventilation studies, ^{133}Xe and $^{99}Tc^m$ aerosols should be exhausted to the exterior of the building. This is desirable but not always necessary with the very short-lived $^{81}Kr^m$, but there should be adequate room ventilation.

Aqueous liquid waste may be disposed of, well diluted with water, via designated sinks or sluices with drains running direct to the foul drain, as long as the levels are within the authorized limits.

Solid waste (swabs, syringes, bottles, etc.) is placed in designated sacks for disposal to authorized incinerators or waste contractors or, if suitably diluted with ordinary waste and within authorized limits, to waste disposal sites. However, there may be other restrictions on disposal, for example with regard to clinical waste, that require this very low activity waste to be incinerated. Used generators are kept in a secure shielded store until they are returned to the manufacturer.

Contaminated clothing and bedding is appropriately bagged and stored in a secure protected area until the activity is sufficiently decayed for release to the laundry.

Records must be kept, for inspection, of all deliveries, stocks, administration, stored waste and disposals of waste.

8.9 SUMMARY

- Comparatively short-lived gamma-emitting radiopharmaceuticals are used for gamma imaging.

- The activity is measured, strictly limited usually to some megabecquerels (MBq), before being administered to the patient, making them temporarily radioactive.

- Most nuclear medicine investigations deliver an effective dose of less than 5 mSv.

- Care is needed to avoid radioactive contamination.

- Once the radiopharmaceutical has time to locate in the organs of interest, the patient is scanned with a gamma camera or tomographic imager for single-photon (SPECT) or positron emitters (PET).

- The camera crystal, usually NaI(Tl), converts the emitted gamma photons to light; these are detected by the photomultiplier tubes and analysed to produce the image.

- Collimator design depends on gamma energy and usually results in a compromise between spatial resolution and sensitivity.

- SPECT cameras need parallel hole collimators.

- The main positron emitter used in PET imaging is ^{18}F.

- PET scanners need detectors, typically bismuth germanate, with high efficiency for the 511 keV annihilation photons.

- High levels of uptake in the image indicate areas of intense functional or pharmacological activity, and low levels correspond to little or no functional activity.

- The uptake can be quantified and followed dynamically.

- Statistical noise is the limiting factor for contrast in the images.

- Images can be fused to anatomical images such as X-ray CT or MRI to make visualization, localization and staging of tumours easier.

- Although data acquisition is different for radionuclides and especially for PET, similar reconstruction techniques to X-ray CT are used to produce images in any two-dimensional plane or, by combination, in three dimensions.

Chapter 9

Imaging with ultrasound

Ultrasound refers to sound waves of such a high frequency (above 20 kHz) as to be inaudible to humans. Whereas audible sound spreads throughout a room, ultrasound with its shorter wavelength can be formed into a narrow beam, although not as well as light with its even shorter wavelength.

Ultrasound, although not electromagnetic radiation, undergoes reflection and refraction at the interface between two different media. It is such reflections or echoes from different tissues that produce the ultrasound images. Diagnostic ultrasound can image soft tissues that are too similar to produce enough X-ray contrast and has a special place in obstetric imaging, as the hazards are perceived to be insignificant compared with X-rays.

Ultrasound waves are produced by a transducer that converts an electrical signal into an ultrasound beam and consists primarily of a piezoceramic disc or rectangular plate. The plate is made of compressed microcrystalline lead zirconate titanate (PZT) or of the plastic polyvinylidine difluoride (PVDF). The two flat faces are made electrically conducting with a very thin coating of silver.

9.1 PIEZOELECTRIC EFFECT

When a direct current (DC) voltage is applied to the flat faces of the disc, it expands (or contracts), and if the voltage is reversed it contracts (or expands). The movement of the faces is proportional to the voltage.

When the disc is compressed, equal and opposite charges and a corresponding voltage appear on the two flat faces; if the pressure is reversed, so is the voltage. The voltage produced is proportional to the pressure.

When an alternating voltage is applied, the disc alternately expands and contracts with the same frequency. When the disc is subjected to an alternating pressure, an alternating voltage is produced of the same frequency.

The same transducer will convert electrical into sound energy and vice versa, and can act as both a transmitter and a receiver.

When heated above a certain temperature (about 350°C for PZT), called its *Curie temperature*, transducers lose their piezoelectric properties. Transducer probes should obviously not be autoclaved (nor should they be immersed in water unless waterproofed). Thin slices of naturally occurring quartz crystals also show the piezoelectric effect and are used in digital timers and computers.

Transducers are used in both pulsed and continuous wave modes.

Pulsed mode

When the transducer is in contact with a patient and a few hundred volts DC are suddenly applied to the disc, it instantly expands, thereby compressing a layer of the material in contact with it (Fig. 9.1a). Because of the elasticity of the material, the compressed layer expands and compresses an adjacent layer of material (Fig. 9.1b). In this way, a layer or wave of compression travels with a *velocity* (*v*) through the material, followed by a corresponding wave of decompression or rarefaction. These short regular pulses of ultrasound are used in imaging.

Continuous wave mode

If, instead of DC, an alternating current (AC) voltage is applied, the crystal face pulses forwards and backwards like a piston, producing successive compressions and rarefactions (Fig. 9.1c). Each compression wave has moved forwards by a distance called the *wavelength* (λ) by the time the next one is produced.

The *frequency* (*f*) with which compressions pass any given point is the same as the frequency at which the transducer vibrates and the frequency of the AC voltage applied to it. It is measured in megahertz (MHz).

The density and therefore the pressure of the material rises and falls above its normal atmospheric value (101 kPa). In a typical diagnostic application, the particles travel to and fro through distances less than 1 μm, with velocities up to 500 mm s^{-1} and accelerations up to 300 000g. The peak of the pressure wave can reach several atmospheres.

The graph of pressure excess p at any point against *time t* is a sine wave (Fig. 9.2a). The interval between successive crests is the period $T = 1/f$. A graph of pressure excess at any instant t_1 against *distance d*

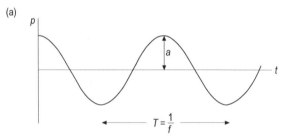

(a)

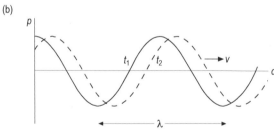

(b)

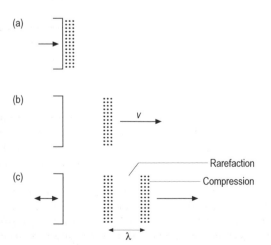

(a)

(b)

(c)

Rarefaction

Compression

Figure 9.1 Production of sound waves by a transducer.

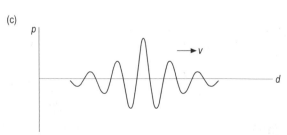

(c)

Figure 9.2 Excess pressure: (a) versus time, continuous wave; (b) versus distance, continuous wave; and (c) versus distance, pulsed wave.

through the material is also sinusoidal (solid curve in Fig. 9.2b). Here, the distance between successive troughs is the wavelength λ. The dashed curve refers to a later instant, t_2. The wave travels forwards with a *velocity v*. As with any sine wave,

$$\text{wavelength} \times \text{frequency} = \text{velocity, or}$$
$$\lambda f = v.$$

For comparison, Figure 9.2c shows the pressure waveform of a pulsed wave, a few periods in duration.

Properties of ultrasound

Unlike light and X-rays, sound requires a material medium in which to travel and is a *longitudinal*, not a transverse, wave. Unlike X- and gamma rays, it can be reflected, refracted and focused, and its wavelength is sufficiently long for its wave properties (interference and diffraction) to predominate. Unlike light, its velocity in a given material is, for practical purposes, a constant, independent of frequency and wavelength.

The *velocity* of ultrasound depends on the material through which it travels. The greater the density, the lower the velocity. The greater the compressibility (or the smaller the elastic modulus), the lower the velocity. Accordingly, velocity depends on temperature.

Some typical figures are given in the first two columns of Table 9.1. Note that sound takes nearly $7\,\mu s$ to travel each centimetre in average soft tissue. The table also lists the product of velocity and density, called the acoustic impedance, as explained in section 9.4.

Air has a much lower density, but it is much more compressible than water or tissue, hence the low velocity.

Because the frequency of a given transducer is fixed, wavelength is proportional to velocity. If a transducer is energized at a frequency of 3.5 MHz, the wavelength of the ultrasound changes as it travels from the transducer (1 mm) through soft tissue (0.4 mm) to bone (0.9 mm).

The intensity of ultrasound, measured in watts per square millimetre (W mm^{-2}), is proportional to the square of the wave amplitude (a in Fig. 9.2a) and is under the operator's control.

9.2 INTERFERENCE

If two sound waves of the same wavelength cross each other, the pressure waves combine. If, as in Figure 9.3a, the two waves, A and B, are exactly in step (in phase), their amplitudes add up; this is called constructive interference. If, as in Figure 9.3b, they are exactly out of step (180° out of phase), they tend to cancel each other out; this is called destructive interference. If they are only partially out of step, they result in a wave of reduced intensity.

Natural or resonant frequency

A transducer can be made to emit sound of any frequency by driving it (in continuous mode) with AC of that frequency. However, a transducer vibrates most violently and produces the largest output of ultrasound when the frequency at which it is made to vibrate produces a wavelength in the transducer equal to twice the thickness (t) of the piezoelectric disc, for the following reason.

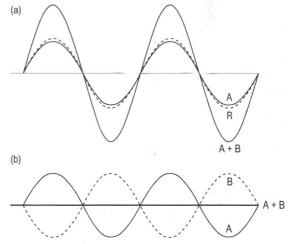

Figure 9.3 Interference: (a) constructive and (b) destructive.

Table 9.1 Velocity of ultrasound in various materials

Material	Velocity (m s^{-1})	Density (kg m^{-3})	Acoustic impedance Z (kg m^{-2} s^{-1})
Air	330	1.29	430
Average soft tissue[a]	1540	1000	1.5×10^6
Typical bone	3200	1650	5.3×10^6
Lead zirconate titanate (PZT)	4000	7500	30×10^6

[a]Range of velocity: 1300–1800 m s^{-1}.

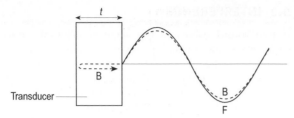

Figure 9.4 Resonance.

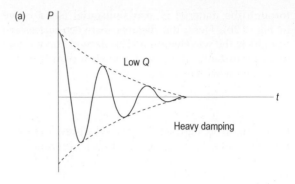

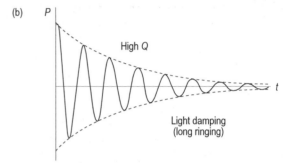

Figure 9.5 Damping: (a) heavy and (b) light.

In Figure 9.4, the front face of the transducer emits sound in both the forwards and the backwards directions. The back wave B is reflected at the back face of the disc. By the time it joins the front wave F, it has travelled an extra distance $2t$. If, as in the diagram, this equals one wavelength (or any exact number of wavelengths), the F and B waves reinforce, for they are exactly in phase. Constructive interference or *resonance* occurs. Otherwise, there will be some destructive interference and loss of output.

The frequency at which the transducer is the most efficient as a transmitter of sound is also the frequency at which it is most sensitive as a receiver of sound. It is called its natural or resonant frequency.

If a large DC voltage is applied briefly (in pulse mode) to the same transducer disc, it will vibrate at its natural frequency. It will emit ultrasound of a frequency that has a wavelength of $2t$. Sound of any other frequency would very quickly die away because of destructive interference, as described above. The thicker the transducer, the lower the natural frequency and the longer the wavelength. The transducer has a natural period $T = 1/f$.

The *natural or resonant frequency* of a transducer disc depends on its dimensions, particularly its thickness, and its material, which affects the velocity of sound in it. To change the frequency, one has to change the transducer. A 3.5 MHz transducer has a disc about 0.5 mm thick.

Pulse duration or length

Once the transducer has been pulsed, it continues to vibrate for a short while with diminishing amplitude as it loses energy in the form of sound. As shown in Figure 9.5, the amplitude of the pressure wave decays exponentially with time. This is called *damping*. If the vibrations continue for an appreciable period, it is called *ringing*. If the damping is heavy (Fig. 9.5a), it has a short time constant or ring-down time. It is said to have a low mechanical coefficient or Q-value, defined below. A transducer that is more lightly damped has a higher Q and, as in Figure 9.5b, produces a longer pulse and a higher output of sound.

Typically, the duration of the ultrasound pulse may be three periods or less (about 1 μs with a 3.5 MHz transducer). The pulse length can equally well be stated as three wavelengths or less (about 1.5 mm in tissue). Ultrasound travels at a nominally constant speed in tissue, which is why time and distance are often used interchangeably.

9.3 SINGLE TRANSDUCER PROBE

Figure 9.6 illustrates the essential features of a single transducer, as used in a mechanical sector scanner (see section 9.8). In the transmitting mode, the energizing voltage is applied between the back face of the piezoelectric disc (3) via an insulated wire (1), and the front face via an earthed metal case (2).

The back face is cemented to a backing block (4) of epoxy resin in which are suspended fine particles of tungsten. The backing block and transducer are 'matched', as described in section 9.4, so as to admit the backwards-travelling waves produced by the back face of the vibrating disc. These waves are scattered and absorbed within the block. Like a tympanist placing a hand on a drum face, this damps the vibration. It results in a short pulse and a low Q. Additional damping and further shortening of the pulse is performed electronically by applying a second, reverse

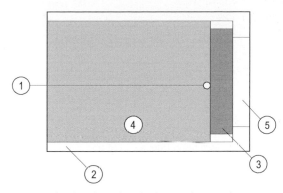

Figure 9.6 Section through a single transducer probe.

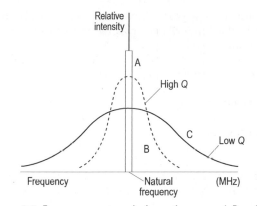

Figure 9.7 Frequency spectrum in A, continuous, and, B and C, pulsed modes.

voltage pulse very shortly after the first. If the block is omitted, so that the disc is backed with air, total reflection takes place, the pulse lasts for 20 or more periods, and the Q and the sound output are increased.

The front face of the disc is fixed to a thin plastic slip (5), which, in addition to protecting the surface of the disc, has other important properties (see section 9.4). In the receiving mode, the signal voltage produced by the returning echo is led away along a wire (1).

Bandwidth
In continuous mode, the transducer emits sound of a single frequency. The frequency spectrum, which plots relative intensity against frequency of sound, is a single line A in Figure 9.7. In pulsed mode, it emits a continuous spectrum of sine waves having a range of frequencies, which combine to form the pulse B or C in Figure 9.7. The bandwidth is the full width at half-maximum intensity (FWHM) of the frequency spectrum. A short pulse C has a wider bandwidth of frequencies than a longer pulse B.

The same graphs (B and C) represent the resonance curve, the response of the transducer as a receiver to waves of different frequencies. The *mechanical coefficient* (Q), referred to above, is the ratio of mean frequency to bandwidth. The greater Q, the narrower the bandwidth both as transmitter and receiver. A transducer with a high Q produces a pure note and responds only to that note, which is good for continuous wave ultrasound. One with a low Q has a short ring-down time, produces short pulses, and responds to a range or band of frequencies, which is good for pulsed ultrasound.

Diameter of the transducer
If the transducer had a diameter equal to one wavelength or less (say 0.5mm), sound would spread out equally in all directions, as spherical waves, and

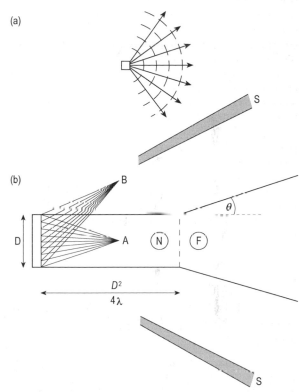

Figure 9.8 Pattern of sound emitted by (a) a very small transducer element and (b) a larger diameter transducer with near (N) and far (F) fields.

would have no directional properties. This is shown in Figure 9.8a, in which dashed lines represent wavefronts and the solid lines show the direction of propagation of the waves.

If, as in Figure 9.8b, its diameter D is, for example, 10 times the wavelength, sound is projected forwards effectively as a plane wave, in a beam of approximately the same diameter as the transducer, for the following reason.

Imagine that the face of the disc is subdivided into 80 small transducers, each 0.5 mm in size, all emitting waves at the same time. For every crest that reaches any point B outside the beam from one minitransducer, a trough arrives simultaneously from another minitransducer, and there is (more or less) total destructive interference of the sound. The separate sound waves that similarly reach any point A inside the beam are, in the main, roughly in phase, and they reinforce each other by constructive interference.

Near and far fields

As a result of the interference described above, the sound energy is largely confined to the beam of diameter D. The nearly parallel part of the beam (N) is called the near field or the Fresnel region, and it extends a distance $D^2/4\lambda$ from the transducer face. In other words, the length of the near zone is proportional to fD^2.

At greater depths in (F), the far field or the Fraunhofer region, the interference effect is lost and the beam diverges. The angle of divergence θ is larger for larger λ/D. In other words, the far zone divergence is larger for smaller fD. Because of vibration of the edges of the transducer disc, there are small beams of low intensity outside the beam in what are called side lobes (S in Fig. 9.8). These may cause image artefacts.

For example, at a frequency of 3.5 MHz, a 12 mm diameter transducer has a near field 80 mm in depth and a divergence angle of between 1° and 2°.

Using a transducer of higher frequency increases the length of the near zone and decreases the divergence of the far zone (for the same diameter of disc). The beam becomes more directional.

Using a transducer of larger diameter increases the length of the near zone and decreases the divergence of the far zone (for the same frequency).

Focusing

Transducers may be designed to focus at a particular depth (or rather a range of depths) corresponding to the region of diagnostic interest. This concentrates the intensity so that it will produce stronger echoes, and improves the lateral resolution. There are several ways to focus the beam.

- Using a *curved* (concave, spherical) *piezoelectric element*. The shape of the beam is shown in Figure 9.9. Being a ceramic, it can be moulded into any shape. The greater the curvature, the shorter the focal length.
- Using a plastic *acoustic lens* cemented to the transducer face in Figure 9.6. (This converging lens will

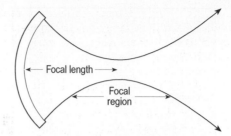

Figure 9.9 Focused beam from a curved transducer.

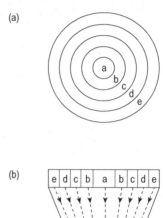

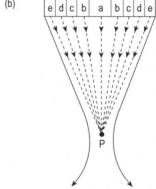

Figure 9.10 Annular array: (a) transducer face and (b) cross-section through the transducer and the ultrasound beam.

be concave or convex according to its material.) Sometimes, a curved mirror is used instead.

Transducers can be made with strong, intermediate or weak focusing. The price of a short focal length is increased divergence of the far field. The shorter the focal length, the narrower and shorter the focal region or depth of focus, over which the beam is reasonably narrow, as depicted in Figure 9.9.

- *Electronic focusing: annular array*, used in mechanical sector scanners.

Figure 9.10a shows the face of a circular piezoelectric disc subdivided into five concentric rings: a, b, c, d and e. If they were all energized simultaneously, they would act as a single transducer and the resulting beam would have the shape depicted in Figure 9.8b. If, however, the outermost ring (e) is energized first, with the subsequent rings (d, c and b) and finally the central element (a) at short time intervals, there will be a point P at which the pulses, travelling along paths of different lengths, all arrive together and so reinforce. The resulting beam shape is shown in Figure 9.10b, the energy being concentrated or focused in the region of P. In compensation, the beam diverges more at greater depths.

The focal length can be altered without changing the transducer: the greater the time delays between energizing successive annular rings, the shorter the focal length. Electronic focusing is considered further in section 9.8.

9.4 BEHAVIOUR OF A BEAM AT AN INTERFACE BETWEEN DIFFERENT MATERIALS

If a beam strikes the boundary between two materials (transducer–skin, tissue–bone, tissue–air, etc.) at right angles, some of the energy is reflected as an 'echo' and some is transmitted.

Acoustic impedance

The proportions of energy reflected and transmitted depend on the acoustic impedances of the two materials. The acoustic impedance (Z) of a material is defined as the product of the density (ρ) of the material and the velocity (v) of sound in it ($Z = v\rho$). It depends on the density and elasticity of the material and, for practical purposes, is independent of frequency. Some values are given in SI units in the third column of Table 9.1.

The fraction of sound energy that is reflected at the interface between two materials depends on the angle of incidence. When the beam strikes the surface at or nearly at right angles, the fraction of sound energy that is reflected (R) at the interface between two materials of acoustic impedance Z_1 and Z_2, respectively, is given by:

$$R = (Z_1 - Z_2)^2 / (Z_1 + Z_2)^2.$$

It is the same whether the sound is travelling from material 1 to material 2 or vice versa. The greater the difference in acoustic impedance, the greater the fraction R reflected. The less the difference in acoustic impedance, the greater $(1 - R)$ the fraction transmitted. In consequence:

- When $Z_1 = Z_2$, there is 100% transmission and no reflection. The two materials are acoustically

matched as, for example, the transducer and the backing block (see section 9.3).

- At an interface between bone ($Z = 5 \times 10^6$) and tissue ($Z = 1.5 \times 10^6$), the fraction reflected is about 30%:

$$R = (5.0 - 1.5)^2 / (5.0 + 1.5)^2.$$

About 70% of the sound energy is therefore transmitted. Generally speaking, it is not possible to image through bone.

- At any interface with air or gas (for which Z is negligible), total reflection occurs, with the following results.
  - Gas-filled organs cast a shadow, and structures underneath cannot be imaged. Normal lung cannot be penetrated. The bowel wall can be visualized but not the lumen itself. Ultrasound is sometimes used to check for air in vessels (e.g. within the liver).
  - It is impossible to get sound from the transducer to the patient and vice versa if there is air trapped between the transducer and the skin; it is all reflected back. For this reason, the transducer is pressed against the patient and a coupling oil or gel is used. Bubbles of air must be avoided.

- Because of the 'mismatch' of acoustic impedance between transducer and tissue, only some 20% of the sound energy would be transmitted in either direction between the transducer and the patient. This is overcome by attaching a *matching plate*, (5) in Figure 9.6, to the front face of the transducer. The plate is a quarter of a wavelength thick and made of a plastic compound having an acoustic impedance intermediate between that of the transducer and the skin – as close as possible to the geometrical mean.

- The figures given so far for 'tissue' refer to average soft tissue. There are subtle differences of density, elasticity and therefore acoustic impedance between different soft tissues (see Table 9.2).

  Small fractions of ultrasound are therefore reflected at interfaces between different soft tissues (e.g. nearly 1% at a fat–kidney interface). Approximate values are given in Table 9.3. Reflections less than 0.01% are unlikely to be detected.

Specular (mirror) reflection

If a beam strikes a large smooth interface at an angle, the same laws of reflection and refraction apply as with light (Fig. 9.11a).

Table 9.2 Acoustic impedances of different soft tissues

Tissue	Acoustic impedance (kg m^{-2} s^{-1})
Muscle	1.70×10^6
Liver	1.64×10^6
Spleen	1.63×10^6
Kidney	1.62×10^6
Fat	1.38×10^6

Table 9.3 Typical reflection factors

Interface	Percentage
Gas–tissue	99.9
Soft tissue–PZT	80
Bone–muscle	30
Plastic–soft tissue	10
Fat–muscle	1
Blood–muscle	0.1
Liver–muscle	0.01

PZT, lead zirconate titanate.

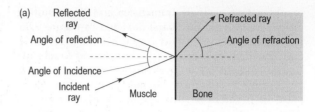
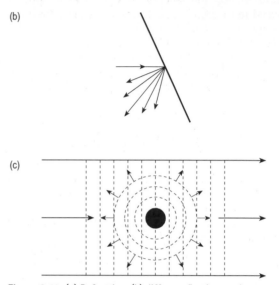

Figure 9.11 (a) Refraction, (b) diffuse reflection, and (c) scattering.

- The angle of reflection equals the angle of incidence.
- The ratio of the sines of the incident and refraction angles is equal to the ratio of sound velocities in the two materials:

$$\sin\theta_1/\sin\theta_2 = c_1/c_2.$$

This is known as Snell's law.

Diffuse reflection

If, as is usually the case, the tissue interface is rough and has undulations equal to a wavelength or so, the reflected beam spreads out over an angle (Fig. 9.11b). The same effect is seen with light and frosted glass. The shorter the wavelength and also the rougher the surface, the wider the spread. On account of this, in imaging the transducer will receive some reflections even if the beam does not strike an interface exactly at right angles.

Scatter

When sound encounters a structure that is much smaller than a wavelength (such as a red blood corpuscle, diameter 10 µm, or tissue parenchyma), it is scattered more or less equally in all directions. This is shown in Figure 9.11c, in which dashed lines represent wavefronts, and solid lines direction of propagation. This effect allows even small structures to be visualized, as some scatter will reach the transducer. The echo signals so produced from the interior of the placenta, liver, pancreas, spleen and

kidney are between about 1 and 10% as strong as those produced by the organ boundaries. Scattering by red blood cells, on which blood flow imaging depends, produces even smaller signals and so necessitates a high frequency (see section 9.13).

9.5 ATTENUATION OF ULTRASOUND

When travelling through a material, sound is attenuated exponentially with the depth of travel for the following reasons.

- Energy is absorbed (and converted into heat) by frictional and viscous forces in the material.
- Energy leaves the forwards-travelling beam due to scattering and to partial reflection by the multitude of interfaces that the beam encounters on route. The higher the frequency, the greater the attenuation.

Attenuation is usually measured in decibels (dB), as this enables a wide range of power or intensity ratios to be expressed in a compact way by using a logarithmic scale as follows:

$10 \times \log$ (power or intensity ratio) = no. of decibels.

Table 9.4 Typical tissue attenuation values (approximate)

Material	Attenuation (dB cm^{-1} at 1 MHz)	Half–value layer (cm)		
		1 MHz	2 MHz	5 MHz
Water	0.0022	1360	340	54
Blood	0.18	17	8.5	3
Average tissue	0.7	4.3	2.1	0.9
Bone	15	0.2	0.1	0.04
Lung	40	0.08	0.04	0.02

Some examples of power ratios:

Ratio	1000/1	100/1	20/1	10/1	2/1	1/1	1/2	1/10	1/100
dB	30	20	13	10	3	0	−3	−10	−20

Note that decibel values are additive. Positive values show amplification and negative values attenuation. The thickness of tissue that reduces the sound intensity to half its original value is called the half-value layer. This ratio of 1/2 results in a loss of 3 dB (see above).

In average tissue, sound of frequency 1 MHz loses about 1 dB cm^{-1}, which corresponds to a half-value layer of 3 cm. The decibel loss in tissue per centimetre is proportional to the frequency. Thus at 3.5 MHz the loss is about 3.5 dB cm^{-1}. In a journey to and fro through 15 cm depth of tissue, the total loss would then be about 100 dB. There is little absorption or scatter in water, and so a full bladder can sometimes aid ultrasound penetration. In bone, the attenuation is much greater: 35 dB cm^{-1} at 2.5 MHz. Air attenuates heavily, and attenuation in the lung is about 40 dB cm^{-1} at 1 MHz. Table 9.4 gives some other typical values.

Penetration

At a certain depth, the intensity of the beam has fallen too low to be useful. The higher the frequency produced by the transducer, the less the effective penetration of the beam. Roughly, penetration (cm) = 40/frequency (MHz).

9.6 A–MODE (AMPLITUDE MODE–ECHORANGING)

A-mode imaging is sometimes used for examining the eye, for identification of cysts in the breast, or for showing midline displacement in the brain. It is the simplest form of ultrasound imaging, which shows only the position of tissue interfaces. As an imaging technique, it has been largely superseded by B-mode imaging or other imaging techniques, such as computed tomography. However, A-mode illustrates the basic principles of ultrasound imaging.

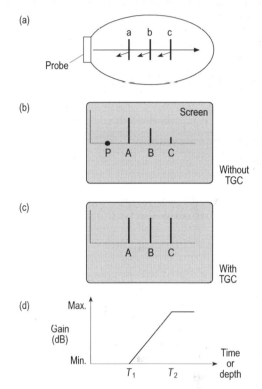

Figure 9.12 A-mode: (a) section through transducer and patient, (b) trace on screen without time gain control, (c) trace on screen using time gain control, and (d) variation of swept gain with depth.

The probe is held stationary against the patient (Fig. 9.12a). It is pulsed (with a voltage of a few hundred volts lasting for a few nanoseconds), and simultaneously the light spot starts to move from the left-hand edge of the display screen (Fig. 9.12b). While the pulse of ultrasound travels with a velocity averaging 1.5 mm µs^{-1} through the patient, the light spot moves at a constant speed, tracing out a horizontal line across the screen.

It takes the ultrasound pulse a time t to reach interface a, by which time the light spot has reached point P on the screen. Some of the energy is reflected back along the path as an echo pulse, which takes a further time t to return to the probe, by which time the light spot has reached A.

The probe now acts as a receiver and, in response to the echo received, generates a small signal voltage that, after amplification, produces at A a short vertical trace ('blip') of height proportional to the echo strength. The other interfaces, b and c, each produce blips at B and C, respectively. The locations of the blips along the trace indicate the depths of the corresponding interfaces along the beam. A 'clock' can be used to superimpose on the horizontal trace a ruler or calliper – a sequence of marker pulses spaced to correspond to 1 cm intervals in the body.

To provide a sustained image, the pulse is repeated, typically 1000 times s^{-1} (the *pulse repetition frequency*, *PRF*, is 1 kHz). After the transducer has been pulsed for about 1 μs (transmit mode), it is then available to receive echoes (receive or listening mode) for about 999 μs before it is pulsed again.

Time gain compensation

Because of attenuation in the tissue, the amplitude of the sound pulse diminishes as it travels into the body, and the echo pulse is similarly attenuated as it travels back towards the transducer. A particular interface, or 'reflector', deep in the body therefore produces a much weaker echo than an identical interface near the surface, as seen in Figure 9.12b.

Attenuation is compensated and the echoes equalized electronically by swept gain or time gain compensation (TGC). As soon as the transducer is pulsed, the decibel gain of the amplifier is steadily and automatically increased, in proportion to the time that has elapsed and thus the distance that has been travelled by the sound. In this way, all echoes from identical interfaces are rendered the same, independent of their depth, as seen in Figure 9.12c.

Swept gain is varied typically from 0 to 50 dB. Figure 9.12d plots the applied gain in decibels against depth in tissue. To make best use of the available TGC in the region of greatest interest (and not waste it while the beam is travelling through, for example, a filled bladder), the decibel gain is not usually applied until the region of interest is reached at the threshold depth T_1. It is then increased linearly through the region of interest until depth T_2. The operator can vary the threshold and the slope of the ramp, and the resulting TGC curve (Fig. 9.12d) can be displayed on the screen.

9.7 B–MODE (BRIGHTNESS MODE IMAGING)

In B-mode, a slice through the patient is imaged. The transducer is pulsed at regular intervals as in A-mode but, unlike A-mode, the following occur.

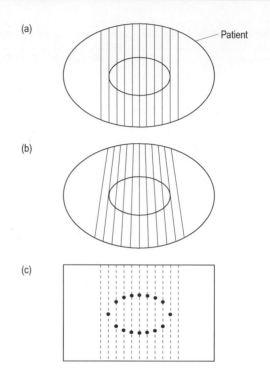

Figure 9.13 B-mode: (a) linear scan, (b) sector scan, and (c) the monitor screen.

- The ultrasound pencil beam scans back and forth across a two-dimensional section of the patient in either a linear, rectangular (Fig. 9.13a) or a sector (Fig. 9.13b) pattern. The diagram shows the scan lines travelled by each ultrasound pulse to produce the image. Only boundaries approximately perpendicular to the scan lines will be imaged.

- Each time the transducer is energized, the ultrasound beam takes a new scan line through the patient, and the trace starts at a point on the monitor screen corresponding to the skin surface and travels in the same direction as the ultrasound wave (Fig. 9.13c).

- The trace itself is suppressed.

- The returning echo pulses are displayed not as blips but as small bright dots corresponding to the amplitude of the signal for each of the interfaces encountered. Figure 9.13c shows the appearance on the screen where the relative signal level and the spatial position of the interfaces are maintained. TGC is used, as described above.

9.8 REAL–TIME IMAGING

In modern B-scanners, the image is automatically scanned in a succession of frames sufficiently rapidly to demonstrate the motion of tissues. Real-time

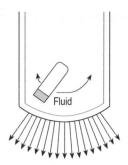

Figure 9.14 Mechanical sector scanner with an oscillating transducer.

imaging also allows a rapid search through a large organ. There are several methods.

9.8.1 Scanners

Mechanical (sector) scanning

The transducer, which is a circular disc and may be an annular array, moves within a fluid-filled plastic dome pressed against the body.

In one design, illustrated in Figure 9.14, the transducer is oscillated by an electric motor. (Alternatively, the transducer may be fixed and the sound reflected by an oscillating acoustic mirror.) Oscillation has the advantage that the wobble or sector angle, and so the field size, can be varied.

In another design, three to five transducers are mounted on a rotating wheel. Only the transducer nearest to the patient at any time is energized.

In either case, the ultrasonic beam sweeps across a sector of the body, each sweep producing one image frame. The rate of oscillation or rotation, and so the frame rate, can be varied.

Electronic scanning: stepped linear array

An elongated transducer, say $10 \times 100\,mm$ (shown in plan and section in Fig. 9.15) is divided into a large number (128 or more) of separate narrow strips, each about a wavelength in width. Individually, they would each give a poor beam, with a short near field and widely diverging far field. The piezoelectric elements are therefore energized in overlapping groups, in succession – say, 1–6, 2–7, 3–8, . . . – so that a well-defined ultrasound beam comes in effect from a small (square) transducer and scans a rectangular area in the body with (say) 120 scan lines.

Electronic focusing In fact, however, the outermost pair of strips in each group are energized first, then after a very short delay the next pair, and finally the innermost pair, so that pulses all arrive at some point

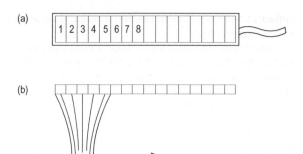

Figure 9.15 Linear transducer array: (a) transducer face and (b) cross-section through transducer and ultrasound beam with electronic focusing in the azimuthal plane.

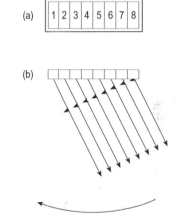

Figure 9.16 Steered beam produced by a phased array: (a) transducer face and (b) cross-section through transducer and ultrasound beam.

(P) at the same time, and reinforce. Figure 9.15 shows the beam shape; it is focused in the region of P. The timing of the applied pulses can be varied in order to change the focal depth P.

Electronic sector scanner: steered or phased array

The similar but shorter transducer (shown in plan and section in Fig. 9.16) contains fewer elements. If they are energized simultaneously, they act as a single transducer and the beam travels forwards. If they are energized separately in rapid sequence – 1, 2, 3, . . . – the pulses reinforce only in one direction. They interfere destructively in all others, and the beam swings to the right. If they are energized in reverse sequence – . . . 3, 2, 1 – the beam swings to the left. By slightly changing the time delay sequence between each pulse, the scan line is swept across the patient, covering a sector field (as with mechanical sector scanning).

Figure 9.16 does not show how, as with the linear array, the beam is in addition focused electronically at a selected depth by an adjustment to the phase delay pattern.

Focal depth

With both types of array, the focal length can be altered electronically by the operator: the greater the time delays between energizing the successive pairs of elements, the shorter the focal length. Unlike the circular annular array, the beam is focused electronically in one plane only, the azimuthal plane, parallel to the length of the array. Focusing in the perpendicular, elevation plane is done by shaping each transducer into a curve or using an acoustic lens, and this effectively defines the slice thickness.

Electronic focusing in the elevation plane is made possible by using a '1.5D transducer', in which up to seven rows of smaller elements replace the single row of a conventional linear array. Inter-row spacing has to be 10λ, and interelement spacing $\lambda/2$. Element selection is used rather than beam steering. These transducers produce better resolution of small lesions with greater uniformity at depth.

Focusing of the beam improves the image in the focal region but generally makes it worse beyond it. This can be mitigated by *multiple zone focusing*. Along each scan line, three (or four) pulses are sent in succession at the usual PRF. Each time, the phase delays are altered to focus at a different depth, for both transmission and reception. Each time, the transducer is gated so that it receives echoes from the corresponding focal zone only. Echoes arriving earlier from nearer points or later from deeper points are blocked. The focal zones overlap slightly so that the image shows no joins. However, three (or four) times fewer frames can be scanned each second.

Aspects of real-time imaging

Scan line density   The patient's tissues are in effect 'sampled' along a number of scan lines or 'lines of sight', depending on the number of elements in a multielement array. To obtain good-quality images with high resolution, each frame must be made up of a sufficiently large number of scan lines. In fact, about 100 lines per frame suffice, because the lateral resolution is in any case limited (see section 9.10).

Frame rate   To follow moving tissues, a sufficiently large number of frames must be scanned each second. The frame repetition frequency depends on the number

of lines per frame and is increased by increasing the PRF:

$$\text{frame rate} \times \text{lines per frame} = \text{PRF}.$$

To take a typical example, 30 frames s^{-1} each of 100 lines per frame require a PRF of 3 kHz.

Depth of view   To image structures at depth, each pulse must have time to make the return journey from the deepest tissue before the next pulse is generated. The depth of view is increased by reducing the PRF:

$$\text{depth of view} = 0.5 \times \text{sound velocity}/\text{PRF}.$$

It is therefore not possible to achieve both a high frame rate (frame repetition frequency) and a high scan line density and at the same time produce an image with a large depth of view. One or more aspects have to be compromised.

Combining the above equations:

$$\text{depth of view} \times (\text{scan lines}/\text{view})$$
$$\times (\text{frame rate}) = \text{constant}.$$

For example, a depth of 20 cm allows 30 frames s^{-1} and 100 lines/frame.

Sector scan versus linear scan

A linear scan needs a larger area of patient contact; gives a better quality image; maintains a wide field of view near the skin; and is used in imaging the whole abdomen, liver, superficial vessels and thyroid, and is also used in obstetrics and gynaecology.

A sector scan is easier to manipulate, requires a smaller acoustic window, has a narrower field near the skin but a wider field at depth, and is used to image the heart through intercostal spaces or subcostally and the infant brain through the fontanel. It is also used in intracavitary probes.

A linear array can be made in a curved format, as in Figure 9.17, to produce a sector-type image with a wide field of view without the complications of beam steering. The lines of sight are perpendicular to the array surface, and there is no loss of focus at the edges. However, beam divergence can limit the useful depth and the line density is reduced with depth.

Sector scan: mechanical versus electronic

A mechanical scanner is generally cheaper and employs a circular transducer focused by a lens or annular array, giving better resolution. An electronic scanner has no moving parts and is more compact.

To avoid the obscuring effects of bone or gas, two types of scanner may be used endoscopically: a linear array or a single high-frequency transducer rotating through 360°. Thus the heart may be imaged via the

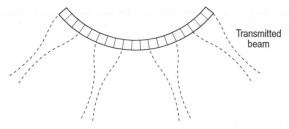

Figure 9.17 Curvilinear array produces a sector-type scan with no loss of focus at the edges.

oesophagus, the prostate via the rectum, and the fetus from the vagina.

Transvascular transducers use very small crystal arrays on the end of a catheter, and miniaturized electronics. They operate at 10–20 MHz and are used in assessing cardiac vessels and stents.

With advances in instrumentation such as multi-element broadband transducers, miniaturized electronics, high-speed digital components and image-processing techniques, signal to noise ratio and image quality are constantly improving.

9.8.2 Contrast agents

Ultrasound contrast agents are used to improve image quality and information. They do this mainly by increasing the reflections from the tissue containing the agent. The agents must have low toxicity and be readily eliminated by the body. They are generally based on microbubbles (less than 4 μm) or nanoparticles (less than 1 μm). Although bubble diameters are very much smaller than the ultrasound wavelength, they can resonate at the ultrasound frequency and at the harmonic frequencies (see section 9.8.3), enhancing echoes from the blood even at very high dilutions. Microbubbles are destroyed by ultrasound of high intensity. This property can be used to study subsequent refill dynamics at lower ultrasound power for reperfusion imaging. After the ultrasound examination, normal static diffusion leads to total bubble destruction within a few hours.

- Air-filled microspheres encapsulated in a thin shell of albumin. Injected intravenously, they increase back-scatter from ventricular borders to improve visualization and flow evaluation. They also adhere to thrombi, thus improving deep venous thrombosis diagnosis.

- Low-solubility gas encapsulated in a lipid shell. They may be used for all vascular applications (especially small vessels in the pancreas, kidney and liver), peripheral vascular disease and tumour vasculature.

- Perfluorocarbon nanoparticles. These stay in the blood for many hours post intravenously and are slowly taken up by the liver and spleen, improving imaging of metastases.

- Gold-bound colloidal microtubes. These may be immunologically targeted. Echo enhancement is possible when antibodies are conjugated with microtubes.

Targeted contrast agents have the potential not only for diagnosis but also eventually for drug and gene therapy.

9.8.3 Harmonic imaging

As ultrasound propagates through tissue, it becomes distorted because the speed of sound varies with tissue type. Consequently, the sound wave changes in shape from a perfect sinusoidal wave into a distorted one, indicating a change in the frequency components. These changes become more pronounced with depth and degrade the normal imaging process, especially, for example, for obese patients. Figure 9.18 illustrates this and shows the breakdown of the pulse, having transferred its high acoustic pressure or energy into its frequency components, or harmonics. The fundamental frequency is the *first harmonic*, and the subsequent harmonics are integral multiples of the first harmonic. Thus if the ultrasound frequency probe operates at 2 MHz, its second, third and fourth harmonics are at 4, 6 and 8 MHz, respectively.

Figure 9.18.c shows that the *second harmonic* can reach a useful magnitude and, if isolated, this can then be used to form an image instead of the fundamental frequency. Two methods are used to do this. Note that the bandwidth of the transducer has to cover the frequencies of both the transmitting and the receiving beams.

Harmonic band filtering

Harmonics start being produced when the transmitted beam has passed a few centimetres through the patient. They exist but are not produced in the returning echo beam (except those harmonics produced by microbubble contrast agents). The fundamental frequency is removed using a filter, leaving the tissue-generated harmonics to be processed for the image. The transmitted pulse should contain none of the higher frequencies, as this could corrupt the received signal. To ensure this, the pulse is stretched to produce a narrow transmission band. This degrades the axial resolution, in part compensated by the improved detection of the second harmonic.

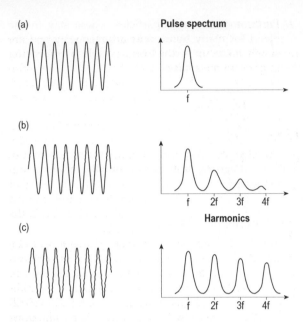

(a)

Pulse spectrum

f

(b)

f   2f   3f   4f

Harmonics

(c)

f   2f   3f   4f

Figure 9.18 Change in sound wave profile with different tissues at depth: (**a**) initial; (**b**) after a few centimetres of tissue; and (**c**) after a few more centimetres of tissue.

Pulse inversion

If every other transmitted pulse has its polarity reversed and the echoes received from each pair of transmitted pulses are summed, all the odd harmonics disappear from the signal, including the initially transmitted frequency. At the same time, the amplitude of each even harmonic is doubled, which enhances the signal to noise ratio for the second harmonic, thus enabling imaging with this signal. This technique preserves axial resolution but takes longer than standard imaging, so motion artefacts can occur.

Advantages of tissue harmonic imaging include the following.

- Reverberation artefacts are reduced, as low-amplitude echoes do not produce harmonics.

- Distortion and scattering from fatty tissues are reduced, as these are at the fundamental frequency and so suppressed, hence contrast resolution is improved.

- Low contrast lesions and liquid-filled cavities are better visualized, as there is reduced acoustic noise.

9.8.4 Three–dimensional imaging

Three-dimensional images are obtained from a set of two-dimensional scans. Either the movement of the probe is controlled electronically in a two-dimensional array so that the position and orientation are linked with the data collection or, while the operator moves the probe, its position and orientation are constantly registered. The images can be a set of parallel slices or a series of wedge shapes. In each case, a three-dimensional volume image can be produced from the data-set. This technique is slower than for two-dimensional scans unless a two-dimensional rectangular array transducer is used, with parallel processing.

Image reconstruction is not trivial, and the images themselves are not always easy to interpret unless they can be viewed as a series of tomographic slices along any angle of orientation within the scanned volume. However, volume rendering can give useful information regarding vasculature and also for fetal imaging.

If the acquisition and display of volume images is in real time, this is called four-dimensional imaging, where the time-varying spatial relationships of structures are displayed.

9.9 IMAGE ACQUISITION AND RECONSTRUCTION

Tissue differentiation is made possible by making the brightness of each 'dot' in the image vary according to the strength of the corresponding echo. The real-time greyscale image is presented on the monitor screen as a matrix of (say) 512 × 512 pixels, corresponding to the matrix of voxels in the body. A digital scan converter is used to improve the greyscale images, to enable freeze frame, to manipulate the data and to archive it if necessary. Consequently, a similar matrix of memory locations, each 6 to 8 bits deep, is located in the computer core memory. Figure 9.19 can be taken to refer equally to any of these matrices.

'Write' mode

As the successive echoes arrive at the transducer, their amplitudes (after digitization) are entered, along the corresponding scan lines of sight (such as W in Fig. 9.19), in memory locations corresponding to the voxels in the body section from which the echoes have arisen. The figures are continually updated.

For any pixel not covered by a scan line, a figure is interpolated from adjacent memory locations. The matrix 512 × 512 is greater than the number of scan lines, so that its pixel structure is not noticeable. The scan lines, however, can be obvious, especially at depth in a sector scan. They may be made less so by mathematically interpolating additional lines between those scanned.

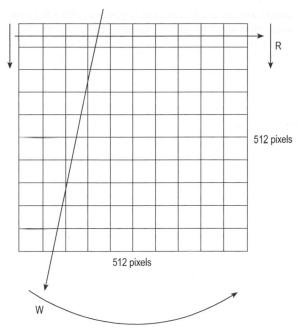

512 pixels

512 pixels

W

Figure 9.19 Digital scan converter, where W corresponds to the write mode for the scan lines of sight and R, the read-out.

'Read' mode

Throughout the scan and for as long as may be required thereafter, the memory locations are scanned along a series of horizontal lines (such as R in Fig. 9.19) in the form of a TV raster, and the numbers read out. After passage through a digital to analogue converter, the signal is used to modulate the brightness of pixels on the monitor screen. Because the memory locations are written in a different order from that in which they are read, the system is called a *digital scan converter*.

The image can be retained in the computer memory while succeeding scans are carried out and stored in other 'frames'. Any frame can then be selected for display. Frame averaging can be carried out, in which 5–10 successive echoes from the same point can be stored in the same memory location, producing a time-average value. Performed pixel by pixel over the whole frame, this smoothes the picture and reduces speckle (temporal averaging).

Images can be stored in the usual ways. Hard copy can be produced from a high-resolution screen with a multiformat camera or using a laser imager. The computer also controls the timing and shaping of the ultrasound pulse and correlates the start and direction of each scan line on the screen with those of the corresponding sound line of sight.

Dynamic range of signals

The smallest signal that can be detected is just greater than the noise, which, in ultrasound, is principally electronic noise: statistical fluctuations in the number of electrons in the very small currents measured. Some additional noise may be caused by reverberations in the patient or in the transducer probe.

The dynamic range of any component of an ultrasound imager is the ratio of the maximum intensity of the signal to the minimum that can be detected. Taking into account the weakness of reflections from some interfaces (Table 9.3) and the attenuation of the beam (Table 9.4), the ratio of the strongest to the weakest echoes is typically 70–80 dB. After TGC, the dynamic range is typically 40–50 dB.

The monitor can display a brightness (greyscale) range of only about 25 dB, within which the eye can distinguish only some 30 grey levels. It is therefore necessary to compress electronically (with a logarithmic amplifier) the signal amplitudes from a 40 to 50 dB range down to a 20 to 30 dB range. This may be done in such a manner as to enhance low-level, medium-level or high-level signals as required.

It is necessary to use a computer that is able to store $2^8 = 256$ different echo levels, corresponding to a dynamic range of 24 dB. Note that the dynamic range of recording film is not as good as that of the monitor, and that of Polaroid film is even worse.

Edge enhancement is used to increase the change in signal level at an interface. Reject control is used to eliminate low-amplitude noise and scatter (signal filtering). Sometimes, noise will exceed the threshold value and be included in the image.

Image processing

Various image processing techniques can be used: digital filtering, temporal averaging and contrast enhancement, as mentioned above.

9.10 RESOLUTION

Axial or depth resolution is the ability to separate two interfaces, A and B, along the same scan line. If, as in Figure 9.20a, they are too close together, the echo pulses A and B will overlap and be recorded as a single interface. The axial resolution is about half the pulse length. The higher the frequency of ultrasound or the shorter the pulse, the better the axial resolution. It would be made worse by omitting the backing block and thereby increasing Q.

Lateral resolution is the ability to separate two structures side by side at the same depth. This depends on the beam width being narrower than the gap. If, as in Figure 9.20b, the structures C and D are too close

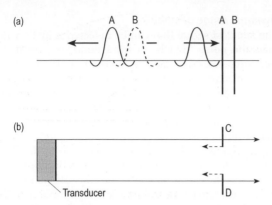

Figure 9.20 (a) Axial and (b) lateral resolution.

together, echoes will continue to be received as the beam, which is a few millimetres wide, sweeps across the gap between them. They will be imaged as a single structure. Resolution in the near field is improved by using a smaller transducer and by focusing.

In the case of a focused transducer, the beam is narrowest and the resolution best in the focal region. There, the approximate beam width = focal length × wavelength/diameter. The shorter the focal length, the narrower (and shorter) the focal region. With any particular diameter, using a higher frequency improves the resolution but reduces the penetration.

In the focal area, axial resolution may be about one wavelength and lateral resolution about three times worse, being about one-third of the transducer diameter.

Resolution and penetration

In choosing a transducer frequency for a particular investigation, it is necessary to compromise between the conflicting requirements of penetration depth (which decreases) and image resolution (which improves) as the frequency is increased. Typical figures are:

3.5–5 MHz	for general purpose abdominal scanning including heart, liver and uterus
5–10 MHz	for thyroid, carotid, breast, testis and other superficial tissues, and for infants
10–15 MHz	for the eye, which is small and acoustically transparent.

Higher frequencies still may be used in dermatology.

9.11 ARTEFACTS

Image formation assumes that sound travels in straight lines, with a constant velocity and (for TGC

purposes) constant attenuation, and is reflected only once from each interface. None of these assumptions hold exactly, and so artefacts appear that can lead to a misdiagnosis. Some of the more common artefacts are listed here.

Speckle Interference between the waves scattered from many small structures, too small and close to be resolved, within tissue (e.g. in liver, kidney, pancreas and spleen) produces a textured appearance. The echo pattern is random and unrelated to the actual pattern of scatterers within the organ, but it may be sufficiently characteristic to assist in tissue differentiation. On the other hand, the interiors of the bladder, cysts, large blood vessels, etc. are largely anechoic.

Reverberation Multiple reflections to and fro between the transducer face and a relatively strongly reflecting interface near the surface (or between two such interfaces) produce a series of delayed echoes equally spaced in time that falsely appear to be distant structures.

Double reflection For example, the diaphragm acts like a mirror, and structures in the liver can appear to lie in the lung. Pacemaker wires can also act as strong reflectors.

Acoustic shadowing Strongly attenuating or reflecting structures (e.g. bowel gas, lung, bone, and gallstones and kidney stones) reduce the intensity of echoes from the region behind them and cast shadows.

Acoustic enhancement Fluid-filled structures (e.g. a cyst or a filled bladder), being weakly attenuating, increase the intensity of echoes from the region behind them, producing a 'negative shadow'. Acoustic shadowing and enhancement are made worse by TGC.

Refraction Refraction of a beam falling obliquely on the two surfaces of bone (e.g. the skull) displaces the beam and the images of structures beyond. It distorts the image. So do variations of velocity, sound traveling significantly faster than the assumed $1540 \, \text{m s}^{-1}$ in some tissues (e.g. gallstones) and more slowly in others (e.g. lung).

Ring-down When a small gas bubble resonates, it emits ultrasound continuously, resulting in a track throughout the scan. This effect can also be caused by air in the stomach.

9.12 M-MODE SCANNING (TIME–MOTION)

The heart valves and heart wall move too quickly to be followed with a normal real-time scanner. Instead, a B-mode image is frozen on the screen and used to

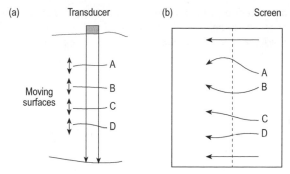

Figure 9.21 M-mode: (a) section through transducer and patient and (b) appearance on monitor screen.

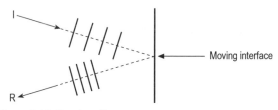

Figure 9.22 Doppler effect.

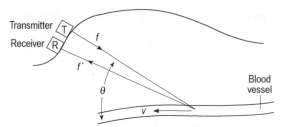

Figure 9.23 Continuous wave Doppler: detection of blood flow in a vessel.

The *change* of frequency is proportional to the velocity of the interface:

$$\frac{\text{change of frequency}}{\text{original frequency}} = 2 \times \frac{\text{velocity of the interface}}{\text{velocity of sound}}.$$

The higher the transducer frequency or the faster the interface moves, the greater the Doppler frequency shift. For example, if the velocity of the interface $v = 30\,\text{cm s}^{-1}$, and the frequency of the transducer $f = 10\,\text{MHz}$, because the velocity of sound $c = 1540\,\text{m s}^{-1}$ then the change of frequency $f - f' = 4\,\text{kHz}$. The Doppler frequency $(f - f')$ is comparatively small and equivalent to an audio frequency, i.e. in the range 0–10 kHz.

The above example refers to motion in the direction of the sound; motion at right angles to the transducer shows no Doppler effect, and that at an angle θ has a reduced effect:

$$(f - f')/f = 2(v/c)\cos\theta.$$

(For the meaning of θ, sometimes called the angle of insonation, see Fig. 9.23.) The maximum Doppler shift is obtained when $\theta = 0$, whereas in imaging the strongest echoes occur when $\theta = 90°$.

The *change* of frequency is measured and shows how *fast* the reflector is moving towards or away from the transducer. It is also possible to detect electronically whether the frequency increases or decreases, and this shows the *direction* of movement.

9.13.1 Continuous wave Doppler

Blood flow velocity is measured by the Doppler shift of ultrasound back-scattered by the blood cells. As shown in Figure 9.23, the probe uses two slightly angled transducers. They are chosen, as regards operating frequency, in the range 2–10 MHz, according to the depth of the vessel. To make the resonant frequency precise and maximize sound output, a high Q is necessary, and no backing block is used. The transmitter T is energized continuously with a radiofrequency alternating voltage of frequency f. The receiver R listens continuously to the back-scattered

direct the beam from a stationary transducer (as in A-mode) along a line of interest, intersecting the moving surfaces of the heart as nearly as possible at right angles (A–D in Fig. 9.21a). Echoes are displayed on the screen (Fig. 9.21b) as a line of (moving) bright dots, as in B-mode. Movement of the heart valves along the line of sight may be displayed by stepping the vertical line of dots slowly and steadily in a horizontal direction across the screen. Quantitative analysis is possible, which is important in echocardiology for the timing of flow across a valve. When combined with two-dimensional Doppler colour information, the line of sight can then be located on the heart.

9.13 DOPPLER METHODS

Doppler effect

The Doppler effect is familiar to those who have heard a siren sounding on an emergency vehicle as it passes by. When incident sound waves I of frequency f are reflected at right angles by a moving interface that is approaching the transducer, the waves are compressed (Fig. 9.22). The wavelength is reduced, and (the velocity being constant) the frequency f of the reflected wave R is increased. With a receding reflector, the frequency is reduced.

waves of frequency f' coming from the crossover area or sensitive volume.

The original frequency f is suppressed, and a Doppler signal, having the difference (or 'beat') frequency $(f - f')$, is extracted electronically. Pulsatile flow involves a range of velocities and produces a spectrum of Doppler frequencies that can be displayed on the screen using a frequency analyser in the manner described below.

The Doppler beat signal can be heard through a loudspeaker or headphones as a rushing sound – an audible indication of the spread of velocities involved in a heartbeat. The higher the pitch, the greater the velocity; the harsher the sound, the greater the turbulence. An audible signal is a useful adjunct to Doppler imaging. It also forms the basis of the ultrasonic stethoscope, used to monitor the fetal heartbeat.

With a continuous wave, it is not possible to locate the moving reflector or to distinguish between the flow in two overlapping vessels at different depths in the beam. On the other hand, with the short pulses used in imaging it is not possible to get accurate Doppler flow information. A compromise using longer pulses allows some information to be obtained about both flow and location.

9.13.2 Pulsed Doppler: range gating

In *duplex* scanning, Doppler measurement is combined with a real time B-scan image. In the simplest case, the scanning head combines a single pulsed Doppler transducer offset to a mechanical or electronic sector scanner. Most of the time is spent in the Doppler mode, the B-scan image being updated once a second. The imaging frequency is chosen to optimize resolution. The Doppler transducer might operate at a lower frequency, which, as described below, allows faster flow to be measured.

A real-time B-mode image is produced, and with its help a line of sight is chosen for the Doppler beam. Along it, cursors are set to identify the *sampling volume* (A in Fig. 9.24a), which is positioned over the vessel in which blood flow is to be measured. If the vessel is clearly defined, the angle θ can be read off to allow measured frequency shifts to be converted into blood flow velocities. The diameter of the lumen of the vessel can also be estimated to allow volume flow rates to be calculated, at least approximately.

The normal short imaging pulses are interspersed with bursts of Doppler ultrasound, each some 10 cycles long. A *range gate* is set to accept only those echoes that arrive within a short interval at a specific time, so that they can have come only from the

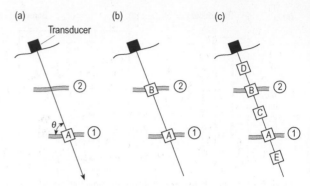

Figure 9.24 Pulsed Doppler: (a) normal and (b and c) high pulse repetition frequency modes; 1 and 2 are blood vessels.

selected sampling volume. The depth of the tissue so 'interrogated' depends on the time at which the gate is opened and its thickness on the time for which it is open. The width of the sampling volume (or gated Doppler acquisition area), which in practice is pear-shaped, is the width of the Doppler beam.

Because ultrasound takes 7 µs to travel 1 cm in average soft tissue, if the gate is opened 70 µs after the transducer is pulsed and closed 7 µs later, blood velocities will be sampled in tissue about 5 mm thick at a depth of 5 cm.

The intervals between pulses must be long enough for the successive Doppler signals not to overlap. A high PRF is chosen for superficial vessels and a lower one for deeper vessels. As the range setting is increased, the PRF is reduced and the TGC automatically increased.

The Doppler signal comprises a wide range of audio frequencies corresponding to the range of blood velocities in the sampling volume. It can be analysed and displayed as a time–velocity spectrum or sonogram. An electrocardiogram trace can be displayed at the same time.

Sonogram

A sonogram is a graph of Doppler frequency against time and displays the variation of blood flow velocity and direction during the heart cycle. It is bounded by an upper curve showing the variation of maximum flow velocity, and a lower curve showing that of minimum flow velocity. As shown in Figure 9.25, the area between the curves is filled with 'pixels', each in practice say 10 ms wide and 100 Hz tall.

The Doppler signal is continuously sampled in a series of 10 ms 'snapshots', during each of which it is analysed into its component frequencies and the spectrum represented as a column of pixels. Each pixel corresponds to a different frequency or flow velocity.

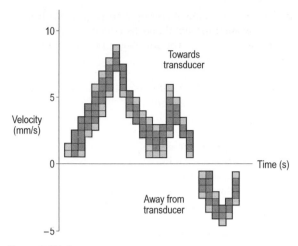

Figure 9.25 Sonogram.

Each pixel has a grey level representing the number of red blood cells in the sampling volume that have that velocity at that instant of time. From the sonogram, parameters such as peak velocity, mean velocity and variance of velocity can be evaluated.

Pressure measurement

Pressures in a stenosed artery or in the jet of blood issuing from a diseased heart valve can be estimated by Doppler measurement of flow velocity. When blood flows through a constriction, the flow velocity increases (to V m s^{-1}, say) and there is a corresponding increase in pressure (P mmHg), given by the modified Bernoulli formula, $P = 4V^2$. This formula is a simplification of the Bernoulli equation, which expresses the facts that blood is incompressible and that energy is conserved but ignores any effects of viscosity and turbulence.

Aliasing

With pulsed Doppler, it is not possible to measure very high-flow velocities with accuracy. If the flow is too fast, it will be shown in the wrong direction and its velocity underestimated. This artefact shows as 'wrap-round' top and bottom in the sonogram and is known as aliasing.

The same artefact can be seen in the cinema when the spoked wheel of a Western stagecoach rotates so fast that it appears to turn backwards, as described in section 9.2. Aliasing is a consequence of the sampling requirement (associated with the names of Shannon and Nyquist) that the waveform being measured (i.e. the Doppler signal) must be sampled at least twice in each period (see Ch. 5.2.1).

In other words, the frequency with which the Doppler pulses are repeated must be at least twice the maximum Doppler shift frequency produced by the flow. Thus the fastest flow that can be measured with accuracy is the velocity that produces a Doppler shift frequency equal to half the PRF being used. A greater flow velocity than this produces aliasing. Aliasing does not occur with continuous wave Doppler.

It is therefore particularly difficult to measure fast flow in deep blood vessels. The deeper the gate has to be set, the smaller the PRF that can be used (see section 9.8) and so the smaller the fastest flow that can be measured without aliasing.

For example, if the Doppler shift frequency produced by the fast blood flow associated with a stenosis is 8 kHz, the PRF must be at least 16 kHz. This allows a listening time of only 60 μs between pulses, in which time the sound can travel to and fro through a depth of view of only 5 cm.

The depth of the sampling volume determines the PRF needed, and the PRF determines the maximum velocity that can be measured without aliasing. Thus:

$$\text{maximum velocity (cm s}^{-1}) \times \text{range (cm)} \times \text{transducer frequency (MHz)} \approx 4000.$$

The risk of aliasing can be reduced by reducing the Doppler effect, either by using a probe of lower frequency f or by increasing the angle θ, but both increase the error in the measured flow. The risk can also be reduced by increasing the PRF, but this causes problems, as we shall now see.

High pulse repetition frequency mode

Suppose that the gate is set to measure the blood velocity in the selected sample volume A (Fig. 9.24a). Normally, the PRF would be set so that there is just time to collect the Doppler echo from A before the transducer is pulsed again. This means that it is not possible to measure the flow velocity if it is very high. This can partially be overcome by the use of a high PRF mode.

Suppose that the PRF is doubled; this will double the maximum measurable blood flow velocity. Unfortunately, at the moment when a Doppler echo from A is being accepted, so is one produced by the next pulse, coming from a sample volume B at exactly half the depth of A (Fig. 9.24b). Sonograms from the two samples would be superimposed on the display. The operator must therefore position the beam in such a way that only sample volume A is placed on a vessel while the nearer sample volume B is placed over an area of little perfusion.

Quadrupling the PRF will further improve the measurement of velocity. It does so at the expense of superimposing velocity data from multiple gated volumes (A–E in Fig. 9.24c). Ambiguity in velocity has been replaced by ambiguity in range. Carrying the idea to the extreme, when the PRF becomes very high, the pulses merge, and we have reinvented continuous wave Doppler with no aliasing but no range data.

9.13.3 Real-time colour flow imaging

Whereas a greyscale (B-mode) image shows the strength of echo coming from each pixel, a *colour-mapped Doppler* image shows the direction and velocity of movement or flow occurring in each pixel by means of an arbitrary colour code, for example:

flow toward the transducer – red
flow away from the transducer – blue
turbulence (i.e. variations in flow direction) – green or
   yellow.

The depth of each colour varies with the velocity of flow, stationary tissues appearing grey. Note that the colour scheme depends on the manufacturer.

A real-time B-mode scanner is used, and the Doppler colour overlay switched on and off at will. Compared with normal B-scan imaging, the Doppler pulse is longer, being a compromise between accurate depth information requiring a short pulse and accurate velocity information requiring a longer pulse. To obtain the latter, a number of Doppler pulses have to be sent in succession along each scan line.

Typically, 25 frames are scanned a second over a 60° sector. In each frame, the beam is steered in succession along 64 scan lines, dwelling on each line long enough for a B-scan pulse followed by a train of, say, eight consecutive Doppler pulses to be sent in and the echoes to return. Along each line the Doppler echoes from 128 separate gated ranges, each 1.5 mm long, are collected and analysed for frequency. The *average velocity* is evaluated in each sample volume, about 3 mm in size, and represented by the depth of colour of the corresponding pixel.

Whereas the sonogram in a gated Doppler image is produced from, say, 100 consecutive pulses (and effectively from an infinite number in continuous wave Doppler), in colour scanning there is time to send only some 4–12 pulses along each scan line. The data acquired are sufficient only to estimate the mean velocity and variance of velocity (as a measure of turbulence) in each sample volume and to colour each pixel accordingly.

To produce the sonogram of any sample volume or to measure peak velocity, a single sample volume is selected on the colour scan and the instrument switched to spectral Doppler mode.

The performance of colour scan Doppler is limited by the small time available to collect the data from each beam position. The following factors can be varied and are interrelated:

- *frame rate*, which should be fast enough to follow changes of flow velocity
- *penetration depth*, which is inversely proportional to PRF
- *field width* or sector size (30–90°)
- *line density*, i.e. scan lines per frame, which should be high enough for good spatial resolution
- *number of pulses in a train*, which should be high enough to give accurate velocity information.

Increasing any one of the above entails reducing one or more of the others. Whenever a high frame rate is desirable, especially for children, the sector size and depth range should be set as small as possible.

To achieve the required number of scan lines and the required frame rate, it may be necessary to restrict colour mapping to a selected part of the B-scan greyscale image.

Aliasing

Aliasing is also a feature of colour scans, because the PRF has to be set low enough to accommodate the deepest sampling volume in the image. Blue-coloured vessels become red, and vice versa. High-velocity laminar flow appears with an aliased blue centre and a non-aliased red edge. High-speed jets with associated turbulence show up as a coloured mosaic. Having located such high-velocity features, the machine can be switched to continuous wave or pulsed Doppler for more accurate measurement and sonogram display.

9.13.4 Power Doppler

Power Doppler images map the amplitude of the Doppler signal without any indication of the velocity. The amplitude of the signal depends on the number of red blood cells within the volume and on attenuation through the tissue. All movement, regardless of phase, contributes to the amplitude, so power Doppler emphasizes the quantity of blood flow. Its main advantage is to differentiate between areas of flow and no flow, so for example vessel walls are also more easily imaged. The power signal is less dependent on the insonation angle but, of course, the colour no longer indicates velocity or flow direction. Weaker signals can be imaged than in colour Doppler, so this increased sensitivity is useful for imaging smaller vessels. As this technique is non-directional, unlike colour Doppler it is not subject to aliasing. However, tissue motion creates artefacts, so power Doppler is best used where such motion is reduced.

9.14 QUALITY ASSURANCE

Ultrasound scanners are generally reliable and stable. However, slight damage to a probe or a drift in the electronics can lead to a slow deterioration of the image. Useful periodic tests include the following.

- Resolution: tested by imaging a test rig composed of parallel wires mounted on a frame and immersed in a Perspex bath containing a fluid in which sound travels at 1540 m s^{-1}.

- Sensitivity, dynamic range and accuracy of the A-scan calliper: using a Perspex block machined with a number of equally spaced vertical rods, some others of different diameters, and of decreasing depth. Figure 9.26 shows a simple example. Because sound travels faster in Perspex than in tissue, each 7 mm of Perspex is equivalent to 4 mm of tissue.

- Greyscale performance and Doppler function, which need more complex objects, usually based on phantoms with tissue-equivalent properties, based on gelatine loaded with different reflecting materials; often called tissue-mimicking phantoms.

- The power output of the transducer is measured by 'weighing' the sound pressure with a force balance, or by measuring the heating effect using a calorimeter. More sophisticated techniques can be used to measure the intensity distribution (beam shape).

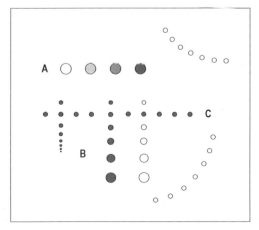

Figure 9.26 Simple Perspex block test object for A, dynamic range; B, sensitivity; and C, calliper verification.

9.15 SAFETY CONSIDERATIONS

Ultrasound is not an electromagnetic radiation and is non-ionizing. Used in diagnosis, it is a low-risk as well as a low-cost method of medical imaging. However, harmful bioeffects have been identified at exposure levels more usually associated with ultrasound therapy.

The intensity of an ultrasound beam is greatest in the focal region, where it is typically 0.1 mW mm^{-2}, averaged over the examination. The peak intensity (during the brief pulse) is likely to be 1000 times greater.

There has been no confirmed evidence of damage from diagnostic ultrasound exposure. However, the output of each probe should be checked periodically, and operators should keep within the agreed safety guidelines:

- the time-averaged intensity should nowhere exceed 100 mW cm^{-2}
- the total sound energy (intensity × dwell time) should nowhere exceed 50 J cm^{-2}.

If either of the above figures were grossly exceeded, there would be risk from:

- local *heating* due to frictional, viscous and molecular relaxation processes, leading to chemical damage but mitigated by blood flow. (This heating effect is used therapeutically.)
- Acoustic *streaming* of cellular contents in the direction of the beam, affecting cell membrane permeability.
- *Cavitation*: the high peak pressure changes causing microbubbles in a liquid or near liquid medium to expand. If they did so to the point of very sudden collapse, there might be an enormous rise of temperature with consequent profound chemical damage to cellular constituents. This is more likely to occur at high pressures and low frequencies and less likely to occur with pulsed beams, as each pulse does not last long enough for resonance to be reached.
- *Mechanical damage* to cell membranes caused by violent acceleration of particles.

As there is a tendency to increase exposure levels to improve image quality, care is needed. The thermal index (TI) is the ratio of the power emitted to that required to increase the temperature by 1°C and gives an indication of the temperature rise in tissue. The mechanical index is a measure of the maximum amplitude of the pressure pulse and is defined as the peak rarefaction pressure divided by the square root of the ultrasound frequency. These calculated indices, which are worst case-based, are indicated on the scanner

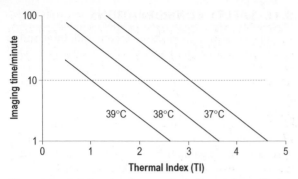

Figure 9.27 Safe imaging times at the indicated thermal index for different body temperatures.

display panel when the equipment itself can exceed an index value of 1. Index values less than 0.5 are below the threshold level for any effect and are considered safe. Above this level, the risks should be considered. The exposure time should be reduced appropriately as the TI increases above the value of 1. The approximation in Figure 9.27 shows that with a TI of 3 indicated, a normal patient may be scanned for 10 min, whereas for a patient running a temperature of 39°C, scanning for even less than 1 min will imply a non-safe situation. Thus particular care is needed when the patient is feverish and when using pulsed Doppler systems.

9.16 SUMMARY

- Ultrasound is inaudible sound (frequencies above 20 kHz).
- Ultrasound waves are produced by a transducer (a piezoceramic) that converts an electrical signal into an ultrasound beam. The transducer also acts as the receiver.
- Clinical ultrasound, having a short wavelength (frequencies from 3.5 to 15 MHz), can be formed into a narrow beam.
- Ultrasound is not electromagnetic radiation, but like light it does undergo reflection and refraction at the interface between two different media.
- Clinical ultrasound produces images from echoes reflected from internal tissue structures and interfaces.
- The echo return time is proportional to the depth of the structure, and the intensity depends on the tissue composition.
- Computer analysis of the transmitted and received signals from sector scanners enables anatomical displays in real time.
- Mechanical scanners generally produce better images, but electronic scanners are easier to handle and are more robust.
- Soft tissues that are too similar to be distinguished by planar X-ray contrast can be imaged.
- Microbubbles or nanoparticles can be used as contrast media.
- Ultrasound does not pass easily across tissue–air or tissue–bone interfaces, so lung and intracranial images are not generally practical.
- The Doppler effect is used to image the direction and velocity of blood flow.
- Signal to noise ratio and image quality improve as better instrumentation is developed.
- Most noise is electronic from the very small currents measured; additional noise comes from reverberations in the patient or in the transducer probe.
- Ultrasound, at normal diagnostic intensity levels, has no known deleterious effects and so is considered safe when indicated for fetal imaging.

Chapter 10

Magnetic resonance imaging

CHAPTER CONTENTS

Magnetic resonance imaging (MRI) uses radiowaves and magnetic fields. Although the nuclei of all atoms contain protons, only those with an odd number possess the property called nuclear magnetic resonance. Hydrogen has a single proton and thus a large magnetic moment, and it is abundant in the body, in water (free or attached to other molecules) and in fat, and so provides the best MRI signals.

The patient is placed in a magnet and a radiowave is sent through the body. The transmitter is turned off and the patient re-emits radiowaves, which are received and used for reconstruction of the image. It is the nuclei of hydrogen atoms that absorb and emit the radio-frequency (RF) energy. MRI measures the hydrogen content of individual voxels in each transverse slice of the patient and represents it as a shade of grey or colour in the corresponding image pixel on the screen.

10.1 THE SPINNING PROTON

Every proton has a positive charge and spins continually like a top around an axis called the spin vector. The circulating charge is like a small loop of current, and each proton acts like a bar magnet or dipole. Its magnetic moment m is represented by a vector joining the north and south poles, drawn as an arrow in Figure 10.1. Normally, all the individual dipoles point in a random fashion, with equal numbers in every direction. The net magnetic effect is then zero. (This ignores the tiny effect on them of the earth's magnetic field of about $50\,\mu T$.)

The patient lies prone or supine in a solenoid coil (see section 10.10 for details of equipment) carrying a direct current (DC). This produces a very uniform and strong magnetic field inside the coil, represented by a vector B pointing along the axis of the coil (and

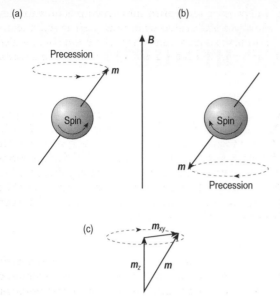

Figure 10.1 The magnetic vectors associated with a spinning proton precessing (a) parallel and (b) antiparallel to a magnetic field, *B*. (c) The transverse and longitudinal components of the magnetic vector.

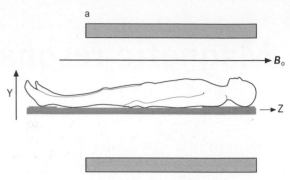

Figure 10.2 The patient on the scanner table inside the main solenoid coil, a, with magnetic field *B* in the horizontal Z-direction from toe to head. The Y-direction is vertical and the X-direction lateral or transverse through the patient.

the length of the patient, see Fig. 10.2). This is taken as the Z-axis; the Y-axis runs vertically from top to bottom and the X-axis horizontally across the machine. The magnetic field strength has a set value usually between 0.15 and 3 T, depending on the machine. By way of example, throughout this chapter we will take a machine with a field strength of 1 T. This is some 20 000 times greater than the earth's magnetic field.

Inside the coil, the patient becomes very slightly magnetized. The static magnetic field *B* causes the magnetic dipoles to turn and point along the Z-axis in one of two stable directions – either, as in Figure 10.1a, in the direction of the field (parallel or 'spin up') or, as in Figure 10.1b, in the opposite direction (antiparallel or 'spin down').

As it takes less energy to align with the magnetic field than to oppose it, slightly more dipoles point spin up than spin down. MRI depends on detecting this small difference, which is proportional to *B* and amounts to about three out of each million protons at 1 T.

Most of the dipoles, each with a magnetic moment *m*, cancel each other out in pairs (parallel and antiparallel), leaving those not so paired to produce a combined, longitudinal net or bulk magnetic vector M_z in the direction of *B*.

Henceforth, the terms *spins* or *protons* will refer only to the *detectable* protons, the excess of spin-up over spin-down protons, and we will ignore the others. For example, in a cubic millimetre of water

there are about 7×10^{19} protons, of which only some 2×10^{14} will be detectable.

Precession

The static field also causes the spinning protons to 'wobble' in a regular manner called precession (Fig. 10.1a,b). The direction of the spin axis tilts and rotates around the direction of the magnetic field *B* with a fixed frequency (millions of revolutions s⁻¹), called the Larmor frequency. Figure 10.1 illustrates the difference between spin, precession and the magnetic moment *m* of a single proton.

This is similar to the way in which the north–south axis of the earth precesses once in 25 000 years because of the gravitational pull of the sun, and a spinning top or gyroscope precesses because of the earth's gravitational field.

The tilting of the spin axis of a precessing proton splits its magnetic vector *m* into a longitudinal component m_z that points in the Z-direction, and a transverse component m_{xy} that rotates in the XY plane (Fig. 10.1c).

Now consider all the detectable protons in a single voxel of tissue (size a few cubic millimetres, illustrated in Fig. 10.3). The m_z vectors all point in the Z-direction and add up to a combined or net longitudinal magnetism M_z (Fig. 10.3a). This cannot be measured directly, as it points in the same direction as *B*. As the protons precess independently, their m_{xy} vectors point in all directions and cancel out. The net transverse magnetism $M_{xy} = 0$.

The stronger the magnetic field, the faster a proton precesses. The frequency of precession (f) or Larmor frequency is proportional to the product of:

- the magnetic field strength, and
- a constant property of the nucleus called the gyromagnetic ratio γ.

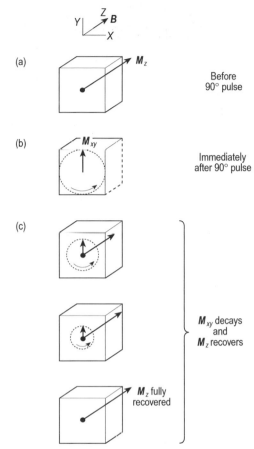

(a)

M$_z$

Before
90° pulse

(b)

M$_{xy}$

Immediately
after 90° pulse

(c)

M$_{xy}$ decays
and
M$_z$ recovers

M$_z$ fully
recovered

Figure 10.3 The net magnetization in a tissue voxel: a time sequence following a 90° pulse.

For hydrogen nuclei in a field of 1 T, $f = 42.6$ MHz. This is an RF and has a very precise value (in water, within ± 0.1 Hz).

In the quantum theory, a frequency of 42.6 MHz corresponds to a quantum energy of 0.2 µeV. The energy of the antiparallel state is therefore 0.2 µeV greater than that of the parallel state. It is because of this small energy difference that slightly more spins line up parallel rather than antiparallel.

Radiofrequency coils
Surrounding and close to the patient are a set of RF coils that inject an RF pulse in a direction perpendicular to *B*. This has two effects:

● some or all of the spin-up protons pick up energy, turn spin down, and are said to be excited. This affects *M*$_z$; it may be reduced, disappear or even reverse, depending on the length and strength of the RF pulse.

● the protons are pulled into synchronism, and they now precess in step or in phase. Their *m*$_{xy}$ vectors add up to a transverse magnetic vector *M*$_{xy}$, which rotates in the *XY* plane (Fig. 10.3b) at the Larmor frequency.

Resonance
It is well known that an opera singer must strike precisely the right note to shatter a wine glass. Similarly, in order to affect the dipoles, the frequency of the RF generator must very accurately match the Larmor precession or resonant frequency of the dipoles. In other words, the photon energy of the radiowaves must be exactly the same as the energy difference between spin-up and spin-down protons.

180° pulse
An RF pulse of a certain total energy will give to each and every dipole exactly the energy (0.2 µeV) required to tip them through 180°. This temporarily reverses the net magnetic vector *M*$_z$.

90° pulse
An RF pulse of half that total energy (i.e. half the intensity or half the duration) will tip half of the dipoles so that equal numbers point spin up and spin down, thus reducing *M*$_z$ to zero. The RF pulse also causes them to move into the same phase and precess together (phase coherence).

This phase coherence of the dipoles produces a transverse magnetism *M*$_{xy}$, perpendicular to *B*, which rotates in the *XY* plane at the Larmor frequency (Fig. 10.3b). It is as if the 90° pulse has tipped the magnetic vector *M*$_z$ through 90°. MRI involves sending a series of many such pulses, repeated at intervals of *TR* seconds, called the repetition time.

10.2 THE MAGNETIC RESONANCE SIGNAL

When the 90° pulse is over, the magnetic vector *M*$_{xy}$ continues for a while to rotate in the transverse *XY* plane. Just like the rotating magnet in a dynamo, it induces in the RF coil an alternating (RF) voltage of a few microvolts. After amplification by an RF amplifier (receiver), tuned like a radio to the resonant frequency, the amplitude or envelope of this signal is sampled, digitized and computer analysed. Using methods of spatial encoding and signal processing described in section 10.4, the magnetic resonance (MR) signal from each individual voxel in the scan matrix can be identified to produce the pixel grey or colour level in the MR image.

Note that only *M*$_{xy}$ produces an MR signal; *M*$_z$ does not. But because *M*$_{xy}$ is produced by tipping *M*$_z$, the signal produced by a 90° pulse depends on the value of M_z immediately before that pulse is applied.

The peak signal is proportional to, and the pixel brightness depends on:

- proton or spin density (PD, number of protons per cubic millimetre) of the voxel
- the gyromagnetic ratio of the nucleus
- the static field strength B, because placing the patient in a stronger magnetic field increases the preponderance of protons that are initially spin up over those that are spin down.

Only mobile protons give signals; those in large molecules or effectively immobilized in bone do not. The greater part of the signal is due to body water, whether free or bound to molecules. Air, in sinuses for example, having no hydrogen, produces no signal and always appears black in the image. Fat has a higher PD than other soft tissues. Grey matter has a somewhat greater PD than white matter. Tissues do not, however, vary greatly in their proton densities.

Free induction decay

The MR signal is greatest immediately after the brief 90° pulse has been switched off. Thereafter, the dipoles are free to return, some earlier than others, to their original orientation. As indicated in Figure 10.3c, M_z regrows or 'recovers' while M_{xy} decreases or 'decays', and, accordingly, the strength of the MR signal induced in the receiver coil also decays, although its frequency remains the same.

At any instant of time, M_z and M_{xy} combine to produce a *sum* vector M. The 90° pulse has tipped the sum vector through 90° into the XY transverse plane. Then, during relaxation, as M_z increases and M_{xy} decreases, the sum vector spirals (beehive fashion, Fig. 10.4) back from the transverse plane to the longitudinal Z-direction. This is caused by two concurrent and quite independent methods of energy loss or 'relaxation': spin–lattice and spin–spin relaxation.

Spin–lattice relaxation or T_1 recovery

The dipoles are continuously jostled by the thermal motion of the rest of the molecule or nearby molecules. The excited protons give up their energy to the molecular lattice. One by one, the dipoles tip back parallel to the Z-axis, and M_z slowly reappears (Fig. 10.3c). This is also called longitudinal relaxation.

In Figure 10.5, the left-hand axis refers to curve A, which shows how, after M_z has been destroyed at time 0 by the first 90° pulse, it increases again relatively slowly and does so exponentially with a time constant T_1 that depends on the type of tissue.

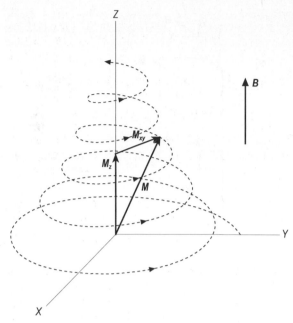

Figure 10.4 Behaviour of the sum magnetic vector M during free induction decay.

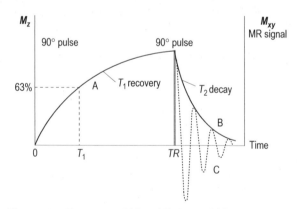

Figure 10.5 T_1 recovery of M_z and T_2 decay of M_{xy}. MR, magnetic resonance.

T_1 is the time for M_z to recover to 63% of its maximum value. After three time constants, recovery is 95% complete:

Time	0	T_1	$2T_1$	$3T_1$
Recovery (%)	0	63	87	95

T_1 has a value of so many hundreds of milliseconds (Table 10.1). If a stronger magnetic field B is used, the protons precess faster and T_1 of tissue lengthens, and M_z reappears more slowly.

Table 10.1 Typical relaxation times of tissues in a field of 1 T

Material	T_1 (ms)	T_2 (ms)
Fat	250	80
Liver	400	40
Kidney	550	60
Spleen	400	60
White matter	650	90
Grey matter	800	100
Cerebrospinal fluid	2000	150
Water	3000	3000
Bone, teeth	Very long	Very short

Causes of spin–lattice relaxation

- Jostling by large molecules that are slow moving and near to the resonant frequency is most effective at removing energy from excited dipoles. Fat (large molecules with low inherent energy) can absorb energy easily and so has a relatively short T_1, as does water bound to the surface of proteins.

- Jostling by small, lightweight molecules with little inertia is rapid and so relatively ineffective at removing energy from the excited dipoles. Consequently, free water, urine, amniotic fluid, cerebrospinal fluid (CSF) and other solutions of salts have a long T_1. The greater the proportion of free water in a tissue, the longer is T_1.

- The atoms in solids and rigid macromolecules are relatively fixed, and they are the least effective at removing energy. Compact bone, teeth, calculi and metallic clips have a very long T_1.

Spin–spin relaxation or T_2 decay

Energy transfer between nuclei produces a loss of phase coherence, resulting in an exponential decay of the transverse magnetic vector, dependent on tissue type.

In a pulse sequence, M_z has not fully recovered when, TR seconds after the first pulse, a second 90° pulse converts the available M_z into M_{xy}. In Figure 10.5, the right-hand axis refers to curve B, which shows how M_{xy} then decays relatively rapidly, for the following reason.

Immediately after the 90° pulse, the dipoles are still all precessing in phase and their m_{xy} vectors simply add up. The large net magnetic vector M_{xy} induces a large MR signal. The dipoles then progressively dephase, as some rotate faster or slower than others. As a result, the net strength of the rotating magnetic vector M_{xy} decreases, and so does the induced signal (dotted curve C in Fig. 10.5).

Much of this dephasing effect is due to field inhomogeneities from machine factors external to the patient, but the clinically important part is related to tissue structure and is called spin–spin or transverse relaxation, or T_2 decay.

As depicted in Figure 10.5, M_{xy} decreases or decays exponentially (curve B), and so does the induced signal (curve C), both with a time constant T_2.

T_2 is the time for the MR signal to fall to 37% of its maximum value. T_2 has a value of so many tens of milliseconds (Table 10.1). After three time constants, only 5% of it remains:

Time	0	$1T_2$	$2T_2$	$3T_2$
Signal (%)	100	37	14	5

Causes of spin–spin relaxation   The dephasing occurs because a spinning proton experiences a tiny additional magnetic field (around 1 μT) produced by each neighbouring proton. Individual protons are affected slightly differently, and the magnetic field B therefore varies a little from place to place and from time to time on the submicroscopic scale. So does the rate of precession; some precess faster and some slower, and energy passes from one proton to another, or spin to spin.

The local variation of magnetic field is greatest in solids and rigid macromolecules in which the atoms are relatively fixed. The dipoles in compact bone, tendons, teeth, calculi and metallic clips dephase quickly. They have a very short T_2 and do not produce a lasting signal.

The effect is least in free water, urine, amniotic fluid, CSF and other solutions of salts. The lighter molecules are in rapid thermal motion, which smoothes out the local field and results in a long T_2. Broadly speaking, the greater the proportion of free water in tissue, the longer is T_2. Spleen has a longer relaxation time than liver, and renal medulla longer than the cortex.

Water bound to the surface of proteins and other large molecules, which move more slowly, has a shorter T_2 than free water, and so does the hydrogen in fat.

Tissue characteristics

T_2 is always shorter than T_1. T_2 is more or less unaffected by, but T_1 of tissue increases with, magnetic field strength, i.e. with resonant frequency. There are no *precise* values of T_1 or T_2 for specific tissues. Figures cover a wide range, and only representative, rounded values are given in Table 10.1. Abnormal tissue tends to have a higher PD, T_1 and T_2 than normal tissue, because of increased water content or vascularity.

Because T_1 and T_2 are properties of the tissues that show a greater variation than PD itself, they are the properties actually used in forming the MR image. Comparing the range of T_1 and T_2 values for brain tissue in Table 10.1 with the limited range of computed tomography (CT) numbers (which depend on the very small differences in X-ray absorption) shows the superior soft tissue contrast resolution of MRI compared with CT.

10.3 SPIN–ECHO SEQUENCE

In practice, the MR or free induction decay (FID) signal is rarely measured because it decays so very rapidly – with a time constant T_2^* of a few milliseconds, much shorter than T_2. This happens because the static field B is not perfectly uniform:

- mainly because of the magnetic field gradient (see section 10.4) deliberately produced across the voxel
- because of unavoidable imperfections in the engineering of the magnet
- because the introduction of the patient unavoidably distorts the static field (due to magnetic susceptibility, see section 10.8).

These systemic effects unfortunately add to the effect of spin–spin interactions in the tissue in causing some dipoles to precess faster than others after a 90° pulse, with consequent dephasing.

To remove the effects associated with the static field but leaving the tissue characteristic T_2 effect, a *spin–echo (SE) pulse sequence* is used. Figure 10.6 depicts one cycle of this sequence, which is repeated hundreds of times in producing one MR image frame. It should be studied in conjunction with the sequence of events (a–d) depicted in Figure 10.7.

In the SE sequence, each 90° pulse is followed, t seconds later, by a 180° pulse. The signal is measured after a further and equal time interval (so that the echo time, TE, is $2t$).

- *Step a.* Immediately after the 90° pulse, the dipoles are all precessing exactly in phase (Fig. 10.7a). M_{xy} is a maximum, and so is the FID signal, but it is not measured at this stage, because it decays so rapidly.

- *Step b.* The m_{xy} vectors begin to dephase, the faster precessing ones (leaders) getting ahead of the slower ones (laggers in Fig. 10.7b). M_{xy} and the FID signal decay with time constant T_2^* (extreme left, Fig. 10.6).

- *Step c.* After time t, the 180° pulse is applied and tips all the dipoles from spin up to spin down. This

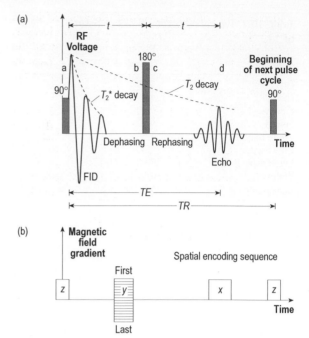

Figure 10.6 One cycle of the spin–echo sequence of (a) radiofrequency pulses and signal and (b) magnetic field gradient switching. FID, free induction decay; RF, radiofrequency; TE, echo time; TR, repetition time.

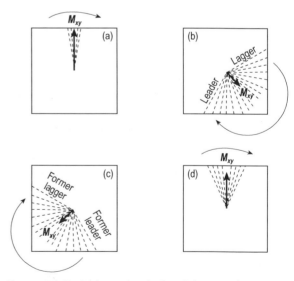

Figure 10.7 Dephasing and rephasing of the m_{xy} vectors of individual protons in a voxel in a spin–echo sequence: (a) dephasing starts immediately after a 90° pulse, (b) just before the 180° pulse; (c) just after the 180° pulse, rephasing begins; and (d) at time TE (echo time), only residual dephasing remains.

turns the individual m_{xy} vectors through 180° in the X-direction (Fig. 10.7c). Laggers become leaders, and vice versa. M_{xy} and the signal are still small. As the m_{xy} vectors continue to rotate in the XY plane, they now rephase. The faster ones catch up with the slower ones, and M_{xy} and the MR signal regrow.

- *Step d*. After a further time t, they are again momentarily in phase (Fig. 10.7d) and M_{xy} and the MR signal are at their peak. Thereafter, they grow out of phase again and M_{xy} and the MR signal decay.

The 180° pulse is often called the rephasing or refocusing pulse. It reverses and eliminates the dephasing effect of systemic magnetic field inhomogeneities. This leaves only the residual dephasing (Fig. 10.7d) due to the random effects of spin–spin interaction, T_2.

The MR signal reappears as an echo of the initial signal (see Fig. 10.6) and is essentially two FID signals back to back. When measured at time $TE = 2t$, it will have been reduced in amplitude by T_2 decay. The longer is TE, the smaller the MR signal.

Tissue contrast

The MR image maps three intrinsic properties (PD, T_1 and T_2) of tissue, and is controlled by two parameters set by the operator: TE (or time to echo) and TR (or time to repeat). These are selected to weight the contrast in the image.

The MR signal arising from a voxel and the brightness of the pixel depends on:

- How many protons there are in the voxel. The greater the PD, the larger the signal and the brighter the pixel.

- How far M_z has recovered from the previous 90° pulse when the next 90° pulse tips it, i.e. the length of T_1 compared with TR.

  Figure 10.8 compares two tissues that differ only in T_1, their PDs being the same. It shows that the shorter T_1 (or the longer TR), the greater the M_z available to be tipped and the larger the MR signal, the brighter the pixel, and the better the signal to noise ratio (SNR). It also shows that the TR can be selected to give a maximum contrast between particular tissues.

- How far M_{xy} has decayed when the echo is formed, i.e. the length of T_2 compared to TE.

  Figure 10.9 compares two tissues that differ only in T_2 (their T_1 and PD being the same). It shows that the longer T_2 or the shorter TE, the larger the MR signal, the brighter the pixel, and the better the SNR. It also shows that the TE can be selected to give a maximum contrast between particular tissues.

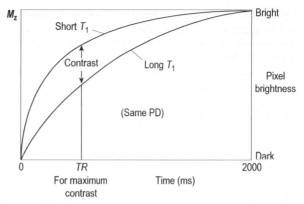

Figure 10.8 T_1 contrast.
PD, proton density; TR, repetition time.

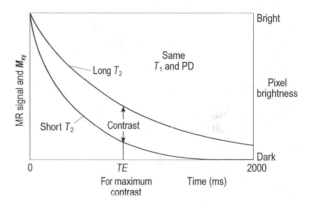

Figure 10.9 T_2 contrast.
MR, magnetic resonance; PD, proton density; TE, echo time.

Weighted images

The TE and TR are chosen so that pixel brightness depends on one of three combinations of PD, T_1 and T_2.

T_1-**weighted image** Figure 10.8 shows that maximum contrast (the difference between the curves) between tissues of different T_1 is produced by a fairly short TR.

A TR of 300–800 ms is used – about the same as the average T_1 of the tissues of interest. A short TE (15 ms) is also used, as this reduces the effect of T_2 on contrast. (It cannot be much shorter, as the system has to apply the 180° RF pulse and a series of gradient pulses before the MR signal can be measured.)

Image contrast is then principally due to the T_1 recovery properties of the tissues. The shorter is T_1, the stronger the signal and the brighter the pixel. *Fat is bright*, as is fatty bone marrow, while *water and CSF are dark*.

T_2-**weighted image** Figure 10.9 shows that the longer is TE, the greater the contrast between tissues of

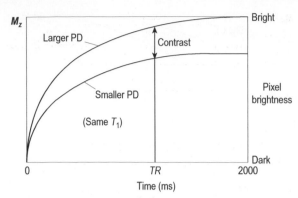

Figure 10.10 Proton density (PD) contrast. *TR*, repetition time.

different T_2. However, it must not be so long that the signal is so small as to be obscured by background noise.

A relatively long *TE* of 90–140 ms is used – about the same as the average T_2 of the tissues of interest. A long *TR* (1000–2000 ms) is also used, as this reduces the effect of T_1 on contrast, although unfortunately it increases the imaging time.

Image contrast is then principally caused by differences in the T_2 decay properties of the tissues. The longer is T_2, the stronger the signal and the brighter the pixel. *Water and CSF appear brighter than fat.*

Proton density–weighted image Figure 10.10 compares two tissues that differ only in PD, their T_1 being the same. It shows that the longer is *TR*, the greater the contrast between tissues of different PDs.

A long *TR* (1000–3000 ms) is used – about $3T_1$ – and this reduces the effect of T_1 on contrast. A short as possible *TE* (15 ms) is used, as this reduces the effect of T_2. Generally speaking, PD weighting produces greater signal strength and less noise.

Image contrast is then principally caused by differences in the proton densities of the tissues. The greater the PD, the stronger the signal and the brighter the image. CSF, fat and indeed most tissues, having a high PD (number of hydrogen protons), appear bright.

Summary A large signal and a bright pixel result from tissues having a large PD and a long T_2. A small signal and a dark pixel result from a long T_1 and (as will be seen later) arterial blood flow. *In all images,* air and cortical bone, having no hydrogen, appear black.

The *TR* controls the amount of T_1 weighting, and *TE* the amount of T_2 weighting in the image, as in Table 10.2.

In practice, matters may not be so clear-cut. It is not possible to rid any image of some T_2 weighting, and relative weighting may differ from tissue to tissue across an image.

Table 10.2 T_1-, T_2- and proton density–weighting effects

Weighting	Properties	Result
T_1-weighted	*TR* and *TE* both short	Short T_1 = bright
T_2-weighted	*TE* and *TR* both long	Long T_2 = bright
PD-weighted	Short *TE* and long *TR*	High PD = bright

PD, proton density; *TE*, echo time; *TR*, repetition time.

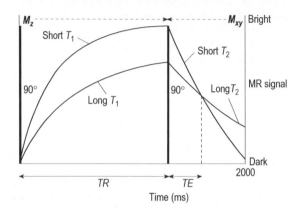

Figure 10.11 Contrast: combined effects of T_1 and T_2. MR, magnetic resonance; *TE*, echo time; *TR*, repetition time.

White and grey matter In a PD-weighted image, grey matter, with its somewhat higher PD, appears brighter than white matter. In a T_2-weighted image, grey matter, with its longer T_2 and higher PD, is brighter than white matter. In a T_1-weighted image, white matter is brighter than grey matter but its shorter T_1 is somewhat counteracted by its lower PD.

The opposing effects of T_1 and T_2
T_1 and T_2 are mutually antagonistic and have opposing effects on image brightness. Generally speaking, tissues with a long T_1 also have a long T_2, and those with a short T_1 have a short T_2. This is why images cannot be weighted for both T_1 and T_2.

Remembering once again that *the signal produced by a 90° pulse depends on the value of* $\mathbf{M_z}$ *immediately before the pulse is applied*, Figures 10.8 and 10.9 can be combined into Figure 10.11. This shows that, with an injudicious choice of *TE* and *TR*, tissues with quite different relaxation times can produce equal signals. Showing no contrast, they will be indistinguishable. With a shorter *TE* than this, the image tends to be T_1-weighted, and with a longer *TE* it tends to be T_2-weighted.

Table 10.3 Factors affecting magnetic resonance signal and contrast

Fixed parameter	Machine settings	Tissue characteristics
Gyromagnetic ratio of nucleus	TR TE –	T_1 T_2 Proton density
Static magnetic field	II (see section 10.5) Tip angle (see section 10.5)	Flow (see section 10.6) Contrast medium (see section 10.6)

TE, echo time; TR, repetition time.

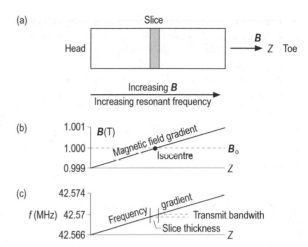

Figure 10.12 Transverse slice selection with a Z-field gradient. (a) sagittal cross-section of the patient, (b) magnetic field gradient, and (c) transmit frequency gradient.

Other factors affecting the magnetic resonance signal and contrast

Table 10.3 shows that there is a more complex state of affairs than in X-ray imaging.

10.4 SPATIAL ENCODING

To produce an image, it is necessary to collect and analyse the signals coming from the patient in terms of their amplitude, frequency and phase, and then to Fourier transform them to produce the individual pixels or voxels in the image. Magnetic field gradients are used to localize the MR signal, which itself is encoded in terms of spatial frequencies using phase-encoding and frequency-encoding gradients. The three basic processes involved are slice selection, phase encoding and frequency encoding. Note that every spatial frequency must be collected and stored before the data can be Fourier transformed to produce the image.

Slice selection

As in CT, an MR image is made up of a series of parallel slices that are imaged in turn. Figure 10.12 represents a sagittal section through the patient with a transverse slice (shaded).

Simultaneously with the 90° RF pulse, DC is sent for a short while through a pair of gradient coils, which are additional to the main RF coil. This current produces a controlled magnetic field gradient, along the Z-axis, within the static magnetic field B_0. The total B is diminished at (say) the head end and augmented at the toe end (Fig. 10.12b) while remaining the same at the isocentre. In this case, it varies from head to toe with a constant gradient of a few milliteslas per metre (mT m^{-1}).

Accordingly, protons at the head end precess more slowly than those in the middle, and those at the

foot do so faster. There is therefore a corresponding gradient, in the Z-direction, of the resonant frequency of the protons, and so the frequency can be used to localize the signal. The protons in a selected slice are all precessing with a narrow range of frequencies (Fig. 10.12c).

The RF transmitter is tuned to generate an RF pulse that contains a small range of frequencies (a narrow bandwidth). Only protons in a certain thin slice of the patient will be excited by it. The magnetic vectors of only those protons will tip and, in due course, produce an MR signal. Note that the slice select gradient field is switched on during the application of the RF pulse. Different slices are selected in turn by simply altering the central frequency of the RF pulse, without having to move the patient.

Slice thickness

The slice thickness may be reduced by either increasing the gradient of the magnetic field or decreasing the RF (or transmit) bandwidth. A thinner slice produces better anatomical detail, the partial volume effect being less, but it takes longer to excite.

A typical slice thickness is 2–10 mm. The RF pulse inevitably contains a certain amount of electromagnetic energy of frequencies slightly higher or lower than the intended bandwidth, thus mildly exciting tissues either side of the desired slice. To prevent this 'cross-talk' affecting the image slice, a gap (say 10% of the slice thickness) may be left between slices, although this is not necessary when the slices are interleaved (see section 10.5).

The slice orientation depends on the physical gradient axis. As described here, using the Z-axis gives a transverse slice. However, using the X-axis would give a sagittal slice, and the Y-axis a coronal slice. Any orientation is actually possible by combining the gradients.

In-slice localization

Having selected the slice, the objects within the slice have to be localized. This is achieved by applying *phase encoding* and *frequency encoding* each orthogonal to the slice, the MR signal being measured during the latter part of the frequency encoding gradient.

The complex MR signal is sampled and computer analysed into a spectrum of component frequencies using a mathematical process called Fourier analysis. The data from every signal in a selected slice are stored in what is known as K space. This space is simply a spatial frequency domain in the computer where the signal spatial frequencies and their origin are stored. The spatial frequencies correspond to the variations in image brightness as the encoding gradients are applied. K space does not correspond to the image but rather has axes corresponding to frequency and phase. The number of lines filled in K space matches the number of encodings in the sequence (e.g. 128, 256 or 512). The central part of K space contains data from shallow encoding gradients, low spatial frequencies and hence less details but stronger signals. The upper and lower parts are filled with data from the steeper gradients, high spatial frequency so better detail but low signal intensity, as indicated in Figure 10.13. Note that K space has to be completely filled with the data from the imaging sequence before the signals can be analysed and processed into the image.

Phase encoding

Immediately after the protons in the slice have been excited by the 90° pulse, but before they are inverted by the 180° pulse, DC is passed for a few milliseconds through a second set of gradient coils. This produces a magnetic field gradient, for example in the Y-direction (Fig. 10.14a,b), from the front to the back of the patient.

For that brief period of time, some of the precessing dipoles and M_{xy} vectors speed up and some slow down. Those in voxels near the top of the column (say) precess more slowly and lag behind those in the middle, while those near the bottom precess faster and get ahead.

When the gradient pulse is over, they all precess again at the same rate, and they again all emit the same frequency signal. However, the *phase differences* remain, and these are dependent on the position. Those near the top are still behind those near the bottom. There is a phase gradient in the MR signals coming from different pixels for the same type of tissue along the selected vertical line (Fig. 10.14c); the nuclei are phase-encoded. With a steep gradient, the spins will be evenly distributed in every direction and the total signal will be zero. With no gradient, the spins are all in phase and the signal will be a maximum. This is referred to as zero spatial frequency and the data are located on the central line of K space.

In order to map, for example, a 512 × 512 matrix, there must be this number of possible spatial frequencies. The phase-encoding pulse must be repeated with the gradient increased a little after each excitation, thus stepping up the phase shifts. By comparing the pattern of increasing phase angles *f*, it is possible to decipher the separate signals across the field of view (FOV). The FOV increases if the phase-encoding step size is made smaller. The pixel size equals the FOV divided by the number of phase-encoding gradient steps used.

Frequency encoding

At the same time as the gradients for phase encoding are applied, DC is passed through the third set of

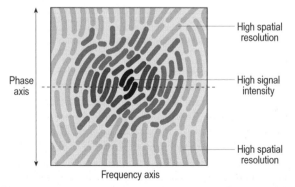

Figure 10.13 K space: each data point in the matrix is a spatial frequency component of the signal.

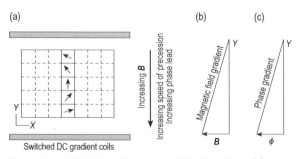

Figure 10.14 Phase encoding using a Y-field gradient: (a) transverse cross-section of the patient, (b) magnetic field gradient, and (c) phase gradient for a given tissue type. DC, direct current.

gradient coils to produce a magnetic field gradient, also orthogonal to the slice selection gradient, for example from side to side in the X-direction (Fig. 10.15).

Protons in each vertical column of Figure 10.15 experience the same magnetic field, precess with the same frequency, and emit MR signals of the same frequency. But those in the left-hand columns (say) precess more slowly than those in the middle, and those on the right precess faster. There is a corresponding frequency gradient from left to right in the MR signals emitted (Fig. 10.15c). This is a bit like the frequency gradient along the keyboard of a piano: the pitch of the note reveals (or 'codes for') the position of the key that was struck. The MR signal produced by exciting the slice therefore consists of a range of RF frequencies either side of the frequency of the applied pulse.

Field of view   The receiver is tuned to accept only a certain range of frequencies, called the receive bandwidth, coming from a corresponding FOV (Fig. 10.15c). The FOV may be increased by either making the field gradient less steep or increasing the receive bandwidth. The voxel width equals the FOV divided by the number of components into which the frequency spectrum has been sampled.

The MR signal emitted by the whole slice therefore comprises a mixture or spectrum of phases as well as of frequencies. At the same time as the computer is analysing the signal for frequency, it is analysing it for phase. This Fourier analysis is analogous to the way the human ear picks out individual instruments from an orchestra. However, because phase angles repeat themselves every 360°, it is impossible to be confident about assigning a particular phase to just one point. Typically, there are several phase cycles across the whole FOV, so the phase angle of, say, 10° is repeated at 370°, 730°, and so on.

Measuring a series of phase angles over 512 repetitions is really the same as measuring a single signal at 512 points all in one go. Figure 10.16 shows how the two methods can be seen as equivalent. By using a Fourier transform along the phase-encoding direction, it is possible to measure the frequencies in this direction, which correspond to position along the phase-encoding axis. The TR is sometimes described as pseudotime, and by analogy the FT of the phase-encoded signals would be called a pseudofrequency. In this sense, it is possible to think of phase encoding as simply frequency encoding over a very long time scale.

Imaging time   The time needed to acquire an image is obtained by multiplying the number of signal averages or excitations N_{ex}, the number of phase-encoding steps, and the pulse repetition time TR, and may total several minutes. Increasing the number of excitations

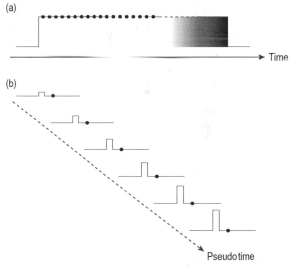

Figure 10.16 Equivalence of frequency and phase encoding, using the concept of pseudotime. Each dot represents an acquired data point. (a) With frequency encoding, all the data points are acquired at microseconds intervals – gradient on all the time; (b) with phase encoding, each data point follows the application of a separate, increasing sized gradient in pseudotime steps equal to repetition time (TR) ms. (Courtesy of E.A. Moore.)

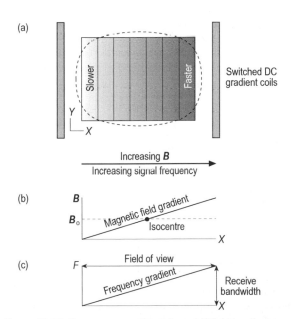

Figure 10.15 Frequency encoding using an X-field gradient: (a) transverse section of the patient, (b) magnetic field gradient, and (c) receive frequency gradient.

reduces noise at the expense of increased imaging time. For example, four repetitions ('excitations') of the foregoing SE sequence that are averaged will improve the SNR by a factor $\sqrt{4} = 2$.

Once all the signals are collected, a fast Fourier transform converts the K-space distribution into an image of the patient. This actually produces a complex image having real and imaginary parts, which are usually combined as a complex magnitude image. Note that a phase image can also be calculated, if required.

If any tissues move during the repetitions, they will be misregistered, i.e. signals will be attributed to the wrong pixels in the phase-encoding direction of K space. Such motion artefacts, described in section 10.8, when seen on an MR image make it clear which is the direction of phase encoding *vis-à-vis* frequency encoding. (Similarly, any chemical shift artefacts, described in section 10.8, reveal the direction of frequency encoding.)

Summary of gradients

The gradient fields are superimposed in pulses on to the static field. One gradient defines the slice and is applied when the RF pulse is turned on. A second orthogonal gradient is used for phase encoding and is applied briefly between the 90° and 180° RF pulses. The third orthogonal gradient is used for frequency encoding, during which the signal is measured. By combining frequency encoding and phase encoding, all the spatial frequencies within a slice can be collected unambiguously as needed to produce the two-dimensional image. Figure 10.6 shows how the field *gradients* are applied during the SE sequence. In practice, the gradient sequences will usually be more complex than described here.

The gradients are used to control the slice thickness and the FOV. The steeper is the slice selection gradient, the thinner the slice. The steeper are the frequency and phase-encoding gradients, the smaller the FOV. The steeper a gradient, the greater the power consumed by the gradient coils.

There is a significant difference between phase and frequency encoding. All the spatial information required in the frequency-encoding direction is obtained in 10–20 ms by sampling a single echo, and increasing the matrix makes no difference to the total scan time (although it may reduce the number of slices possible within the *TR*). In the phase-encoding direction, the spatial information is not complete until all the gradient steps (e.g. 512) have been completed. This can lead to the appearance of motion artefacts (see section 10.8).

10.5 OTHER PULSE SEQUENCE AND IMAGING TECHNIQUES

So far, we have considered imaging in the transverse plane using a single SE sequence. The following gradient sequences are those most often encountered, although they may have different acronyms depending on the MR scanner manufacturer.

Multislice techniques

Most of *TR* is 'wasted' if the scanner has to wait up to 2 s before repeating pulses on a given slice. This time can be used to deliver a succession of 90° and 180° RF pulses, each of a different frequency, exciting a series of up to 32 separate slices before repeating the first slice (Fig. 10.17). The shorter that *TE* is compared with *TR*, the more slices can be interleaved in this way. If *TR* = 1000 ms and *TE* = 60 ms, in principle 1000/60 = 16 slices, but in practice about 13 slices can be excited.

By acquiring the slices out of sequence, the need for gaps due to cross-talk when slices are acquired sequentially is avoided.

Multiecho techniques

This is another way of making use of the long *TR*. Following each 90° pulse, two or more successive 180° pulses produce successive echoes with increasing *TE*. Their peak amplitudes decrease with the time constant T_2. The first echo may produce a PD-weighted image, while successive echoes produce images that are increasingly T_2-weighted (and increasingly noisy). A dual echo sequence can be written as 90, 180, 180 and produces two images per slice. The first echo has a short *TE* (20 ms) and long *TR* (2000 ms), which produces a PD-weighted image. The second echo has a longer *TE* (80 ms) and produces a T_2-weighted image. There may also be time during a single *TR* to interleave a number of slices.

Fast (or turbo) spin–echo

The 90°, 180°, 180°, … sequence can be modified by phase encoding each of the 4–16 echoes (echo spacing 20 ms apart, say) with a different phase-encoding gradient. This reduces by a factor of 4–16 the time

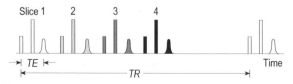

Figure 10.17 Multislice imaging. *TE*, echo time; *TR*, repetition time.

(i.e. the number of TR intervals) needed to acquire a complete image. However, fewer slices can be interleaved. Fat produces an extremely high (bright) signal on fast SE (FSE or TSE) T_2-weighted images, because the rapid succession of $180°$ pulses reduces the spin–spin interactions, thus increasing T_2. Fat suppression techniques are sometimes needed. Conversely, muscle is often darker than in single SE T_2-weighted images, as the succession of pulses increases the transfer of magnetization and results in saturation.

As scan time is reduced, matrix size can be increased to improve spatial resolution (smaller voxels). Note that FSE is incompatible with respiratory compensation techniques, but the use of powerful gradients can enable an image to be obtained in a single breath hold.

Inversion recovery

To accentuate T_1 weighting, an initial $180°$ pulse is used (Fig. 10.18a). This tips the spins antiparallel to the Z-axis and inverts M_z. The spins progressively return to parallel, due to spin–lattice relaxation. M_z recovers, passing through zero and reversing direction after a time of $0.69 \times T_1$.

After a variable time (TI is the time to inversion, e.g. 500 ms), a $90°$ pulse is applied that tilts the available M_z. The M_{xy} vector so produced rotates in the transverse XY plane (Fig. 10.3), producing an MR signal (FID). A second $180°$ pulse is then used to develop an echo signal. The whole ($180°$, $90°$, $180°$) cycle is repeated after TR (Fig. 10.18a). Typical parameters might be $TR = 1000$ ms and $TE = 20$ ms.

Consider two tissues of different T_1. If $TI = 0.69 \times$ the longer T_1, that tissue gives no signal, as there is no available M_z to convert, whereas the tissue with the shorter T_1 does. The image is T_1-weighted, and tissues with longer T_1 are suppressed. The longer TI is or the shorter T_1 is, the greater the MR signal produced. TE controls the T_2 decay and must be short for T_1 weighting.

The TI is used as a T_1 contrast control. TR is about $3T_1$ to ensure nearly total recovery between pulses. This technique is time-consuming, especially at higher field strengths, which makes T_1 and so TI long but gives good grey–white matter discrimination.

Short-TI inversion recovery sequence: for fat suppression

In SE sequences, the very bright signal produced by fat may obscure contrasts in other tissues. There are several ways of dealing with this. One is to remove the signal from fat by using an inversion recovery sequence, with its initial $180°$ pulse, followed rapidly by a $90°$ pulse.

The $180°$ pulse tips both fat and water protons antiparallel, but they recover more quickly in fat, with its short T_1, than in water. This is shown in Figure 10.19, which may be compared with Figure 10.18. After a certain time TI (about 125 ms), half the spins in fat have reverted to parallel, and its $M_z = 0$. Few of the spins in water have so reverted, and it still has some M_z. A $90°$ pulse at this instant produces a signal from water and other tissues but none from fat.

Tip angle

There are several ways of reducing scan times. One method is to reduce TR to 200 ms or even 20 ms. This would give M_z little time to recover and result in rather small signals from the usual $90°$ RF pulse. Instead, an RF pulse of shorter duration (smaller tip angle or flip angle) is used, which inverts only a small fraction of the dipoles.

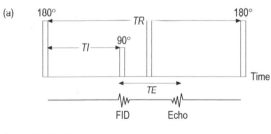

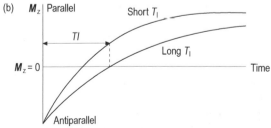

Figure 10.18 (a) Inversion recovery sequence. (b) Recovery of tissue having different T_1 values.
FID, free induction decay; TE, echo time; TI, time to inversion; TR, repetition time.

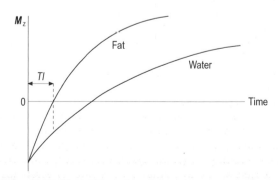

Figure 10.19 Short-TI inversion recovery.

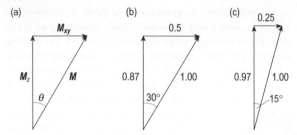

Figure 10.20 (a) Meaning of tip angle. Relative values of M_z and M_{xy} at tip angles (b) 30° and (c) 15°.

Table 10.4 Effect of tip angle

Weighting	Properties	Result
T_1-weighted	TR and TE both short	Tip angle >70°
T_2-weighted	TR and TE both long	Tip angle 5–10°
PD-weighted	Short TE and long TR	Tip angle 5–10°

PD, proton density; *TE*, echo time; *TR*, repetition time.

Figure 10.20a (which may be compared with Fig. 10.4) shows how M_z, M_{xy} and the tip angle θ are related through a right-angled triangle. Figure 10.20b shows that a 30° pulse produces only half of the usual M_{xy} and the consequent MR signal. However, it leaves 87% of M_z, which does not take long to recover fully. This ensures a good signal following the next RF pulse. Similarly (Fig. 10.20c), a 15° pulse produces 25% of the usual M_{xy} but leaves 97% of M_z.

The stronger the initial RF pulse and the longer its duration, the greater the tip angle. The greater the tip angle, the greater the T_1 weighting (Table 10.4).

The *optimum tip angle*, which gives the greatest signal, is a balance between leaving sufficient M_z and producing sufficient M_{xy}. The shorter TR is, compared with T_1, the smaller is the optimum tip angle:

TR/T_1	3	1	0.14	0.03
θ (°)	87	68	30	15

Gradient (recalled) echo (GRE)

With *TE* typically 15 ms, there is time within the short *TR* for very few slices to be imaged. If *TR* is as short as 20 ms, the image must be acquired one slice at a time. Some 15 separate slices can be taken in 30 s, a sufficiently short time for patients to hold their breath but not rapid enough to produce real-time images (see *Echo planar imaging* and *Parallel imaging*).

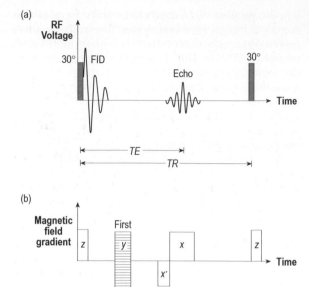

Figure 10.21 Gradient echo. (a) Radiofrequency (RF) pulses and signal and (b) magnetic field gradients.
FID, free induction decay; *TE*, echo time; *TR*, repetition time.

With such short *TE*, there is no time for a 180° pulse as used in SE sequences. Instead, rephasing is achieved using *a gradient echo* (Fig. 10.21). The gradient field is reversed to refocus the out-of-phase spins. This compensates for the dephasing produced by the change of magnetic field across the voxel produced by the gradient field (see section 10.3). Unlike SE, however, it does not eliminate the effect of inhomogeneities in the static field, and so the image is T_2^*-weighted; nor does it compensate for magnetic susceptibility effects (see section 10.8).

The usual frequency-encoding gradient pulse X is preceded by a reverse pulse X' (of half the duration). During the first, negative, part of the gradient pulse, the dipoles at one side of each voxel are made to precess faster than and get ahead of those at the other. Then the gradient current reverses and the latter begin to catch up with the former, coming into phase again to produce the echo signal. The peak of the MR signal appears at the middle of the X-gradient pulse (Fig. 10.21b).

To summarize: compared with the SE sequence, in a GRE sequence the RF pulse is of reduced strength and tips the magnetic vector through a smaller angle than 90°, thus allowing a short *TR*. The negative gradient pulse X' dephases the spins, and the positive gradient pulse X, which is twice as long, rephases them.

An important characteristic of GRE scans is that *moving blood appears bright* (see *Magnetic resonance angiography*).

Echo planar imaging

A 50-ms 'snapshot' may be produced by an extremely fast form of GRE called echo planar imaging (EPI). Following a standard (90°, 180°) SE sequence and slice selection gradient, the polarity of a frequency-encoding gradient is continually reversed, as fast as possible, each time inducing a gradient echo. The phase-encoding gradient is also switched on and off, briefly, just before each echo, thus encoding each of the echoes with a different phase-encoding gradient. Multiple echoes can be collected before M_{xy} has decayed too far, to give a complete image in the 50 ms following the SE 90–180° pulses. PD or T_2 weighting is obtained by using short or long effective *TE*. T_1 weighting is possible if an inverting pulse is applied before the excitation pulse to produce saturation. The whole brain can be imaged in about 2–3 s. However, resolution, echo strength and the signal to noise are all compromised.

The strong field of a superconducting magnet is necessary, and artefacts may be a problem. As very high gradients and very fast switching are needed, this will induce small, unwanted currents in nearby metallic structures, and these may cause blurring and artefacts in the image (see section 10.8). They can be reduced by active shielding of the gradient coils (see section 10.10).

This ultrafast technique can be used for functional imaging, real-time cardiac imaging and perfusion or diffusion imaging.

Imaging in other planes

Any desired image plane can be selected without moving the patient.

To image in the coronal plane, the Y-gradient is used for slice selecting and the other two for frequency and phase encoding. To image in the sagittal plane, the X-gradient is used for slice selecting and the other two for frequency and phase encoding. To image in the coronal oblique plane, slice selection is applied to the X- and Y-gradients simultaneously.

Generally speaking, the phase-encoding gradient is best applied along the shorter dimension of the patient's anatomy.

Three-dimensional Fourier imaging (volume imaging)

This is an alternative method of spatial encoding. A shallow Z-gradient is used to select a thick slice, thick enough to include the whole volume to be imaged. As usual, frequency encoding is used along one axis, but phase encoding is used along both of the others. The data-processing requirements are increased accordingly; so is the scan time, but this may be mitigated by using GRE with a short *TE*. A three-dimensional Fourier transform is used to decode the information. Because the slice selection direction is phase encoded, it is also subject to motion artefacts and to phase wraparound artefacts, just like the normal in-plane phase encoding. The three-dimensional data can be 'reformatted' to produce images of a series of very thin contiguous slices (no gaps) in any orientation, with no cross-talk.

Parallel imaging

Most MR techniques need high temporal and spatial resolution. Before parallel imaging techniques were available, multiple slice techniques and increasing the gradient strength were the only way to do this, although the latter is expensive and has unwanted side effects (peripheral nerve stimulation).

Simultaneous acquisition of spatial harmonics (SMASH) and *sensitivity encoding (SENSE)* each use an array of RF detection coils to perform some of the phase encoding usually done by magnetic field gradients. Conventional spatial encoding with gradients is a serial process, whereas SMASH and SENSE are partially parallel imaging techniques. Each coil in an array is connected to a separate RF receiver, resulting in parallel streams of data, each of which produces a separate image. SMASH and SENSE use the information from both the localized sensitivities of the individual coils and their independent signals. Thus images are obtained with fewer phase encode steps, the limiting factor in MRI. Most existing fast-imaging sequences such as EPI can be used with SMASH and SENSE in half the normal image acquisition time.

If each RF coil *transmits* as well as receives the signal, better separation of the signals is obtained. The pulse duration is reduced, enabling short *TE*–short *TR* sequences, optimizing the SNR with reduced scan time in transmit SENSE.

This field is developing constantly and is enabling techniques such as radial or spiral scanning to become available.

10.6 SPECIALIZED IMAGING TECHNIQUES

Magnetic resonance angiography

The effect on the MR image of the flow of blood depends on many factors, including its velocity, flow profile, and direction relative to the slice (it is greatest for flow perpendicular to the slice), as well as the

(a)

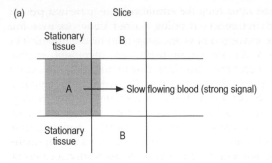

(b)

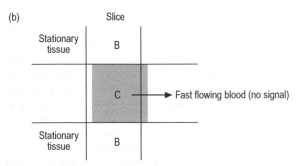

Figure 10.22 Appearance of blood during spin–echo: **(a)** slow-flowing and **(b)** fast-flowing.

pulse sequence and its parameters. In multislice imaging, the appearance depends on whether the slices are acquired in the same or opposite direction to the flow. A few simple principles can be identified regarding the SE sequence.

- *Vessels containing slow-flowing blood (e.g. in a vein) may appear bright (flow enhancement).* Previously unexcited blood (A in Fig. 10.22a) that enters the slice during a 90° pulse is more affected by the pulse and produces a stronger echo than stationary tissue (B) in which M_z has not yet fully recovered from the previous 90° pulse. The effect is most noticeable when the pulses are repeated rapidly, with a short TR.

- *Vessels containing fast-flowing blood (e.g. in the aorta) appear dark or void.* Some of the blood (C in Fig. 10.22b) excited by the 90° pulse has already left the slice before the 180° pulse occurs, and so produces no echo signal. Conventional T_1 weighting with presaturation pulses produces 'black blood' flow, and so any signals from a vessel indicate stagnant flow or an occlusion.

- *Turbulent flow produces a rapid loss of coherence, thus reducing M_{xy}, and usually appears dark* – for example, turbulence downstream of a stricture in a vessel.

In a GRE scan, *flowing blood and CSF usually appear bright*, for the following reason. The RF pulses, which are rapidly repeated, excite spins only in the selected slice, but the gradient pulse (unlike the 180° pulse in SE, Fig. 10.22) rephases all spins whether in the slice or outside it. Even if (as in the second principle above) some of the excited blood has left the slice, the gradient pulse will rephase it, and it will still produce a signal. Flowing blood does not therefore appear black. On the contrary (as in the first principle above), the in-flowing blood will give a larger signal and appear brighter than stationary tissues, which have previously been repeatedly excited as long as TR is well below the T_1 recovery of the stationary tissues.

To image only the blood vessels in GRE, moving blood is recognized either by its increased brightness in 'time of flight angiography', or by the phase change caused by movement along the magnetic field gradient ('phase contrast angiography'). Stationary tissue shows no net phase change. No contrast medium is required because of the large difference in the MR signals from flowing blood and tissue. In two-dimensional angiography, a series of images, stacked in the direction of the vessel, is produced, analysed for maximum intensity related to each voxel; this is projected on to a single image plane to produce the angiogram. The same construction technique is used for CT angiography (Ch. 7.4.2). For good three-dimensional (volume) angiography with high signal to noise, high-velocity flow is needed (e.g. intracranial flow).

Perfusion imaging

Perfusion imaging uses a paramagnetic contrast agent to measure the rate at which blood is delivered to the capillary bed of tissues and thus metabolic activity. There are two main methods – either using a bolus of contrast agent or arterial spin labelling – usually needing EPI techniques.

Gadolinium (as the ion Gd^{3+}) is a highly suitable material to use as, having seven unpaired electrons, it is strongly paramagnetic. Being very toxic, it is chelated with diethylenetriaminepenta-acetic acid (DTPA), which is water-soluble and to which it remains bound until excreted. However, it is contraindicated in patients with renal dysfunction.

Used as an intravenous contrast medium, Gd-DTPA is not itself visible on the MR image. Tumbling at around the Larmor frequency, the paramagnetic molecules shorten both T_1 and T_2 of the hydrogen nuclei in their vicinity as a magnetic susceptibility effect. As the effect on T_1 is greater than on T_2, it is called a positive contrast agent. The area of uptake is made brighter in a T_1-weighted image. T_1 weighting is therefore generally used after gadolinium injection.

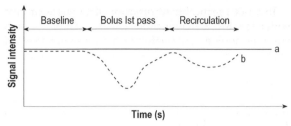

Figure 10.23 Signal intensity during bolus transit through different tissues: a, no change in signal, no perfusion; b, strong change, normal perfusion.

However, during the first pass of the agent, the gadolinium remains in the blood vessels and causes a large susceptibility effect in perfused tissues. T_2^* weighting with a gradient echo is sensitive to these changes. Because the transit of the bolus through the tissue lasts only a few seconds, fast imaging techniques must be used. Analysis of the signal decay gives information on blood volume and a measurement of perfusion in terms of millilitres of blood per 100 g tissue per minute, the tracer concentration being roughly proportional to the relaxation rate in normally perfused tissues (Fig. 10.23).

As Gd-DTPA is water-soluble, it may produce increased contrast between pathological and normal tissue. It does not cross the normal blood–brain barrier and so is used to reveal breakdown of the barrier. The protons in water are more affected than those in fat. Water may appear equally bright as fat, and fat suppression techniques may have to be used.

The greater the concentration of Gd-DTPA, the shorter the relaxation times. Because T_1 and T_2 shortening have opposite effects, the concentration of Gd-DTPA must not be so great that the T_2 effect cancels out the T_1 effect.

In *arterial spin labelling*, two images are generally obtained, one in which the blood water magnetization is different, obtained by spin inversion techniques (*spin-labelled* image), from that of tissue water, and the *control* image, in which they are in the same state (no inversion is applied). Subtracting the two images gives the perfusion image from which the blood flow can be measured.

Applying the off-resonance RF pulse for inversion can cause magnetization transfer between free and bound water, resulting in a decrease of the expected contrast. To mitigate the effect in the subtracted image, an off-resonance RF pulse is usually applied before acquisition of the control image so that the magnetization transfer effects cancel.

Diffusion imaging

Diffusion-weighted imaging requires combining EPI or fast GRE sequences with two large gradient pulses applied after each RF excitation. The gradient pulses effectively cancel if spins do not move (are static), while moving spins undergo a phase shift. Tissue water with normal random thermal motion (diffusion) attenuates the signal due to the destructive interference of all the phase-dispersed spins, while a high signal appears from tissues with restricted movement or diffusion. Subtle changes in the restriction of movement are reflected in the signal attenuation that is directly related to the apparent (or effective) diffusion coefficient multiplied by a sensitivity weighting factor that depends on the time and the amplitude of the diffusion gradient.

Diffusion gradients must be strong and are applied in X-, Y- and Z-directions to obtain the diffusion-weighted image. Although the images themselves provide visual information on, for example, tissues damaged because of oedema, much more can be obtained only by post-processing of the data to provide parameters that enable quantitative assessment of tissue integrity and connectivity, for example.

Functional imaging (functional MRI)

Functional MRI techniques acquire images of the brain during an activity or stimulus and compares them with at-rest images. The physiological effect that produces the greatest change in MR signal between stimulus and rest is the blood oxygenation level. Haemoglobin contains iron and transports oxygen bound to the iron in the vascular system and so into the tissues. Oxyhaemoglobin is diamagnetic (magnetic properties are weakly opposed to the main field), while deoxyhaemoglobin is paramagnetic and produces magnetic field inhomogeneities in neighbouring tissues, increasing T_2^*. At rest, tissues have roughly equal amounts of oxy- and deoxyhaemoglobin. When metabolic activity is increased, more oxygen is extracted from the capillaries, increasing blood flow and causing a change in deoxyhaemoglobin and thus the MR signal. The effects are very short-lived and so need very rapid sequences such as EPI or fast GRE. Typically, low-resolution volume images are acquired with long TE (about 50 ms) every few seconds while the physiological stimulus is applied. The areas of the subtracted images (stimulus minus rest) that show increased signal intensity correspond to the brain area activated by the stimulus. The subtracted images can then be overlaid on to a normal high-resolution image of the area to provide the functional map.

Magnetic resonance spectroscopic imaging

Magnetic resonance spectroscopy provides a frequency spectrum fingerprint of the tissue based on its molecular and chemical composition. Peak intensities and

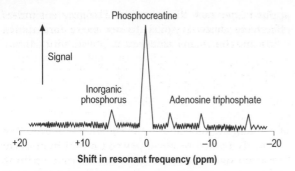

Figure 10.24 Magnetic resonance spectroscopy.

position indicate how an atom is bonded to a molecule. Most clinical spectroscopy studies hydrogen, but other MR-active nuclei are possible.

Nuclei with even numbers of protons and even numbers of neutrons (even Z and even A) cannot show MR ($\gamma = 0$). Those with an odd number of protons or an odd number of neutrons can do so. Different nuclides have different gyromagnetic ratios.

For MRI to be feasible, a nuclide must have a high gyromagnetic ratio, the isotope must be abundant in the element, and the element must be abundant in the human body. Of the four most abundant elements in the human body, ^{1}H is, on all three counts, the easiest to image. ^{16}O, ^{14}N and ^{12}C possess no nuclear magnetism. ^{13}C has an odd number of neutrons but accounts for only 1% of carbon atoms. Naturally abundant ^{31}P has a lower gyromagnetic ratio (17.2 MHz at 1 T) than ^{1}H, but it can be imaged using a sufficiently strong magnetic field and appropriate surface coils. Although the MR signal is several orders of magnitude less than for ^{1}H and so the images have lower spatial resolution (see below), the metabolism of phosphorus is of significant interest as an indicator of energy metabolism and is also used as a monitor of therapy outcome.

Because of chemical shift, phosphorus nuclei have different resonant frequencies when bound in inorganic salts, adenosine triphosphate, phospho monoester, phospho diester and phosphocreatine. Using a broadband RF pulse, all these can be made to resonate. The MR signals from a defined volume of tissue can be analysed as a frequency spectrum (Fig. 10.24), and each of the metabolites can be imaged separately. Sequential imaging allows the study of their metabolism in vivo.

A high magnetic field (2 T or more) is needed to give sufficient signal strength and sufficiently good *spectral* resolution. The field must be uniform to better than 1 ppm. As spectroscopy depends on frequency, only phase-encoding gradients can be used in imaging. Accordingly, to reduce imaging time, much larger pixels in a coarser matrix of 1 cm pixels must be used.

It is not practicable to produce MR images in vivo with other MR active nuclides (such as ^{19}F or ^{13}C) and other metabolites, although they are routinely assessed in vitro, as their low SNR implies very long scan times.

Dixon method for chemical shift imaging

Spinning protons are affected to some extent by the magnetic fields of atomic electrons circulating in nearby atoms. The resonant frequency of a proton is therefore affected by its chemical environment. Measurement of this 'chemical shift' can give information about molecular structure.

The valence electrons in the H–O bond in water produce a slightly smaller magnetic field in the region of the proton than do those in the H–C bond in lipids. As a result, the resonant frequency of the proton is about 3 ppm greater in fat than in water.

The difference in resonant frequencies can be exploited to produce separate images of water and fat:

- After the 90° pulse in a conventional MR scan, the dipoles in water and fat precess at slightly different rates and are continually going in and out of phase with each other every few milliseconds. A (water plus fat) image is obtained by setting the *TE* when they are exactly in phase, and a (water minus fat) image is obtained by slightly delaying the *TE* until they are exactly out of phase. Adding these two images produces a water-only image, and subtracting them gives a fat-only image.

10.7 MAGNETIC RESONANCE IMAGE QUALITY

Image quality depends on many parameters, such as the magnetic field strength, the pulse sequence and its timing, number of excitations, slice thickness, slice separation, dimensions of the image matrix and FOV, inherent or injected contrast, and the use of surface coils. In this section, their effect on the signal, noise, image contrast, spatial resolution and scan times are considered. Section 10.8 looks specifically at image artefacts.

Signal to noise ratio

Noise is a random variation in the MR signal, occurring at all frequencies and all the time, due to the following.

- *Patient.* Noise is principally due to the presence of the patient. Random thermal movement of the hydrogen atoms in the tissues induces in the receiver coils currents having a wide range of RFs, called white noise.

- *Scanner*. Electronic noise comes from the statistical fluctuations in the numbers of electrons in the currents flowing in the electronic circuits.

- *Environment*. Some noise can come from RF interference, either outside the scanner room or inside from ancillary equipment.

All noise reduces and obscures contrasts between tissues. It appears worst in the areas of low PD and low signal. The SNR can be improved by any of the following measures, although each needs to be optimized for the image required:

- *Increasing the signal* by:
  — increasing voxel size by increasing the FOV or slice thickness or by decreasing the number of phase-encoding steps, although at the expense of spatial resolution
  — decreasing *TE*
  — increasing *TR* or the tip angle.
  SE sequences generally give a bigger signal than gradient echo (GRE). The signal strength would also be increased by using a machine with a higher field strength.

- *Reducing the noise* by:
  — increasing N_{ex} (the number of excitations)
  — reducing the bandwidth of the receiver so that it picks up less of the spectrum of noise frequencies, although unfortunately this increases the chemical shift and motion artefacts, described below
  — reducing cross-talk by having larger gaps between slices or by using multislice techniques
  — reducing the volume of tissue from which noise is picked up by using well-positioned surface coils of good design such as a phased array with multiple small coils.
  Three-dimensional imaging can give a better SNR than two-dimensional multislice imaging, but at the expense of increased imaging times.

Contrast

Contrast is the difference in the SNR between adjacent tissues and is controlled similarly to the SNR, as above. It can, however, be enhanced, either by using MR techniques to weight PD, T_1 and T_2, depending on the tissue to be imaged (as in section 10.3), or by using a contrast agent.

- *Magnetization transfer contrast* uses off-resonant frequency RF pulses to transfer magnetization to free protons to suppress the signal from protons bound to macromolecules.

- *Fat suppression* can be achieved using a short-*TI* inversion recovery (STIR) sequence to enhance the contrast between lesions and adjacent fatty tissue.

- T_2 *weighting* specifically increases the contrast between normal and abnormal tissue, the latter being brighter, as it contains water and is more evident than on T_1- or PD-weighted images.

- *Paramagnetic contrast media* such as gadolinium shortens T_1 of nearby hydrogen nuclei in adjacent tissues and thus enhances the inherent contrast. Manganese (as the ion Mn^{3+}), with five unpaired electrons, and iron (as the ion Fe^{2+}), with four, have also been used as paramagnetic or positive contrast agents but are not in such wide clinical use.

- *Superparamagnetic contrast media*. Minute (30 nm) particles of the iron oxide Fe_3O_4 with an inert coating are too small to be ferromagnetic but, being very easily magnetized, they are referred to as superparamagnetic. So too is dysprosium (as the ion Dy^{3+}) DTPA, with five unpaired electrons. Used as contrast agents, they produce local magnetic field gradients that are sufficiently large to shorten T_2^* and T_2. Areas of uptake appear black. They are also called bulk susceptibility or negative contrast agents.

- *Hyperpolarized gas as a new contrast agent*. Hyperpolarized (by laser) xenon (^{129}Xe) is starting to be used for imaging and spectroscopy. Xenon dissolves in blood and shows a large chemical shift. It can be used at very low fields, giving good SNR. It has good potential for MRI of the lungs and for low-field angiography. It is also capable of transferring polarization to ^{13}C for future spectroscopic imaging.

Spatial resolution

Spatial resolution depends on the pixel size, which in turn depends on the matrix and the FOV chosen. A representative value would be 1 mm. Using a larger matrix, reducing the FOV and using a local coil reduce the pixel size and improve resolution. Using a thinner slice also improves resolution, on account of the partial volume effect. Three-dimensional data (volume) acquisition, described above, has high resolution and better SNR than a two-dimensional (multislice) scan of the same voxel size.

Scan time

Scan time is a function of *TR*, the phase matrix (number of encodings), and the number of excitations (N_{ex}). Short scan times obviously help to reduce motion artefacts and thus improve image quality, but a compromise is needed.

- *Reducing the* TR:
  — reduces SNR
  — reduces the number of slices per acquisition
  — increases T_1 weighting (tissues more likely to be saturated).
- *Reducing the phase matrix*:
  — reduces resolution.
- *Reducing the* N_{ex}:
  — reduces SNR
  — increases motion artefact.

10.8 ARTEFACTS

Aliasing

Aliasing is a sign that the FOV is too small. It occurs if that part of the patient which is excited by the RF overlaps the chosen FOV. Then signals picked up by the body coil from tissues outside the FOV are falsely allocated to pixels within the matrix. This can produce image wrap-round *in the phase-encoding direction*. Part of the image is shifted bodily to the opposite side from its true anatomy.

The electronic circuits are designed to suppress aliasing in the frequency-encoding direction. Aliasing in the phase-encoding direction can be reduced by:

- An anti-aliasing or over-sampling technique; for example, doubling the FOV in the phase-encoding direction and at the same time doubling the number of phase-encoding steps (to keep the same pixel size), halving N_{ex} to keep the same imaging time and SNR, and displaying only the central half of the image (i.e. covering the original FOV).
- Using a surface coil that more closely matches the FOV, or increasing the FOV to match the coil.

Motion artefacts

Patients may find it hard to keep still during the long imaging time. As well as causing blurring or smearing of the image, motion can be responsible for ghost images. Frequency encoding takes place so quickly and phase encoding so slowly that the effects of motion are usually apparent only *in the phase-encoding direction*. Note that the ghosts appear in this direction even if the motion is through the slice or in the frequency direction. Swapping the frequency and phase direction sometimes displaces the artefact from the area of interest. Cyclical motion of tissues due to heart motion or breathing can produce multiple images in the phase-encoding direction of, for example, the abdominal aorta or any pulsating vessel.

Cardiac triggering can be used to reduce cardiac motion artefacts. The pulse sequence is triggered by the R-wave and *TR* made equal to the R–R interval. The acquisition of data is thereby synchronized with cardiac motion. Respiratory triggering is also possible but more difficult because the motion is slower. Reliance is usually placed on a fast scan with breath holding.

Pulsatile flow in arteries and the chambers of the heart can also produce multiple ghost images (e.g. of the aorta), again in the phase-encoding direction. The faster the motion, the wider is the spacing of the ghosts. Techniques such as the *motion artefact suppression technique* removes artefacts caused by phase changes resulting from movement (e.g. of blood and CSF). It does so by modifying the field gradients and is generally described as gradient moment rephasing.

Magnetic susceptibility

When an iron core is inserted in a DC solenoid, it becomes magnetized and increases the magnetic field. A patient inserted inside a DC solenoid similarly becomes very slightly magnetized. This is an atomic and not a nuclear effect. The patient disturbs the static magnetic field very slightly, especially:

- at the interfaces between tissue (susceptible) and air (not susceptible to magnetization) in lungs, sinuses, etc.
- because of the concentration of haemoglobin that may occur following bleeding, as this is slightly ferromagnetic due to its iron content.

Such unavoidable inhomogeneities of, typically, 2 ppm in the local magnetic field lead to an increase or a decrease in the MR signal and are responsible for certain artefacts. They are likely to be more noticeable on GRE than on SE images.

Chemical shift artefact

The imaging system cannot distinguish whether changes in resonant frequency are due to chemical shift or to the frequency-encoding gradient. Both are interpreted as a displacement *in the frequency-encoding direction*. Compared with water, fat, with its slightly higher resonant frequency, is falsely allocated to locations a few pixels up the gradient. For example, kidney is displaced relative to perinephric fat (Fig. 10.25). A white band is produced where the signal from fat is superimposed on that from water, and a black band where neither produces a signal. Similar effects are seen with fat around the optic nerve and at the margins of vertebral bodies. The stronger the static field of the machine, the greater the shift in terms of pixels.

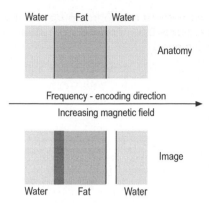

Figure 10.25 Chemical shift artefact.

It can be reduced by using a steeper gradient or a wider receiver bandwidth (although the latter lets through more noise). Alternatively, two chemical shift images can be superimposed with perfect registration between fat and water, thus eliminating chemical shift artefacts.

Other artefacts

A *central line* or 'zipper' artefact is produced across the middle of the image (usually *in the phase-encoding direction*) when RF leaks from the transmitter to the receiver. Line artefacts can also be produced by RF interference from outside, with the patient acting as an aerial (e.g. when the shielded door is ajar).

Implants of *ferrous materials* distort the local magnetic field and can distort or even black out quite a large surrounding area of the image.

Truncation or 'ringing' refers to the parallel striations that can appear at high contrast interfaces (e.g. between fat and muscle or between CSF and the spinal cord). This is similar to the artefact encountered in CT and is due to a low sampling rate. This is more likely *in the phase-encoding direction*. It can be reduced by increasing the matrix or reducing the FOV.

Methods to reduce the more common artefacts are summarized in Table 10.5.

10.9 QUALITY ASSURANCE

As for other imaging modalities, MRI requires a regular quality assurance programme. The homogeneity of the magnetic field is crucial, and it can be measured directly at different positions within the magnet using a special nuclear MR probe or, indirectly, by using imaging test devices.

Table 10.5 Common artefacts and solutions

Artefact	Possible solution
Aliasing	Enlarge the FOV or better match surface coils
Chemical shift	Increase frequency bandwidth, reduce FOV or superimposition
Motion	Counsel, immobilize or sedate patient, or swap phase and frequency
Magnetic susceptibility	Remove metal object or use spin–echo
Phase mismapping	Exchange phase and frequency directions, or use gating
Truncation	Increase phase encodings or reduce the FOV

FOV, field of view.

The same general quality assurance factors as for CT need to be considered: contrast, resolution, noise, artefacts (ghosting) and geometrical distortion. Quality assurance tests should include verification of slice thickness, image uniformity and linearity, SNR, spatial resolution and contrast (using phantoms), RF pulse parameters, and the video display characteristics. Test devices are available designed to fit into the coils to measure each of parameters listed.

Emergency equipment and safety features regarding the special hazards of MRI should also be part of standard checks. Box 10.1 gives a short checklist of quality assurance tests.

10.10 MAGNETS AND COILS

The patient is placed inside the magnet bore and is surrounded by a set of coils (the innermost coils in Fig. 10.26) connected to an RF generator (transmitter or oscillator), which sends through them a pulse of RF current lasting 1 ms or less.

There are three types of main magnet.

- A *permanent magnet* consists of two opposing flat-faced highly magnetized pole pieces (iron and alloys of aluminium, nickel and cobalt are commonly used) fixed to an iron frame. It is large and can weigh some 80 tonnes. It is expensive to buy but the cheapest to run. It requires no power but cannot be shut down and will only give low-strength, vertical fields, up to about 0.3 T. This magnet is used for claustrophobic patients, children, obese adults and interventional procedures.

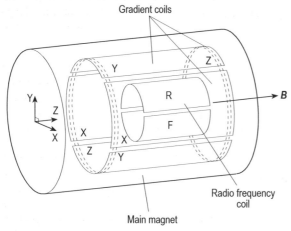

Figure 10.26 Arrangement of the coils in a magnetic resonance machine.

- A *resistive electromagnet* is a set of DC coils with copper or aluminium conductors, which consume some 50–100 kW of power. The heat produced is removed by cooling water, pumped rapidly through the hollow coils. The vertical or horizontal magnetic field is limited by heating to 0.5 T, and has significant fringe fields. It can be switched off at will, at the end of the day or in an emergency. It

then takes 15–30 min to 'ramp up', i.e. re-establish the field. It is the cheapest and smallest, weighing some 2 tonnes.

- A *superconducting electromagnet* is a DC solenoid, about 1 m in diameter, with conductors made of a rather brittle niobium–titanium alloy in a copper matrix. They are supercooled by a 'cryogen': liquid helium at 4 K ($-269°C$). At this temperature, they have negligible resistance, and large (DC) currents can be used without overheating, producing horizontal fields up to at least 3 T but with significant fringe fields. The machine is correspondingly large and expensive and weighs some 6 tonnes. Its tunnel configuration is unsuitable for very large or claustrophobic patients. Small-bore machines up to 7 T are also in use for brain imaging.

It takes several hours for the coil to cool down and the current to build up. The coil is then short circuited and the power removed. The current continues to flow while using virtually no power, but liquid gas is consumed to maintain the low-temperature need for negligible resistance. If and when the machine is shut down, the electro-magnetic energy (some 20 kWh) stored within the superconducting coil has to be removed carefully to avoid a 'quench' (see section 10.11).

The expensive liquid helium is contained within a fragile cryostat (vacuum, Dewar or Thermos vessels) and replenished periodically. A refrigerator system is used to reduce helium losses. Care must be taken when replenishing the cryogen. Air entering the system would solidify like a plug.

The coolant level must be logged daily. If it falls too low, quenching occurs; the temperature rises, superconductivity is lost and the stored energy released. If the temperature rises, the liquid gas boils off rapidly and must be vented outside the building. As the superconductivity disappears, the copper matrix takes over the conduction of current.

The magnetic field

The main field must be stable, unaffected by ambient temperature, and uniform to 5 ppm over a large volume for imaging (1 ppm for spectroscopy). In the case of a permanent magnet, the field is usually aligned vertically, from front to back of the supine patient, while in a solenoid it points horizontally along the length of the patient.

The magnetic field lines form closed loops and crowd together within a solenoid but spread widely outside it as a *fringe field* (Fig. 10.27). This effect is reduced by an iron shroud weighing many tonnes or by additional large shimming coils. The fringe field of

(a)　　　　　　　　　　　　　　　　　　　　(b)

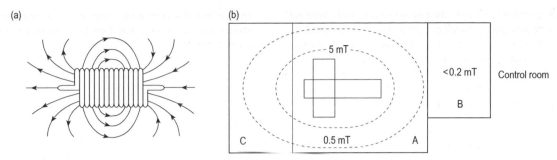

Figure 10.27 Fringe fields (a) and field contour plots (b) showing controlled areas. A, scanner room; C, equipment room; B, operator control area/room.

a permanent magnet is negligible, as it is concentrated within the iron yoke.

Optimum field strength The static magnetic field should be large enough to produce an adequate signal but not so large that it exceeds the safety guidelines (see section 10.11). Opinions differ about the optimum field strength for MRI. *Against a high field* is an increased T_1, necessitating a longer TR and imaging time and the greater cost of the magnet. The static field is harder to make uniform, and there is a stronger fringe field, which can affect equipment in adjacent areas. Chemical shift artefacts are increased unless a higher field gradient is also used. Motion and susceptibility artefacts are worsened. Potential hazards to the patient, including RF heating, are greater. *In favour of a high field* is a larger MR signal and improved SNR producing optimum images, and special applications become possible.

Coils

Working inwards from the outer main magnet coils (see Fig. 10.26), there are the following.

- The *shim coils* (not shown) carrying DC, which are fine tuned to make the main magnetic field as uniform as possible throughout the imaging volume.

- The three sets of *gradient coils*, carrying DC, which are varied to alter the slope of the magnetic field, typically $20\,\mathrm{mT\,m^{-1}}$. The coils are connected to gradient amplifiers that control the rise time and maximum value of the gradients. The currents must be switched off rapidly, in 1 ms or less, which causes the coils to emit a loud bang. The direction the current is passed through the coil determines the increase or decrease in the field strength relative to the centre. The slice select or Z-axis gradient field is switched on during the application of the RF pulse. The steeper the gradient, the thinner the slice.

During the few milliseconds that the MR echo signal is being received, DC is passed through a second set of gradient coils (XX in Fig. 10.26). This produces a magnetic field gradient from side to side, in the X-direction (Fig. 10.15b), for example for frequency encoding. Steep frequency encoding gradients are needed for small FOV.

Immediately after the protons in the slice have been excited by the 90° pulse, but before they are inverted by the 180° pulse, DC is passed for a few milliseconds through a third set of gradient coils (YY in Fig. 10.26). This produces a magnetic field gradient from the front to the back of the patient, in the Y-direction (e.g. for phase encoding). Steep-phase encoding gradients produce fine-phase matrices.

- RF (transmitter/receiver) coils, which are tuned like a radio to the resonant frequency. They produce a magnetic field at right angles to the main field. To maximize the signal, the coil should be as close as possible to the part being imaged. The RF coils are of several types.
  - The standard *body coil* is usually a permanent part of the scanner. It is used to transmit the RF pulse for all types of scan and to receive the MR signal when imaging large parts of the body (e.g. the chest and abdomen). The patient should be positioned so that the coil includes the anatomy to be imaged.
  - The *head* (transmit/receiver) *coil* is part of the helmet used in brain scanning.
  - *Surface* or local (receiver) *coils* are separate coils designed to be applied as close as possible to image parts close to the surface, the lumbar spine, knee, orbit, etc., before the patient is inserted into the machine. They receive signals effectively from a depth equal to the coil radius. They allow smaller voxels and give better resolution but have a smaller FOV and less

uniformity. They are harder to use and must be positioned carefully. Being closer to the patient than body coils, they pick up a larger signal. Having a smaller FOV and limited penetration, they pick up less noise, thus improving the SNR. Intracavity (e.g. rectal) coils can also be used to give greater resolution of small structures deep in the body.

— *Phased array coils* are multiple (four or more) receiver coils whose signals are received individually (less noise) and then combined to increase SNR but with a large FOV. All data are acquired in a single sequence. The greater the number of independent coils, the more difficult it is to keep them decoupled without losing the signal. Geometrical and electrical methods are needed for this. With a 64-channel array, MR cine at 125 frames s^{-1} has been achieved at 1.5 T.

— *Transmit phased array coils* produce a current on each element. Special amplifiers are needed to define this current. Careful control of the relative amplitude and phase of each element enables them to be mutually independent. With reduced pulse duration, higher SNR, improved field homogeneity and, incidentally, reduced specific absorption rate (see section 10.11) at high field strengths, parallel MRI can be used in the excitation phase as in Transmit SENSE.

The complete magnetic resonance system

In addition to the magnet, coils and their controllers in Figure 10.24, there is a pulse control unit. The pulse sequences are selected at the operator console, and the control unit synchronizes the gradients and RF pulses

for the selected parameters. The main computer has an array processor (for the Fourier transforms) and sends the data to the image processor (Fig. 10.28).

Siting of the machine should take account of:

● steel girders and reinforced concrete, which may become magnetized in the fringe field, and moving elevators and vehicles, all of which can distort the main field
● lifts and power cables, which may cause RF interference and so distort the image and also produce linear artefacts.

The walls of the room incorporate wire mesh (a Faraday cage) to screen the scanner from such external RF interference. Doors are similarly screened and also interlocked to ensure that they are properly closed during imaging.

10.11 HAZARDS AND SAFE PRACTICE

Magnetic resonance imaging does not involve ionizing radiation. As at present practised, following (in the UK) Medicines and Healthcare products Regulatory Agency (MHRA) guidelines based on the Health Protection Agency advice and implementing European directives, the threshold for the following potential hazards do not appear to be exceeded; certainly, no acute ill effects have been noted.

Static magnetic field (always present)

Voltages might be induced in flowing blood, which could cause depolarization, and, in moving heart muscle, changes may be seen in the electrocardiogram. No adverse effects are expected if fields do not

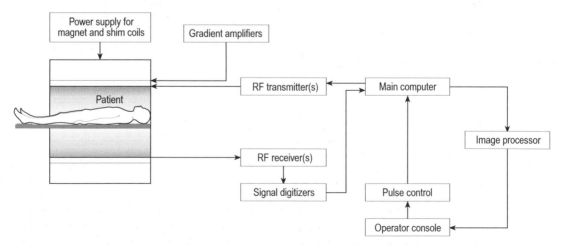

Figure 10.28 Typical system configuration. RF, radiofrequency.

exceed the following MHRA guidelines for whole body exposure of patients:

Normal mode:	less than 2.5 T
Controlled mode:	between 2.5 T and 4 T
Research or experimental mode:	more than 4 T

Pregnant patients should not be exposed above 2.5 T. In the **controlled** mode, patients must have a panic button and be monitored with constant visual contact with the possibility of verbal contact. Using a pulse oximeter (fibre-optic) is also recommended. Note that the patient's electrocardiogram is affected above 0.3 T but returns to normal after exposure. Ethics committee approval is required above 4 T, as adverse bioeffects may occur.

Staff should not be exposed to more than 2 T whole body and 5 T for limbs. Over 24 h, the average exposure should not exceed 0.2 T. Manufacturers supply field plots around their machines to show 200 mT field lines (0.2 T). Table 10.6 gives the restricted exposure times.

Note that MRI is contraindicated if the patient has an implanted pacemaker. Anyone with a cardiac pacemaker should be excluded from MR areas and where stray fields are greater than 0.5 mT. Consequently, this defines the controlled area for safety purposes around the scanner installation.

Time-varying gradient fields (dB/dt)

Electric fields are produced perpendicular to the gradient field, inducing eddy currents in conductive tissues and causing stimulation, for example peripheral nerve stimulation, involuntary muscular contraction, breathing difficulties and even ventricular fibrillation. Peripheral nerve stimulation has the lowest threshold, about $60 \, T s^{-1}$ for a rise time less than 1 ms, but it does vary between patients.

Particular care should be taken of patients with heart disease. Other effects are flashes of light (magnetophosphenes) on the retina, vertigo, nausea and sensations of metallic taste all experienced with dB/dt for fields greater than 3 T.

Symptoms associated with time-varying gradient fields do not seem to occur below $20 \, T s^{-1}$. There is not thought to be any effect on fetal development but, as a precaution, MRI is usually not carried out during the first trimester of a pregnancy and pregnant staff may be redeployed.

Implanted devices and monitoring equipment may be affected by dB/dt-induced voltages (e.g. cochlear implants, cardiac pacemakers and electrocardiography monitors). Devices need to be specified as **MR compatible** or **MR safe** to be unaffected by the MR scanner and safe to use. This specification also indicates they do not affect the image quality. Note that **MR conditional** labels indicate equipment that may be taken into the scanner room but may be affected by the fields and may cause image distortion.

Acoustic noise associated with fast-switching magnetic fields (GRE) increases with field strength and with higher gradient amplitudes (e.g. shorter *TR*, *TE*, high resolution, thin slices). The machine limit is 140 dB, although most do not exceed 120 dB. However, hearing protection is required to prevent irreversible damage at 90 dB. Earplugs reduce noise by 10–30 dB and alleviate patient discomfort and distress. Hearing protection should be matched to the frequency spectrum of the noise produced. Note also that low-frequency sounds are transmitted to the fetus and, although not yet proven, damage to hearing development is of concern.

Radiofrequency fields

Microwave heating may occur, especially at the higher frequencies associated with strong static fields. It is usually compensated by vasodilation. The cornea, with no blood supply, and the testes, with little, may be at risk. Heating of metallic implants may also present a problem. Skin and rectal temperature rise may be monitored and should not exceed 1°C.

The *specific absorption ratio* (SAR) is the RF energy deposited per mass of tissue expressed as watts per kilogram. Restricting whole body SAR in the body to an average of $1 \, W kg^{-1}$ restricts the whole body temperature rise to 0.5°C. Table 10.7 gives recommended exposure limits. The patient's weight is needed to calculate the temperature rise and control pulse sequences to ensure safe heating levels.

The SAR is greater for large body parts than for small, for high static fields than for low, for a 180° pulse than for a 90° pulse, for SE than for GRE, and for high-conductivity tissues (brain, blood, liver and CSF) than for low-conductivity tissues (fat and bone marrow). There may be some hotspots, and some combination of imaging parameters may not be allowed.

Table 10.6 Restricted whole body exposure times

Exposure time (h)	Average field strength (T)
24	0.2
8	0.6
4	1.2
2	2.0
1	2.0 (limit)

Table 10.7 Recommended specific absorption ratio whole body exposure limits

Exposure time (t, min)	SAR limit (W kg^{-1})	
	<0.5°C	<1.0°C
<15	2.0	4.0
15–30	30/t	60/t
>30	1.0	2.0

Only MR-compatible monitoring equipment should be used in the imaging room, and special care taken over the disposition of leads to minimize induced currents. The majority of reported adverse incidents concern burns to the patient, often from monitoring leads and electrodes.

Other hazards

Protocols for the operation of the MR machine take account of other potential hazards, such as the following.

Mechanical attraction of ferromagnetic objects varies as the square of the magnetic field and the inverse cube of the distance (projectile effect). The fringe field, which can extend for a few metres (as in Fig. 10.27b), may convert scissors and scalpels into potentially lethal projectiles. Oxygen cylinders, patient beds, fire-fighting apparatus, etc. have all caused major incidents and injury. Aneurysm clips may be displaced or rotated in the tissues when the patient is inserted into the magnet. Non-magnetic, MR-compatible materials should always be used. MRI may be contraindicated in case of ferrous foreign bodies, especially near the eye. Joint and dental prostheses are firmly fixed and should present no problem.

The *fringe field* can also affect some watches, destroy data on computer disks and credit cards, distort nearby video displays, and affect photomultipliers. It is minimized by the design of the coil and the use of iron shielding. The area around the main magnet is designated as *controlled* (see Fig. 10.27) and must be carefully supervised. On account of the effect on implanted pacemakers, free access of the public is limited to areas outside the controlled area where the field is less than 0.5 mT.

Safety procedures

Patient screening   Patients must be screened or interviewed before any examination, in accordance with the local imaging protocol. Safety questions must cover implants (especially pacemakers), surgical history, functional disorders, allergies (contrast agents), presence of metallic objects (internal, fixed externally or removable) and weight (for the SAR). Much advice is available on implantable devices, metallic foreign bodies and transdermal patches, tattoos, etc. Appropriate clothing should be provided, and patients should remove hairpins, jewellery and even eye make-up (as this can contain iron oxide, creating artefacts in brain images).

Requirements for safe imaging   Once cleared for imaging, patient comfort, safety and confidence are crucial. Successful and safe imaging requires:

- positioning equipment leads to avoid RF burns
- using MR-compatible foam pads for comfort while ensuring that pillows and covers do not inhibit heat loss
- providing music, human contact or even light sedation, as appropriate, to minimize claustrophobia
- hearing protection against the loud percussive noise produced by the repeatedly switching gradient – essential for anaesthetized patients
- visual monitoring and, when appropriate, physiological monitoring using MR-compatible equipment.

Note that only appropriately trained and experienced anaesthetists should attend the patient, as special equipment and procedures are necessary.

Emergencies

Written procedures to cover emergencies and avoid panic reactions include the following.

Cardiac arrest   The procedure comprises resuscitation to keep airways open and cardiac massage while the patient is removed from the magnet on to an MR-compatible trolley and taken quickly to the resuscitation area outside the controlled area, where the resuscitation team will take over. Or, if the scanner has a resistive magnet, it is switched off to enable prompt access by the resuscitation team. All equipment is removed before switching the magnet on again.

Fire   Resistive magnets should be switched off. Permanent magnets have lower fringe fields, but fire-fighting equipment should be used only at a distance of 1 m or more from the bore. Superconducting magnets should be quenched only if the firemen need to enter the inner controlled area. Note that non-ferrous carbon dioxide extinguishers should be used.

Quench   Before initiating a controlled quench in the event of a fire or when someone is trapped to the magnet by a metal object, the door should be fixed open to avoid a build-up of pressure in the scan room. All scan rooms contain an oxygen monitor and a gas-venting system. External venting channels should be checked periodically to ensure that they function. Accidental quenching, releasing helium cooling gas

Table 10.8 Favourable effects of changing imaging parameters

Parameter	Effect of parameter when increased	when decreased
TR	SNR increases / Allows more slices	Scan time shortens / T_1 contrast may increase
TE	T_2 contrast may increase	SNR increases / Allows more slices
Slice thickness	SNR increases / Larger volume scanned	Spatial resolution increases / Partial volume effects lessen
Slice interspace	Larger volume scanned / Cross-talk reduces	Less chance of pathology escaping detection
Matrix	Smaller pixels / Spatial resolution improves	Larger pixels / SNR increases / Scan time shortens
N_{ex}	SNR increases	Scan time shortens
FOV	Image covers larger area / SNR improves / Aliasing artefacts less likely	Spatial resolution improves
	when body or head coil used	when local coil used
Coils	Gives large FOV	SNR increases / Motion artefacts less likely / Aliasing artefacts less likely

FOV, field of view; SNR, signal to noise ratio.

into the room, might cause suffocation or produce frostbite. The glass window between the scanner and the control room should be broken to equalize the pressure if necessary.

10.12 SUMMARY

- Table 10.8 lists the favourable effects of changing imaging parameters.

- MRI measures the hydrogen content of individual voxels in each transverse slice of the patient and represents it as a shade of grey or colour in the corresponding image pixel on the screen.

- The patient is placed in a strong electromagnetic field for an MRI scan.

- Hydrogen nuclei (protons) in the body align themselves parallel or antiparallel with the magnetic field.

- For each transverse image slice, a short, powerful radiosignal is sent through the patient's body, perpendicular to the main magnetic field.

- The hydrogen atoms, which have the same frequency as the radiowave, resonate with the RF wave.

- The hydrogen atoms return to their original energy state, releasing their excitation energy as an RF signal (the MR signal) when the input radiowave is turned off. The time this takes, relaxation time, depends on the type of tissue.

- The time and signals are computer-analysed and an image is reconstructed.

- The favourable effects of increasing each MRI parameter are also the drawbacks of decreasing it, and vice versa.

- Soft tissue contrast is high. The range of T_1 and T_2 values in soft tissue is even wider than the range of CT numbers.

- Bone and air do not produce artefacts.

- MRI is non-invasive, contrast media being required only for specialized techniques.

- Images can be obtained simultaneously in a number of planes at any angle.

- MHRA guidelines should be incorporated into safety protocols to avoid potential hazards to patients and staff.

- Ionizing radiation is not involved.

Bibliography

British Institute of Radiology (2003) *Assurance of Quality in the Diagnostic Imaging Department*, 2nd edn. BIR, London.

Cherry SR, Sorenson J, Phelps M (2003) *Physics in Nuclear Medicine*, 3rd edn. Saunders, Philadelphia.

Curry TS, Dowdey JE, Murry RC (1990) *Christensen's Physics of Diagnostic Radiology*, 4th edn. Lea & Febiger, Philadelphia.

Dendy PP, Heaton B (1999) *Physics for Diagnostic Radiology*, 2nd edn. Institute of Physics Publishing, Bristol.

Health and Safety Commission (2000) *Work with Ionising Radiation L121 (Ionising Radiations Regulations 1999, Approved Code of Practice and Guidance)*. Health and Safety Executive, London.

Hendee WR, Ritenour ER (2002) *Medical Imaging Physics*, 4th edn. Wiley-Liss, New York.

Hendrick WR, Hykes DL, Starchman DE (2005) *Ultrasound Physics and Instrumentation*, 4th edn. Elsevier, Philadelphia.

Institute of Physics and Engineering in Medicine (2002) *Medical and Dental Guidance Notes: a good practice guide on all aspects of ionising radiation protection in the clinical environment*. IPEM, York.

Institute of Physics and Engineering in Medicine (2005) *Recommended Standards for the Routine Performance Testing of Diagnostic X-ray Imaging Systems*, report 91. IPEM, York.

Kalender WA (2005) *Computed Tomography: fundamentals, system technology, image quality, applications*, 2nd edn. Publicis, Erlangen.

Khanna M, Menezes L, Gallagher D (2004) *MCQs for the FRCR, Part 1*. Greenwich Medical Media, London.

Martin CJ, Dendy PP, Corbett RH (2003) *Medical Imaging and Radiation Protection for Medical Students and Clinical Staff*. British Institute of Radiology, London.

Martin CJ, Sutton DG (eds) (2002) *Practical Radiation Protection in Healthcare*. Oxford University Press, Oxford.

McRobbie DW, Moore EA, Graves MJ, Prince MR (2006) *MRI from Picture to Proton*. Cambridge University Press, Cambridge.

Saha GB (2004) *Basics of PET imaging*. Springer, New York.

Tolan D, Hyland R, Taylor C, Cowen A (2004) *FRCR Part 1: MCQs and mock examination*. Royal Society of Medicine Press, London.

Westbrook C (2002) *MRI at a Glance*. Blackwell Science, Oxford.

Subject index

Notes: Page references in *italics* indicate figures, tables and boxed material. Page references in **bold** refer to major discussions.